Published by Hayle Medical,
30 West, 37th Street, Suite 612,
New York, NY 10018, USA
www.haylemedical.com

Selected Topics in Chronic Obstructive Pulmonary Disease
Edited by Michael Glass

International Standard Book Number: 978-1-63241-352-9 (Hardback)

Contents

Preface

This book has been an outcome of determined endeavour from a group of educationists in the field. The primary objective was to involve a broad spectrum of professionals from diverse cultural background involved in the field for developing new researches. The book not only targets students but also scholars pursuing higher research for further enhancement of the theoretical and practical applications of the subject.

A few years back, many clinicians had a negative view regarding the cure of Chronic Obstructive Pulmonary Disease (COPD), which has changed over the due course of time. This book on COPD is a medium to present researches and theories on this disease from experts from around the globe. It presents the readers with an array of topics related to treatment and care of patients with COPD challenges, the entire range of respiratory medicine, testing the limits of pulmonary function (and exercise) testing, bronchology, chest physiotherapy, thoracic surgery and radiologic imaging. Also, valuable inferences from specialty fields such as cardiology, geriatric medicine and neuropsychiatry are often required for comprehensive management of COPD. The recent researches regarding COPD hold bright future prospects.

It was an honour to edit such a profound book and also a challenging task to compile and examine all the relevant data for accuracy and originality. I wish to acknowledge the efforts of the contributors for submitting such brilliant and diverse chapters in the field and for endlessly working for the completion of the book. Last, but not the least; I thank my family for being a constant source of support in all my research endeavours.

Editor

Treatment

Management of Acute Exacerbations

Cenk Kirakli
Izmir Dr. Suat Seren Chest Diseases
and Surgery Training Hospital
Turkey

1. Introduction

American Thoracic Society (ATS) and European Respiratory Society (ERS) define an exacerbation as an acute change in a patient's baseline dyspnea, cough, or sputum that is beyond normal variability, and that is sufficient to warrant a change in therapy(Celli MacNee 2004). Exacerbations have a negative impact on mortality and morbidity and as the disease progress, the frequency and severity of exacerbations increase, leading to a fall in the quality of life of COPD patients. There is no standard method or tool for the diagnosis of an exacerbation. The changes in the clinical status of the patient should be taken into account.

The most important parameters predicting mortality in patients who are hospitalized due to an acute exacerbation are; severity and stage of COPD, advanced age, co morbidities such as diabetes mellitus or cardiovascular disease, need of intubation and mechanical ventilation, high APACHE II score, presence of sepsis and multi organ failure (Groenewegen et al. 2003).

2. Etiology of exacerbations

Tracheobronchial infections (40-50% bacterial, 30-40% viral, 5-10% atypical bacteria) are involved in 50-70% of COPD exacerbations. Another factor is air pollution that is thought to be involved in 10% of exacerbations. In about 30%, the etiologic factor cannot be identified(Sapey Stockley 2006). Other medical problems, such as congestive heart failure, nonpulmonary infections, pulmonary embolism, and pneumothorax, can also lead to a COPD exacerbation.

Infections:

Bacterial: (Streptococcus pneumonia, Haemophilus influenza, Moraxella catarrhalis, Chlamydia pneumoniae, Pseudomonas aeruginosa, Staphylococcus aureus)

Viral: (Rhinovirus, influenza, adenovirus, parainfluenza, coronavirus, respiratory cincitial virus)

Environmental factors:

Indoor and outdoor air pollution

Patients who are known to have COPD are defined as an exacerbation when they are admitted to the emergency departments with increased dyspnea during fall and winter. The main issue is the underestimation of non-infectious causes such as pulmonary embolism, pleural effusion, pneumothorax, thoracic traumas, inappropriate use of sedatives, narcotics and beta blockers, arrhythmias, cardiac failure or problems in the use of long term oxygen therapy. Therefore, in a COPD patient with increased dyspnea, first the diagnosis of exacerbation should be established correctly and then the etiology should be identified as infectious or non-infectious.

Potentially pathogen bacteria are identified in 30% of sputum cultures in mild exacerbations, while this rate can be up to 70% in severe exacerbations in patients who need ventilatory support (Sapey Stockley 2006; Siddiqi Sethi 2008).

3. Initial evaluation of an exacerbation

There are two main steps in the evaluation of a COPD exacerbation. The first step is the determination of severity of the disease that will guide the physician about the treatment approach and hospitalization decision. The second step is the identification of the etiologic cause and decide whether to initiate antibiotherapy or not.

The Global Initiative for Chronic Obstructive Lung Disease (GOLD) classifies COPD exacerbations as mild, moderate or severe, based on the intensity of the medical intervention required to control the patient's symptoms (Table 1)(Rabe et al. 2007).

Clinical history	Mild (home treatment)	Moderate (hospital treatment)	Severe (ICU treatment)
Comorbidity	+	+++	+++
Frequent exacerbation history	+	+++	+++
COPD stage	Mild/Moderate	Moderate/Severe	Severe
Hemodynamic status	Stable	Stable	Stable/Unstable
Accessory respiratory muscle use, cyanosis, paradoxal breathing, cyanosis, tachypnea	No	++	+++
Change in neurologic status	No	No	Yes
Symptoms of right heart failure	No	++	+++
Persistence of symptoms despite drug therapy	No	++	+++

+: probably doesn' t exist, ++: probably exists, +++: strongly may exist, ICU: intensive care unit

Table 1. Classification of COPD exacerbations

Another classification approach is suggested by Anthonisen and colleagues (Anthonisen et al. 1987). According to this approach, severe exacerbations requiring antibiotheraphy are characterized by the presence of increase in all of the 3 criteria: dyspnea, sputum production and sputum purulence. Moderate exacerbations show only the 2 of these criteria, while in mild exacerbations, only one of these criteria is present with a recent history of upper airway infection or fever or symptoms like wheezing, cough, tachypnea and tachycardia.

Diagnostic evaluation of a suspected COPD exacerbation varies whether the patient will be treated in the hospital or at home. Routine sputum culture evaluation is not recommended for mild exacerbations. In case of a severe exacerbation, oxygen saturation must be measured by a pulse oxymeter. Patients who are referred to a hospital must be evaluated by advanced diagnostic tests such as arterial blood gas analysis, chest x-ray, sputum gram staining and cultures, electrocardiography and blood drug levels if possible (Table 2).

Diagnostic procedures	Mild	Moderate	Severe
Oxygen saturation	Yes	Yes	Yes
Arterial blood gas analysis	No	Yes	Yes
Chest X-ray	No	Yes	Yes
Blood tests *	No	Yes	Yes
Serum drug concentrations**	If possible	If possible	If possible
Sputum gram staining and cultures	No	Yes	Yes
ECG	No	Yes	Yes
BNP †	No	No	Yes
Cardiac enzyme measurement ‡	No	No	Yes

*: blood cell count, serum electrolytes, urea, creatinine, liver function tests.
**: theophylline, warfarin, carbamazepine, digoxin
†: One third of dyspnea in chronic lung disease may be attributable to congestive heart failure.
‡: Cardiac ischemia (myocardial infarction is underdiagnosed in patients with COPD).

Table 2. Diagnostic evaluation of patients with suspected COPD exacerbation

About 50% of COPD exacerbations are not reported to physicians(Seemungal et al. 2000). This suggests that half of the exacerbations are mild and do not require hospitalization. Indications for hospitalization of a patient with COPD exacerbation are as follows:

1. Onset of new physical signs such as cyanosis, peripheral edema, detoriation in the neurological status, arrhythmias etc.
2. Having severe or very severe COPD and being under long term oxygen therapy at home.

3. No response to initial drug therapy.
4. Pulmonary (pneumonia), or non-pulmonary (cardiac disease, diabetes mellitus) comorbidities with high risk.
5. Having exacerbations often.
6. Newly diagnosed arrhythmias.
7. Diagnostic uncertainty.
8. Advanced age.
9. Detoriation in the arterial blood gas analysis results
    (pH< 7.35 or PaO_2< 60mmHg or SaO_2< 90%)
10. Insufficient home support

4. Treatment of COPD exacerbations

All moderate and severe exacerbations must be evaluated in the hospital and in all severe exacerbations; arterial blood gas analysis must be performed. The patient must be evaluated immediately in terms of respiratory failure and oxygen therapy must be initiated if needed. Life threatening exacerbations should be followed up in the ICU. Respiratory failure with hypercapnia and respiratory acidosis is related with high mortality both at the time of admission and also during the 12 months follow up. While carbon dioxide retention is possible in moderate and severe exacerbations under oxygen therapy, arterial blood gas analysis must be performed every 30-60 minutes in order to detect the $PaCO_2$ and pH levels.

The inhaled oxygen concentration must be titrated to achieve a SaO_2> 90% or a PaO_2> 60 mmHg. High-flow oxygen devices deliver oxygen more effectively than nasal canulas but nasal canulas may be tolerated better. If adequate oxygenation cannot be achieved by high flow masks or if the acidosis begins worsening (pH<7.35 and/or $PaCO_2$> 50mmHg), noninvasive ventilation (NIV) is indicated. Success rates of NIV in COPD exacerbations are reported as 80-85% (Mehta&Hill 2001). The effect of NIV must be evaluated at the end of first and second hour by an arterial blood gas analysis. If there is worsening in the arterial blood gas result or if the patients cannot tolerate NIV, has worsening hypoxemia or has severe comorbidities such as myocardial infarction, hemodynamic instability, severe arrhythmias or sepsis, intubation and invasive mechanical ventilation must be initiated immediately.

Short acting inhaled β-2 agonists are the first line preferred drugs for COPD exacerbations. The dosage and frequency of these drugs must be increased. Another option is to add an inhaler short acting anticholinergic drug or increase the dosage if the patient is already taking the drug. Nevertheless, the effectiveness of this combination still remains controversial. If there is a long acting bronchodilator the patient is not using, it can also be added to the therapy even though there is no clinical evidence showing the benefit of these drugs during an exacerbation. In severe exacerbations if the patient cannot inhale effectively, nebulised forms must be used. The role of theophylline in COPD exacerbations is controversial. If there is not enough response to short acting inhaled β-2 agonists, it can be used as a second choice drug. Serum levels must be obtained and patients must be followed carefully because of its cardiovascular side effects.

Characteristics of the patient and exacerbation	Possible causes	Oral therapy choices	Parenteral therapy choices
Mild exacerbation (no signs of respiratory failure and severe obstruction, no comorbidities, 3 or less exacerbations in the last one year, no antibiotic use in the last 3 months)	• H.Influenza • S.Pneumoniae • M.Catarrhalis • C.Pneumoniae • Viruses	• β-lactam (Penicilin,Ampicillin/ Amoxicillin) • Tetracycline • Trimethoprim/ Sulfhamethoxazole • β-lactam/ β-lactamase inhibitors (Co-amoxilav) • Macrolides (Azithromycin, Clarithromycin, Roxithromycin) • 2nd or 3rd generation cephalosporins • Ketolides (Telithromycin)	
Moderate/ Severe exacerbation (complicated exacerbation, risk factors for treatment failure but not for P. Aeruginosa	Added to above; • β-lactamase producing enteric gram (-) bacteria (K.Pneumonia, E.Coli e.g)	• β-lactam/ β-lactamase inhibitors (Co-amoxilav) • 2nd or 3rd generation cephalosporins • Floroquinolones (Gemifloxacin, Levofloxacin, Moxifloxacin)	• β-lactam/ β-lactamase inhibitors (Co-amoxilav, ampicillin/ sulbactam) • 2nd or 3rd generation cephalosporins • Floroquinolones (Levofloxacin, Moxifloxacin)
Severe exacerbation with a high risk of P. Aeruginosa*	Added to above; • P. Aeruginosa	• Floroquinolones (Ciprofloxacin, Levofloxacin-high dose)	• Floroquinolones (Ciprofloxacin, Levofloxacin-high dose) • β-lactams with antipseudomonal activity

*Hospitalization in the last one month, frequent antibiotic use in the last one year, exacerbation causing severe respiratory failure, isolation of *P. Aeruginosa* in the sputum culture during stable state or prior exacerbations.

Table 3. Antibiotherapy options in infectious exacerbations of COPD

Adding systemic (oral or intravenous) glucocorticosteroids to other therapies in the hospital management of exacerbations of COPD is recommended (Niewoehner et al. 1999). Systemic use of corticosteroids may lead to fast recovery and improvement in hypoxemia and lung functions in COPD exacerbations. The recommended dosage of prednisolon is 30-40 mg/day for 7-10 days if the patient has an initial FEV1 value below 50%. Prolonged treatment does not have a positive affect, besides it may increase the risk of side effects (e.g. muscle atrophy, hyperglycemia).

Bronchoscopic studies showed that the amount of bacteria is increased nearly in 50% of COPD patients during an exacerbation when compared to the stable state(Sethi 2004). The decision to use antibiotics and the choice of antibiotic should be guided by the patient's symptoms (e.g., presence of purulent sputum), recent antibiotic use, and local microbial resistance patterns. Prophylactic or continuous use of antibiotics does not improve outcome in patients with COPD (Rabe, Hurd et al. 2007).

Even though the most common bacteria responsible for the exacerbations are H.influenzae, S. pneumoniae and M. Catarrhalis; some enteric Gram (-) bacteria and Pseudomonas aeruginosa are also isolated in most of the patiens with hypoxemia, severe airway obstruction, malnutrition, frequent hospitalization and antibiotic use history and comorbidity(Incalzi et al. 2006). There are some studies suggesting that atypical bacteria can also be an etiologic reason for an exacerbation but antibiotherapy targeting these bacteria showed no positive affect on clinical outcomes(Diederen et al. 2007; Tasbakan et al. 2007). Viruses can also be responsible in 15-40% of all exacerbations. Most of these are present with a bacterial infection.

Antibiotherapy reduces the mortality rates and treatment failure especially in severe exacerbations of COPD(Puhan et al. 2007). Antibiotics also decrease the relapse rates of exacerbationsin outpatients(Adams et al. 2000). Therefore, antibiotherapy is strongly indicated expecially if the patient has purulant sputum and increase in dyspnea. Treatment options according to clinical status is summarized in Table 3.

5. Preperation for hospital discharge

In order to qualify for a discharge, the patient must have stable clinical conditions and a stable or improving arterial PaO_2 of greater than 60mmHg. The patient should not require short acting β-agonist more often than every 4 hours. If the patient is stable and can use a metered dose inhaler, there is no extra benefit of using nebulised forms (Jenkins et al. 1987). Patient education including topics such as medical treatment, nutrition, rehabilitation and physiotherapy programs and when to seek for professional medical help may improve the response to future exacerbations. Home support such as home mechanical ventilation, long term oxygen therapy, nebulisers or similar equipments should be arranged before discharge.

6. Preventing future exacerbations

Pulmonary rehabilitation, smoking cessation and immunization against influenza and pneumonia have been shown to improve health quality and reduce exacerbations in COPD patients. There are also some data showing that long term oxygen therapy reduces the risk of hospitalization and shortens hospital stays in severely ill COPD patients. Long-acting inhaled bronchodilators and inhaled corticosteroids to improve symptoms and reduce the risk of exacerbations in patients with stable COPD are reviewed elsewhere with promising results.

7. References

Adams, S. G., et al. (2000). "Antibiotics are associated with lower relapse rates in outpatients with acute exacerbations of COPD." Chest 117(5): 1345-1352.

Anthonisen, N. R., et al. (1987). "Antibiotic therapy in exacerbations of chronic obstructive pulmonary disease." Ann Intern Med 106(2): 196-204.

Celli, B. R. and W. MacNee (2004). "Standards for the diagnosis and treatment of patients with COPD: a summary of the ATS/ERS position paper." Eur Respir J 23(6): 932-946.

Diederen, B. M., et al. (2007). "The role of atypical respiratory pathogens in exacerbations of chronic obstructive pulmonary disease." Eur Respir J 30(2): 240-244.

Groenewegen, K. H., et al. (2003). "Mortality and mortality-related factors after hospitalization for acute exacerbation of COPD." Chest 124(2): 459-467.

Incalzi, R. A., et al. (2006). "Use of antibiotics in elderly patients with exacerbated COPD: the OLD-chronic obstructive pulmonary disease study." J Am Geriatr Soc 54(4): 642-647.

Jenkins, S. C., et al. (1987). "Comparison of domiciliary nebulized salbutamol and salbutamol from a metered-dose inhaler in stable chronic airflow limitation." Chest 91(6): 804-807.

Mehta, S. and N. S. Hill (2001). "Noninvasive ventilation." Am J Respir Crit Care Med 163(2): 540-577.

Niewoehner, D. E., et al. (1999). "Effect of systemic glucocorticoids on exacerbations of chronic obstructive pulmonary disease. Department of Veterans Affairs Cooperative Study Group." N Engl J Med 340(25): 1941-1947.

Puhan, M. A., et al. (2007). "Exacerbations of chronic obstructive pulmonary disease: when are antibiotics indicated? A systematic review." Respir Res 8: 30.

Rabe, K. F., et al. (2007). "Global strategy for the diagnosis, management, and prevention of chronic obstructive pulmonary disease: GOLD executive summary." Am J Respir Crit Care Med 176(6): 532-555.

Sapey, E. and R. A. Stockley (2006). "COPD exacerbations . 2: aetiology." Thorax 61(3): 250-258.

Seemungal, T. A., et al. (2000). "Time course and recovery of exacerbations in patients with chronic obstructive pulmonary disease." Am J Respir Crit Care Med 161(5): 1608-1613.

Sethi, S. (2004). "Bacteria in exacerbations of chronic obstructive pulmonary disease: phenomenon or epiphenomenon?" Proc Am Thorac Soc 1(2): 109-114.

Siddiqi, A. and S. Sethi (2008). "Optimizing antibiotic selection in treating COPD exacerbations." Int J Chron Obstruct Pulmon Dis 3(1): 31-44.

Tasbakan, M. S., et al. (2007). "[Role of atypical pathogens in infectious exacerbations of COPD]." Tuberk Toraks 55(4): 336-341.

2

Adherence to Therapy in Chronic Obstructive Pulmonary Disease

Tamas Agh and Agnes Meszaros
Semmelweis University
Hungary

1. Introduction

Chronic obstructive pulmonary disease (COPD) is a major public health problem for both industrialised and developing countries (Viegi et al., 2001). The prevalence of COPD is increasing worldwide, resulting in a substantial economic burden, including direct and indirect health-care costs (Chapman et al., 2006).

Non-adherence in COPD is common and poses a significant barrier to optimal disease management. According to the World Health Organization (WHO), adherence to long-term therapies averages only 50% (WHO, 2003). Patient adherence in chronic diseases can result in poor health outcomes and increased health-care expenditures (WHO, 2003). Discontinuation of COPD therapy contributes to increasing the frequency of exacerbations, the number of hospitalisations and the mortality rate (Bourbeau & Bartlett, 2008; Regueiro et al., 1998; Vestbo et al., 2011).

Clinical trials may overestimate the level of adherence to medication regimens. Adherence rates in clinical trials have been expected to be approximately 70%–90% among patients with COPD (Kesten et al., 2000; van Grunsven et al., 2000; Rand et al., 1995). In clinical practice, these rates are only in the range of 20%–60% (Agh et al., 2011; Bosley et al., 1994; Dolce et al., 1991; Krigsman et al., 2007a). This difference reflects the fact that patient adherence may be an important explanatory factor of the difference between the efficacy of treatment under experimental conditions and the real-world effectiveness of the treatment (Revicki & Frank, 1999).

Non-adherence in patients with COPD has a number of causes, including factors related to the characteristics of the patient, the disease, the therapies and the health-care provider–patient relationship (Baiardini et al., 2009; Restrepo et al., 2008; WHO, 2003). Physicians should understand the factors and the strategies that facilitate adherence to improve the effectiveness of the therapy.

The goals of this chapter are as follows: to highlight the importance of adherence in the management of COPD; to introduce the reader to the concepts of adherence, compliance and persistence; to address different methods of measuring adherence; to identify factors related to adherence; and to emphasise strategies to enhance adherence in patients with COPD.

2. General overview of adherence

There are a number of terms used to describe the extent to which a patient undertakes the recommendations (medication regimens, lifestyle changes, etc.) of health-care providers. The most commonly used terms are compliance, adherence and persistence.

2.1 Terminology: Compliance, adherence and persistence

The definitions used to describe the concepts of compliance, adherence and persistence are not standardised, which causes many difficulties when comparing or combining results of different studies. The definitions from the International Society for Pharmacoeconomics and Outcomes Research (ISPOR) and the WHO are the most widely accepted in the literature.

Medication compliance, as defined by the ISPOR, "refers to the act of conforming to the recommendations made by the provider with respect of timing, dosage and frequency of medication taking" (Carmer et al., 2008). Compliance is expressed as an index number, which is typically given as a percentage and refers to a specified time interval. One of the most commonly used models for calculating medication compliance is the medication possession ratio (MPR). In the model of the MPR, the number of days of medication supplied within the refill interval is divided by the number of days in the refill interval (Peterson et al., 2007). Medication compliance may also be reported as a dichotomous variable, classifying patients into good and poor (or non-) compliance categories (Table 1). The cut-off point of compliance should be determined according to medication and type of disease. However, it is generally set independently at 80%, whether this compliance rate is adequate for disease control or not (Carmer et al., 2008).

Drugs	Months (1 month = 30 days)												Supply (days)	MPR
A	x	x	x	x	x	x				x	x	x	9x30=270	270/360=0.75
B		x	x	x	x		x	x	x	x			8x30=240	240/360=0.66
C			x		x		x	x		x	x	x	7x30=210	210/360=0.58

$\sum$ **MPR**: ((270+240+210)/3)/360 = 0.66 → 66%*
*:Patient is non-compliant (cut-off point: 80%).
| x |: medication supplied, | |: medication not supplied

Table 1. Calculation of medication compliance: medication possession ratio (MPR)

According to the definition of ISPOR, medication persistence may be described as "the duration of time from initiation to discontinuation of therapy" (Carmer et al., 2008). Persistence analyses must also define a permissible gap period, which specifies the maximum allowable time period between refills without discontinuation of the therapy. Persistence may be counted in days. However, it can also be given as the percentage of the number of persistent patients at the end of a predefined time period (Patricia et al., 2006) (Table 2). A patient's drug taking behaviour can best be quantified using both parameters: medication compliance and persistence (Carmer et al., 2008).

Although most research in the field has focused on medication compliance and persistence, therapeutic adherence certainly includes other non-drug therapeutic recommendations

Patients	Months (1 month = 30 days)												Days persistent (gap: 30 days)*	Persisted 180 days**
A	x	x	x	x			x	x	x				120	no
B	x	x	x	x	x	x			x		x		180	yes
C	x	x			x	x			x		x		60	no

*: Patients persisted an average of 120 days ((120+180+60)/3)
**: 33% (1/3) of the patients were persistent for 180 days
|x| : medication supplied, | | : medication not supplied

Table 2. Calculation of medication persistence

(following diets, executing lifestyle changes, etc.) as well. Explanation of adherence by the WHO also reflects this concept. The WHO definition of adherence is the following: "the extent to which a person's behaviour—taking medication, following a diet, and/or executing lifestyle changes—corresponds with agreed recommendations from a health-care provider" (WHO, 2003). This definition accurately highlights the importance of the patient's active role in their own health-care, which emphasises that the relationship between the patient and the health-care provider should be based on a partnership, instead of a one-sided paternal relationship.

Recently, medication adherence has become the preferred term instead of medication compliance. The primary difference between compliance and adherence is that compliance reflects the patient as a passive recipient of medical advice. Furthermore, compliance has also been viewed as a judgmental term when applied to patient behaviour. Thus, medication adherence will be the preferred term from this point forward.

2.2 Methods of measuring adherence

Most studies in adherence research have focused on medication-taking behaviour. Therefore, the following is a brief overview of the methodology of the assessment of medication adherence in COPD. There are a number of ways to assess adherence; nevertheless, there is not a gold standard because each method has strengths and limitations (Table 3).

The easiest way to assess medication adherence within clinical settings is to collect information from the patient themselves through questionnaires or patient diaries (Agh et al., 2011; Dolce et al., 1991; George et al., 2005, 2006a; Laforest et al., 2010). However, it should be mentioned that self-reporting methods may overestimate a patient's drug-taking behaviour (Dompleing et al., 1992; Rand et al., 1992, 1995). Using postal administration can help to obtain data that are more objective because patients are normally intimidated by their health-care providers and tend to give them the expected answers (Agh et al., 2011). Another commonly used method is the analysis of electronic pharmacy records (Breekveldt-Postma et al., 2007; Cramre et al., 2007; Jung et al., 2009). Retrospective database analysis is rapid and inexpensive. Nevertheless, this approach may also be inaccurate. It evaluates the prescriptions written by physicians or the prescriptions filled by patients, but not the medication intake directly.

	Advantage	Disadvantage
Indirect methods		
Patient self-report: adherence questionnaire, patient diary	Easy to obtain	Unreliable
Pharmacy refill data	Rapid Inexpensive	Inaccurate: • Pharmacy database can be incomplete • No indication of ingestion
Pill count, inhaler weighing	Easy to obtain Inexpensive	Inaccurate: • No indication of ingestion • "Dumping"*
Electronic adherence monitoring	Accurate measure of dosing history	Expensive No indication of ingestion
Therapeutic outcome	Easy to obtain	Clinical outcomes can depend on other factors
Direct methods		
Direct observation of the medication intake	Accurate indication of the ingestion	Unpleasant for the patient Require large human resources
Biological assay	Confirm drug use	Expensive Unpleasant for the patient Limited information regarding use over time Insensitive to inhaled drugs

*"Dumping": removing most of the medication at one time.

Table 3. Methods of measuring adherence

Pill count (Dompleing et al., 1992; van Grunsven et al., 2000) and canister weighing (Rand et al., 1995; Simmons et al., 2000) are widely used methods of adherence assessment in clinical trials. Pill counts are limited to oral medications, but canister weighing can also be used to monitor inhaled drugs. These approaches assess only the quantity of the medication removed from the canister without indication of ingestion, dose or dose frequency. Electronic compliance monitoring devices can provide more objective information about medication use than the aforementioned methods (Corden et al., 1997; Simmons et al., 1996, 2000). The cap of the pill bottles can be equipped with a microchip that stores data about each opening. Electronic recording devices (chronologs) can be fitted to metered-dose inhalers and nebulisers as well. Electronic monitors provide an accurate measure of dosing history but also cannot confirm ingestion. The major disadvantage of this method is the price; it is relatively costly.

Medication compliance can also be estimated based on direct assessments, such as direct observation of the medication intake or evaluation of blood levels or urinary excretion of the drug or its metabolite or drug-marker (Clark et al., 1996; Hatton et al., 1996). These methods are unpleasant for the patient and expensive. Interestingly, therapeutic drug monitoring may overestimate the actual adherence rate because patients tend to comply shortly before the drug test but not during the whole observation period. Another limitation is that a biochemical drug test is insensitive to inhaled medication.

The assessment of therapeutic adherence seems to be more complicated. However, clinical outcomes can be used to evaluate adherence, as these depend largely on the extent to which a patient undertakes the recommendations of health-care providers.

3. Adherence with COPD therapy

3.1 Adherence to medication

Medication non-adherence can take many forms: failure to fill prescriptions (primary non-adherence) or overuse, underuse or alteration of schedule or doses of medication (secondary non-adherence) (Bourbeau et al., 2007; George et al., 2007; Rand et al., 2005).

Only a limited number of studies have evaluated adherence in patients with COPD. Jung et al. (Jung et al., 2009) examined medication adherence and persistence among a sample of COPD patients during their last year of life. The study reviewed the use of inhaled corticosteroids (ICS), long-acting β_2 agonists (LABA), anticholinergics (AC) and methylxanthines (MTX), alone and in combination. The overall MPR to COPD medication was 44%. Approximately 30% of the patients persisted with the therapy, and the overall time to discontinuation was 94.2 days. These rates of cooperation are much lower than the drug-taking rates in other chronic diseases. Adherence in hypertension, dyslipidaemia and diabetes is, on average, 72% (MPR), and persistence is 63% (Cramer et al., 2008). In the previously mentioned study, Jung et al. (Jung et al., 2009) found differences between the mean MPRs of COPD drug classes (MTX: 52%, AC: 38%, ICS: 35%, LABA: 34%). Medication adherence was the highest with MTX. One possible explanation of this finding could be that elderly patients may have more difficulty using inhaled medications; therefore, they prefer oral drugs.

Breekveldt-Postma et al. (Breekveldt-Postma et al., 2007) evaluated medication persistence among COPD patients in the first therapy year; new users of tiotropium, ipratropium, LABA and a fixed combination of LABA and ICS (LABA + ICS) were included in their study. The persistence was the highest, 37%, with tiotropium. The COPD patient's drug-taking behaviour was found to be significantly lower with other inhaled medications (ipratropium: 14%, LABA: 13%, LABA + ICS: 17%). Subgroup analysis of persistence data in patients with prior hospitalisation for COPD indicated that hospitalisation may have an enhancing effect on patient cooperation. The one-year persistence rates were increased by 2–3 times in the first year after hospitalisation (tiotropium: 61%, ipratropium: 37%, LABA: 41%, LABA + ICS: 33%). A similar study by Cramer et al. (Cramer et al., 2007) examined trends in patient persistence with inhaled COPD medication. They monitored the refill data of ipratropium, ipratropium + salbutamol, formoterol, formoterol + budesonide, salmeterol, salmeterol + fluticason and tiotropium in a cohort of 31,368 COPD patients. The one-year persistence was considerably higher with tiotropium (53%) compared with other treatments (7%–30%). The significant differences in levels of adherence and persistence between inhaled medications could be partially the result of dosing frequency.

All of the aforementioned studies examined primary adherence, which is based on prescription refill rates. These results represent the maximum possible level of patient cooperation because refill adherence cannot confirm ingestion and does not provide any information on the frequency of medication use. Studies evaluating secondary adherence can provide data about medication use that is more reliable.

The Lung Health Study (Rand et al., 1995) was a double-blind, multicentre, randomised, controlled trial on smoking intervention and bronchodilator therapy (ipratropium or placebo) as early interventions of COPD. Satisfactory adherence was reported by 70% of the participants at the first 4-month follow-up visit, but this rate declined to 60% over the next 18 months. The overall adherence estimated by canister weighing was 72% in the first year and 70% in the second year. Nevertheless, in the first year, only 48% of the participants were classified as adherent with both methods. In an ancillary study within the Lung Health Study, medication adherence rates measured by both self-report and canister weighing were compared with data from electronic medication monitoring (Rand et al., 1992). This study found that self-reporting and canister weighing significantly overestimate adherence: only 15% of the participants used their inhaler 2.5 or more times per day (when three puffs per day were prescribed). In addition, 14% of the patients seemed to be "dumping" medication prior to the clinic visit by removing most of the medication at one time (i.e., actuating inhaler more than 100 times in a 3-h interval) to hide non-adherence. The level of adherence with the prescribed medication regimen was best immediately following each follow-up visit and declined during the interval between follow-up visits. The adherence after each visit was lower for each successive follow-up. These trends could be observed only with electronic medication monitors; self-reporting or weighing could not detect these changes (Simmons et al., 1996).

Studies also suggest that while the underuse of medication seems to be one of the largest problems in the management of COPD, overuse is also common. Symptom-relieving drugs, such as short-acting β_2 agonists (SABA), are more often overused than maintenance therapies (Dekker et al., 1993). Krigsman et al. (Krigsman et al., 2007a) evaluated the primary adherence in patients with asthma and COPD. The obtained results indicated that 53% of the patients underused and 18% overused their prescribed medication regimens. In another study by Krigsman et al. (Krigsman et al., 2007b), it was found that 59% of COPD patients had an undersupply and 12% had an oversupply of ICS medication.

Eighty-four percent of COPD patients have one or more co-morbidity (Yeo et al., 2006). For this reason, a question arises about whether the level of a patient's adherence is the same with therapies for different chronic diseases. Krigsman et al. (Krigsman et al., 2007c) investigated refill adherence in patients who suffered from diabetes and COPD. Participants showed higher adherence for their diabetes drugs (68%) than their COPD medications (42%).

Long-term oxygen therapy (LTOT) plays an important role in the management of COPD (Würtemberger & Hütter, 2000). The daily duration of oxygen administration is crucial in the effectiveness of LTOT. Pepin et al. (Pepin et al., 1996) found that only 45% of the COPD patients who were prescribed oxygen therapy for an average of 16 hours per day (16±3 h/d) used oxygen for 15 hours or more per day. Another study reported that 23% of the patients who had been prescribed LTOT refused to use liquid oxygen away from home and that 12% underused their oxygen (Würtemberger & Hütter, 2000).

Immunisation with both the influenza and pneumococcal vaccines may produce a number of acute exacerbations, hospitalisation and COPD mortality (Nichol et al., 1999; Varkey et al., 2009). However, the vaccination rates in patients with chronic lung diseases are low (Nichol et al., 1999; Tuppin et al., 2011), and the willingness to vaccinate differs by age group. The influenza vaccination status is significantly higher in patients aged 65 years or older (86.2%) than in the younger population (65.7%) (Mehuys et al., 2010).

3.2 Adherence to non-drug therapy

Adherence to non-drug therapies, such as respiratory rehabilitation, exercise programs, healthy lifestyle or smoking cessation, is crucial in the management of COPD. Approximately 60% of the patients refuse to take part in rehabilitation programs, and out of those who join, 30% fail to complete the program (Nici et al., 2006). The most important barriers to rehabilitation adherence include exacerbations and progression of COPD (Bourbeau et al., 2007; Brooks et al., 2002). The literature in this field is quite weak; there is a clear need for further research to find out more about the suboptimal adherence to non-drug therapies in patients with COPD.

4. Factors associated with adherence in patients with COPD

Non-adherence in patients with COPD is a multidimensional phenomenon. The factors include the characteristics of the patient, the disease, the therapies and the health-care provider–patient relationship; many of these are potentially modifiable (Baiardini et al., 2009; Restrepo et al., 2008; WHO, 2003) (Table 4).

COPD	Treatment
• Progressive nature of the disease ↓*	• Polypharmacy ↓
• Poor prognosis ↓	• Higher dosing frequency ↓
• Lack of clinical symptoms ↓	• Higher medication cost ↓
• Disease severity —	• Side effects ↓
• Lung function —	• Oral administration ↑
Patient	**Health-care provider–patient relationship**
• Gender -	• Higher quality of communication ↑
• Demographic factors: old age ↑	• Type of caregiver: specialist ↑
• Improved quality of life ↓	• Closer follow-up ↑
• Social support ↑	• Hospitalisation ↑
• Psychiatric co-morbidities ↓	

*Influence on adherence: decrease (↓), improve (↑), no effect (—)

Table 4. Factors associated with adherence in patients with COPD

4.1 Factors related to the characteristics of COPD

COPD is a progressive chronic disease. Adequate cooperation with COPD therapy can improve the patient's quality of life and reduce the frequency of exacerbations but cannot fully control the disease symptoms. A progressive decline in lung function is often interpreted by patients as the medication not helping, so they stop following the recommendations (Chambers et al., 1999). In contrast, a lack of clinical symptoms could also be a reason for suboptimal adherence (DiMatteo, 2004). As implied above, the negative impact of COPD severity or lung function on a patient's adherence is not obvious. Prior studies have shown that disease severity or the post-bronchodilator forced expiratory volume in one second (FEV_1) percentage may be either not (Agh et al., 2011) or negatively (Turner et al., 1995) related to adherence. The pathologic characteristics of COPD influence adherence to non-drug therapy as well; a poor COPD prognosis has been identified as one of the most demotivating factors to quit smoking (George et al., 2006b).

4.2 Factors related to the characteristics of the patient

Most prior studies have found that gender does not influence the level of patient cooperation (Agh et al., 2011; Apter et al., 1998; Corden et al., 1997; Turner et al., 1995). Adherence differences between men and women reported in the literature may be caused by psychological factors (Laforest et al., 2010). The prevalence of anxiety and depression are higher in women with COPD, and these psychiatric comorbidities have been independently linked with non-adherence (Bosley et al., 1995; DiMatteo et al., 2000).

In general, drug-taking behaviour is related to age; older patients seem to be more adherent. Patients of advanced age are more likely to adhere to therapy that requires adjustments in daily life (Agh et al., 2011). However, memory loss and cognitive impairment, which are associated with both age and COPD duration, may adversely affect adherence (Incalzi et al., 1997).

Social support can also influence patient adherence. Stable family life has been found to improve adherence to medication regimens (Tashkin, 1995; Turner et al., 1995). Furthermore, the study by George et al. (George et al., 2006b) indicates that patients with a good relationship with family and friends may live longer and may quit smoking with a higher success rate.

Better quality of life has been considered a trigger for non-adherence (Agh et al., 2011). Decision-making regarding patient adherence is a personal trade-off between the efficacy of the therapy and the negative effects that it generates. Adherence to COPD therapy can reduce the clinical symptoms and improve the patient's quality of life. However, COPD treatment regimens require adjustments in daily life, such as smoking cessation and exercise programs, and can cause side effects as well. Therefore, the interruption of drug therapy can temporarily also increases the patient's quality of life. Therapy in newly diagnosed COPD patients may significantly improve quality of life; however, the change in quality of life may be much smaller in patients treated previously for longer durations (Soumerai et al., 1991). From the patient's perspective, the benefits from the increase in the quality of life during the complication-free period can outweigh the effects of the worsening disease symptoms (Agh et al., 2011).

4.3 Factors related to the characteristics of the therapy

The number of medications and the dosing frequency have been linked with adherence. According to our evaluations, the dosing frequency of respiratory drugs is one of the most important factors affecting non-adherence in patients with COPD (Agh et al., 2011; WHO, 2003). As a partial result of the daily drug doses, a significant difference has been shown in the adherence rates between the different respiratory drug classes (Apter et al., 1998; Breekveldt-Postma et al., 2007; Laforest et al., 2010). Tiotropium, a once-daily inhaled drug, may enhance adherence compared with other inhaled respiratory medications that are dosed more times daily. We also found that polypharmacy is another common cause of poor adherence (Agh et al., 2011); complicated treatment regimens may frustrate the patients, which may lead to non-adherence (van der Palen et al., 1999).

Patient cooperation is better with oral medication than with inhaled drugs (James et al., 1985; Tashkin et al., 1991). Adherence with inhaled drugs may be compromised by inadequate inhaler technique (Garcia-Aymerich et al., 2000; Shrestha et al., 1996). Furthermore, better adherence with oral theophylline can also be due to the simplicity of the dosing regimens (Kelloway et al., 1995).

Other factors, such as adverse effects and medication costs, are also important. Medication cost is one of the greatest barriers to achieving adequate adherence (Cramer et al., 2007, Jung et al., 2009). Side effects or concerns about side effects from medications can reduce adherence as well (Dolce et al., 1991; Rand et al., 1995). For example, patients with COPD often confuse the side effects of ICS with those of anabolic steroids, which may decrease their cooperation willingness (Boulet, 1998).

4.4 Factors related to the characteristics of the health-care provider–patient relationship

Effective COPD management requires a good relationship between health-care providers and the patients. Quality of communication is related to adherence. Adherent patients report better overall communication with their providers (Blais et al., 2004). Education during the consultation and providing more information about the therapy may improve adherence (Raynor, 1992), as it reduces the risk of forgetting the providers' recommendations and the likelihood of misunderstandings between providers and patients. Previous studies suggest that immediately after the consultation, patients recall less than 50% of the information conveyed by their provider (DiMatteo, 1991).

The type of caregiver also influences adherence. Medication adherence may increase if the prescribing physician is a specialist instead of a general practitioner (Lau et al., 1996). Furthermore, periodic visits, closer follow-up and hospitalisation may also have increasing effects on patient cooperation (Breekveldt-Postma et al., 2007).

5. Adherence enhancing interventions

Strategies for improving patient adherence have to be formulated based on factors related to adherence. Seventy-six adherence interventions were evaluated in the systematic review by Petrilla and Benner (Petrilla & Benner, 2003).

They identified the following main categories of adherence-enhancing interventions:

- coordination of healthcare: improved linkages between primary care physicians, clinicians and other health professionals;
- live consultation and education;
- changes to the therapy dose, dosage and packaging to enhance the drug-taking convenience;
- patient education materials;
- disease management programs by clinicians;
- reminders: medication refill reminders delivered by mail or telephone;
- self-monitoring;
- social support programs;
- and combinations of these interventions.

Successful adherence-enhancing programs include simplified treatment regimens, facilitation of the physician–patient relationship and patient education methods (Petrilla & Benner, 2003).

While many studies have evaluated strategies to enhance adherence, few of these have focused on COPD. Strategies for improving adherence in COPD include simplifying treatment regimens, improving communication between providers and patients, disease education, optimising inhaler technique, reinforcement and self-management (self-monitoring of symptoms and medication use).

It may be important to prescribe drugs with a fixed combination and/or a low dosing frequency to enhance adherence to COPD medication. Furthermore, the recommended treatment should fit into the patient's limitations and lifestyle. Because many COPD patients are elderly, with the dual risk of cognitive impairment and complex medication regimens, the use of dosing aids and adherence devices, such as medication lists, dosette boxes and timers, should be promoted.

Health-care providers must help their patients understand the progressive nature of COPD and the goals of the comprehensive treatment regimens. Physicians should actively involve patients in decisions regarding their therapy and give strong weight to their personal preferences and concerns. Periodic monitoring, understanding the patient's beliefs and positive reinforcement could also enhance adherence to therapy (Dunbar et al., 1979).

6. Conclusion

Suboptimal adherence to medication regimens and to other non-drug therapies are both major problems in the management of COPD. Poor adherence poses a significant health and economic burden in patients with COPD. Non-adherence seems to be influenced by many individual reasons, such as factors associated with the characteristics of the disease, the patient, the therapy and the physician-patient relationship. Among other things, simplified treatment regimens, adequate patient education methods and better communication between caregivers and patients have been found to be critical for overcoming the barriers of poor adherence. However, further research is needed to identify factors related to patient cooperation to develop more effective strategies that can improve adherence.

7. References

Agh, T.; Inotai, A. & Mezsaros, A. (2011). Factors Associated with Medication Adherence in Patients with Chronic Obstructive Pulmonary Disease. *Respiration,* Vol.82, No.4, (September 2011), pp. 328–34, ISSN 0025–7931f

Apter, A.J.; Reisine, S.T.; Affleck, G.; Barrows, E. & ZuWallack, R.L. (1998). Adherence with twice-daily dosing of inhaled steroids. Socioeconomic and health-belief differences. *American Journal of Respiratory and Critical Care Medicine,* Vol.157, No.6, (June 1998), pp. 1810–1817, ISSN 1073–449X

Baiardini, I.; Braido, F.; Bonini, M.; Compalati, E. & Canonica, G.W. (2009). Why do doctors and patients not follow guidelines? *Current Opinion in Allergy and Clinical Immunology,* Vol.9, No.3, (June 2009), pp. 228–233, ISSN 1528–4050

Blais, L.; Bourbeau, J.; Sheehy, O. & LeLorier, J. (2004). Inhaled corticosteroids in COPD: determinants of use and trends in patient persistence with treatment. *Canadian Respiratory Journal*, Vol.11, No.1, (January 2004), pp. 27–32, ISSN 1198–2241

Bosley, C.M.; Parry, D.T. & Cochrane, G.M. (1994). Patient compliance with inhaled medication. Does combining beta agonists with corticosteroids improve compliance? *European Respiratory Journal*, Vol.7, No.3, (March 1994), pp. 504–509 ISSN 0903–1936

Bosley, C.M.; Fosbury, J.A. & Cochrane, G.M. (1995). The psychological factors associated with poor compliance with treatment in asthma. *European Respiratory Journal*, Vol.8, No.6, (June 1995), pp. 899–904, ISSN 0903–1936

Boulet, L.P. (1998). Perception of the role and potential side effects of inhaled corticosteroids among asthmatic patients. *Chest*, Vol.113, No.3, (March 1998), pp. 587–592, ISSN 0012–3692

Bourbeau, J. & Bartlett, S.J. (2008). Patient adherence in COPD. *Thorax*, Vol.63, No.9, (September 2008), pp. 831–838, ISSN 0040–6376

Breekveldt-Postma, N.S.; Koerselman, J.; Erkens, J.A.; Lammers, J.W. & Herings, R.M. (2007). Enhanced persistence with tiotropium compared with other respiratory drugs in COPD. *Respiratory Medicine*, Vol.101, No.7, (July 2007), pp. 1398–1405, ISSN 0954–6111

Brooks, D.; Krip, B.; Mangovski-Alzamora, S. & Goldstein, R.S. (2002). The effect of postrehabilitation programmes among individuals with chronic obstructive pulmonary disease. *European Respiratoy Journal*, Vol.20, No.1, (July 2002), pp. 20–29, ISSN 0903–1936

Caetano, P.A.; Lam, J.M. & Morgan, S.G. (2006). Toward a standard definition and measurement of persistence with drug therapy: Examples from research on statin and antihypertensive utilization. *Clinical Therapeutics*, Vol.28, No.9, (September 2006), pp. 1411–1424, ISSN 0149–1918

Chambers, C.V.; Markson, L.; Ciamond, J.J.; Lasch, L. & Berger, M. (1999). Health belief and compliance with inhaled coritcosteroids by asthmatic patients in primary care practices. *Respiratory Medicine*, Vol.93, No.2, (February 1999), pp. 88–94, ISSN 0954–6111

Chapman, K.R.; Mannino, D.M.; Soriano, J.B.; Vermeire, P.A.; Buist, A.S.; Thun, M.J.; Connell, C.; Jemal, A.; Lee, T.A.; Miravitlles, M.; Aldington, S. & Beasley, R. (2006). Epidemiology and costs of chronic obstructive pulmonary disease. *European Respiratoy Journal*, Vol.27, No.1, (January 2006), pp. 188–207, ISSN 0903–1936

Clark, D.J.; Tan, K.S. & Lipworth, B.J. (1996). Evaluation of plasma and urinary salbutamol levels in COPD. *Eurpean Journal of Clinical Pharmacology*, Vol.51, No.1, (September 1996), pp. 91–93, ISSN 0031–6970

Corden, Z.M.; Bosley, C.M.; Rees, P.J. & Cochrane, G.M. (1997). Home nebulized therapy for patients with COPD: patient compliance with treatment and its relation to quality of life. *Chest*, Vol.112, No.5, (November 1997), pp. 1278–1282, ISSN 0012–3692

Cramer, J.A.; Bradley-Kennedy, C. & Scalera, A. (2007). Treatment persistence and compliance with medications for chronic obstructive pulmonary disease. *Canadian Respiratory Journal*, Vol.14, No.1, (January 2007), pp. 25–29 ISSN 1198–2241

Cramer, J.A.; Roy, A.; Burrell, A.; Fairchild, C.J.; Fuldeore, M.J.; Ollendorf, D.A. & Wong, P.K. (2008). Medication compliance and persistence: terminology and definitions. *Value in Health*, Vol.11, No.1, (January 2008), pp. 44–7, ISSN 1098–3015

Cramer, J. A.; Benedict, A.; Muszbek, N.; Keskinaslan, A. & Khan, Z.M. (2008). The significance of compliance and persistence in the treatment of diabetes, hypertension and dyslipidaemia: a review. *International Journal of Clinical Practice*, Vol.62, No.1, (January 2008), pp. 76–87, ISSN 1368–5031

Dekker, F.W.; Dieleman, F.E.; Kaptein, A.A. & Mulder, J.D. (1993). Compliance with pulmonary medication in general practice. *European Respiratory Journal*, Vol.6, No.6, (June 1993), pp. 886–890, ISSN 0903–1936

DiMatteo, M.R. (1991). *Psychology of Health Illness and Medical Care: An Individual Perspective*, Brooks/Cole, ISBN 978–053–4150–48–8, Pacific Grove, California, United States

DiMatteo, M.R.; Lepper, H.S. & Croghan, T.W. (2000). Depression is a risk factor for noncompliance with medical treatment: meta-analysis of the effects of anxiety and depression on patient adherence. *Archives of Internal Medicine*, Vol.160, No.14, (July 2000), pp. 2101–2107, ISSN 0003–9926

DiMatteo, M.R. (2004.) Variations in patients' adherence to medical recommendations: a quantitative review of 50 years of research. *Medical Care*, Vol.42, No.3, (March 2004), pp. 200–209, ISSN 0025–7079

Dolce, J.J.; Crisp, C.; Manzella, B.; Richards, J.M.; Hardin, J.M. & Bailey, W.C. (1991). Medication Adherence Patterns in Chronic Obstructive Pulmonary Disease. *Chest*, Vol.99, No.4, (April 1991), pp. 837–841, ISSN 0012–3692

Dompeling, E.; van Grunsven, P.M.; van Schayck, C.P.; Folgering, H.; Molema, J. & van Weel, C. (1992). Treatment with inhaled steroids in asthma and chronic bronchitis: long-term compliance and inhaler technique. Family Practice, Vol.9, No.2, (June 1992), pp. 161–166, ISSN 0263–2136

Dunbar, J.; Marshall, G. & Hovel, M. (1979). Behavioral strategies for improving compliance. In: *Compliance in health care*, R. Haynes, D. Wayne, D.L. Sackett, (Eds.), pp. 174–190, Johns Hopkins University Press, ISBN 0–8018–2162–2, Baltimore, United States

George, J.; Kong, D.C.; Thoman, R. & Stewart, K. (2005). Factors associated with medication nonadherence in patients with COPD. *Chest*, Vol.128, No.5, (November 2005), pp. 3198–3204, ISSN 0012–3692

George, J.; Mackinnon, A.; Kong, D.C. & Stewart, K. (2006a). Development and validation of the Beliefs and Behaviour Questionnaire (BBQ). *Patient Education and Counseling*, Vol.64, No.1-3, (December 2006), pp. 50–60, ISSN 0738–3991

George, J.; Kong, D.C.; Santamaria, N.; Ioannides-Demos, L. & Stewart, K. (2006b). Smoking cessation: COPD patients' perspective. *Journal of Pharmacy Practice and Research*, Vol.36, No.2, (June 2006), pp. 107–10, ISSN 1445–937X

George, J.;Kong, D.C. & Stewart K. (2007). Adherence to disease management programs in patients with COPD. *International Journal of COPD*, Vol.2, No.3, (October 2007), pp. 253–262, ISSN 1176–9106

Garcia-Aymerich, J.; Barreiro, E.; Farrero, E.; Marrades, R.M.; Morera, J. & Anto, J.M. (2000). Patients hospitalized for COPD have a high prevalence of modifiable risk factors for exacerbation (EFRAM study). *European Respiratory Journal*, Vol.16, No.6, (December 2009), pp. 1037–1042, ISSN 0903–1936

Hatton, M.Q.; Allen, M.B.; Vathenen, S.V.; Feely, M.p. & Cooke N.J. (1996). Compliance with oral corticosteroids during steroid trials in chronic airways obstruction. *Thorax,* Vol.51, No.3, (March 1996), pp. 323–324, ISSN 0040–6376

Incalzi, R.A.; Capparella, O.; Gemma, A.; Landi, F.; Bruno, E.; DiMeo, F. & Carbonin, P. (1997). The interaction between age and comorbidity contributes to predicting the mortality of geriatric patients in the acute-care hospital. *Journal of Internal Medicine,* Vol.242, No.4, (October 1997), pp. 291–298, ISSN 0954–6820

James, P.N.; Anderson, J.B.; Prior, J.G.; White, J.P.; Henry, J.A. & Cochrane, G.M. (1985). Patterns of drug taking in patients with chronic airflow obstruction. *Postgraduate Medical Journal,* Vol.61, No.711, (Januar 1985), pp. 7–10, ISSN 0032–5473

Jung, E.; Pickard, A.S.; Salmon, J.W.; Bartle, B. & Lee, T.A. (2009). Medication adherence and persistence in the last year of life in COPD patients. *Respiratory Medicine,* Vol.103, No.4, (April 2009), pp. 525–534, ISSN 0954–6111

Kelloway, J.S.; Wyatt, R.A. & Adlis, S.A. (1994). Comparison of patients' compliance with prescribed oral and inhaled asthma medications. *Archives of Internal Medicine,* Vol.154, No.12, (June 1994), pp. 1349–1352, ISSN 0003–9926

Kesten, S.; Flanders, J.; Serby, C.W. & Witek, T.J. (2000) Compliance with tiotropium, a once daily dry powder inhaled bronchodilator, in one year COPD trials. *Chest,* Vol.118, No.4, (October 2000), pp. 191S–192S, ISSN 0012–3692

Krigsman, K.; Nilsson, J.L. & Ring, L. (2007a). Refill adherence for patients with asthma and COPD: comparison of a pharmacy record database with manually collected repeat prescriptions. *Pharmacoepidemiology & Drug Safety,* Vol.16, No.4, (April 2007), pp. 441–448, ISSN 1053–8569

Krigsman, K.; Moen, J.; Nilsson, J.L. & Ring, L. (2007b). Refill adherence by the elderly for asthma/chronic obstructive pulmonary disease drugs dispensed over a 10-year period. *Journal of Clinical Pharmacy and Therapeutics,* Vol.32, No.6, (December 2007), pp. 603–611, ISSN 0269–4727

Krigsman, K.; Nilsson, J.L. & Ring, L. (2007c). Adherence to multiple drug therapies: refi ll adherence to concomitant use of diabetes and asthma/COPD medication. *Pharmacoepidemiology & Drug Safety,* Vol.16, No.10, (October 2007), pp. 1120–1128, ISSN 1053–8569

Laforest, L.; Denis, F.; Van Ganse, E.; Ritleng, C.; Saussier, C.; Passante, N.; Devouassoux, G.; Chatte, G.; Freymond, N. & Pacheco, Y. (2010). Correlates of adherence to respiratory drugs in COPD patients. *Primary Care Respiratory Journal,* Vol.19, No.2, (June 2010), pp. 148–154, ISSN 1475–1534

Mehuys, E.; Boussery, K.; Adriaens, E.; van Bortel, L.; de Bolle, L.; van Tongelen, I.; Remon, J.P. & Brusselle, G. (2010). COPD management in primary care: an observational, community pharmacy-based study. *Annals of Pharmacotherapy,* Vol.44, No.2, (February 2010), pp. 257–266, ISSN 1060–0280

Nici, L.; ZuWallack, R.; Wouters, E. & Donner, C.F. (2006). On pulmonary rehabilitation and the flight of the bumblebee: the ATS/ERS Statement on Pulmonary Rehabilitation. *European Respiratory Journal,* Vol.28, No.3, (September 2006), pp. 461–462, ISSN 0903–1936

Nichol, K.L.; Baken, L. & Nelson, A. (1999). Relation between influenza vaccination and outpatient visits, hospitalization, and mortality in elderly persons with chronic lung disease. *Annals of Internal Medicine*, Vol.130, No.5, (March 1999), pp. 397–403, ISSN 0003–4819

Pepin, J.L.; Barjhoux, C.E.;Deschaux, C. & Brambilla, C. (1996). Long-term oxygen therapy at home. Compliance with medical prescription and effective use of therapy. ANTADIR Working Group on Oxygen Therapy. *Chest*, Vol.109, No.5, (May 1996), pp. 1144–1150, ISSN 0012–3692

Peterson, A.M.; Nau, D.P.; Cramer, J.A.; Benner, J.; Gwadry-Sridhar, F. & Nichol, M. (2007). A checklist for medication compliance and persistence studies using retrospective databases. *Value in Health*, Vol.10, No.1, (January 2007), pp. 3–12, ISSN 1098–3015

Petrilla, A.A. & Benner, J.S. (2003). Critical evaluation of interventions to enhance patient compliance with chronic medications. *Value in Health*, Vol.6, No.3, (May 2003), pp. 200, ISSN 1098–3015

Rand, C.S.; Wise, R.A.; Nides, M.; Simmons, M.S.; Bleecker, E.R.; Kusek, J.W.; Li, V.C. & Tashkin, D.P. (1992). Metered-dose inhaler adherence in a clinical trial. *American Review of Respiratory Disease*, Vol.146, No.6, (December 1992), pp. 1559–1564, ISSN 0003–0805

Rand, C.S.; Nides, M.; Cowles, M.K.; Wise, R.A. & Connett, J. (1995). Long-term metered-dose inhaler adherence in a clinical trial. The Lung Health Study Research Group. *American Journal of Respiratory and Critical Care Medicine*, Vol.152, No.2, (August 1995), pp. 580–588, ISSN 1073–449X

Rand, C.S. (2005). Patient adherence with COPD therapy. *European Respiratory Review*, Vol.14, No.96, (December 2005), pp. 97–101, ISSN 0905–9180

Raynor, D. (1992). Patient compliance: the pharmacist's role. *International Journal of Pharmacy Practice*, Vol.1, No.3, (March 1992), pp. 126–135, ISSN 0961–7671

Regueiro, C.R.; Hamel, M.B.; Davis, R.B.; Desbiens, N.; Connors, A.F. & Phillips, R.S. (1998). A comparison of generalist and pulmonologist care for patients hospitalized with severe chronic obstructive pulmonary disease: Resource intensity, hospital costs, and survival. *American Journal of Medicine*, Vol.105, No.5, (November 1998), pp. 366–372, ISSN 0002–9343

Restrepo, R.D.; Alvarez, M.T.; Wittnebel, L.D.; Sorenson, H.; Wettstein, R.; Vines, D.L.; Sikkema-Ortiz, J.; Gardner, D.D. & Wilkins, R.L. (2008) Medication adherence issues in patients treated for COPD. *International Journal of Chronic Obstructive Plumonary Disease*, Vol.3, No.3, (October 2008), pp. 371–384, ISSN 1178–2005

Revicki, D.A. & Frank, L. (1999). Pharmacoeconomic evaluation in the real world: Effectiveness versus efficacy studies. *Pharmacoeconomics*, Vol.15, No.5, (May 1999), pp. 423–434, ISSN 1170–7690

Shrestha, M.; Parupia, M.; Andrews, B.; Kim, S.; Martin, T.; Park, D. & Gee, E. (1996). Metered-dose inhaler technique of patients in an urban ED: Prevalence of incorrect technique and attempt at education. *The American Journal of Emergency Medicine*, Vol.14, No.4, (July 1996), pp. 380–384, ISSN 0735–6757

Simmons, M.S.; Nides, M.A.; Rand, C.S.; Wise, R.A. & Tashkin, D.P. (1996). Trends in compliance with bronchodilator inhaler use between follow-up visits in a clinical trial. *Chest*, Vol.109, No.4, (April 1996), pp. 963–968, ISSN 0012–3692

Simmons, M.S.; Nides, M.A.; Rand, C.S.; Wise, R.A. & Tashkin, D.P. (2000). Unpredictability of deception in compliance with physician-prescribed bronchodilator inhaler use in a clinical trial. *Chest*, Vol.118, No.2, (August 2000), pp. 290–295, ISSN 0012–3692

Soumerai, S.B.; Ross-Degnan, D.; Avorn, J.; McLaughlin, T. & Choodnovskiy, I. (1991). Effects of Medicaid drug-payment limits on admission to hospitals and nursing homes. *New England Journal of Medicine*, Vol.325, No.15, (October 1991), pp. 1072–1077, ISSN 0028–4793

Tashkin, D.P.; Rand, C.; Nides, M.; Simmons, M.; Wise, R.; Coulson, A.H.; Li, V. & Gong, H. Jr. (1991). A nebulizer chronolog to monitor compliance with inhaler use. *American Journal of Medicine*, Vol.91, No.4, (October 1991), pp. 33S–36S, ISSN 0002–9343

Tashkin, D.P. (1995). Multiple dose regimens. Impact on compliance. *Chest*, Vol.107, No.5, (May 1995), pp. 176S–182S, ISSN 0012–3692

Tuppin, P.; Samson, S.; Weill, A.; Ricordeau, P. & Allemand, H. (2011). Seasonal influenza vaccination coverage in France during two influenza seasons (2007 and 2008) and during a context of pandemic influenza A(H1N1) in 2009. *Vaccine*, Vol.29, No.28, (June 2011), pp. 4632–4637, ISSN 0264–410X

Turner, J.; Wright, E.; Mendella, L. & Anthonisen, (1995). Predictors of patient adherence to long-term home nebulizer therapy for COPD. The IPPB Study Group. Intermittent Positive Pressure Breathing. *Chest*, Vol.108, No.2, (August 1995), pp. 394–400, ISSN 0012–3692

van der Palen, J.; Klein, J.J.; van Herwaarden, C.L.; Zielhuis, G.A. & Seydel, E.R. (1991). Multiple inhalers confuse asthma patients. *European Respiratory Journal*, Vol.14, No.5, (November 1999), pp. 1034–1037, ISSN 0903–1936

van Grunsven, P.M.; van Schayck, C.P.; van Deuveren, M.; van Herwaarden, C.L.; Akkermans, R.P. & van Weel, C. (2000). Compliance during longterm treatment with fluticasone propionate in subjects with early signs of asthma or chronic obstructive pulmonary disease (COPD): results of the Detection, Intervention, and Monitoring Program of COPD and Asthma (DIMCA) Study. *Journal of Asthma*, Vol.37, No.3, (May 2000), pp. 225–234, ISSN 0277–0903

Varkey, J.B.; Varkey, A.B. & Varkey, B. (2009). Prophylactic vaccinations in chronic obstructive pulmonary disease: current status. *Current Opinion in Pulmonary Medicine*, Vol.15, No.2, (March 2009), pp. 90–99, ISSN 1070–5287

Vestbo, J.; Anderson, J.A.; Calverley, P.M.; Celli, B.; Ferguson, G.T.; Jenkins, C.; Yates, J.C. & Jones, P.W. (2011). Bias due to withdrawal in long-term randomised trials in COPD: evidence from the TORCH study. *Clinical Respiratory Journal*, Vol.5, No.1, (Januar 2011), pp. 44–49, ISSN 1752–6981

Viegi, G.; Scognamiglio, A.; Baldacci, S.; Pistelli, F. & Carrozzi, L. (2001). Epidemiology of Chronic Obstructive Pulmonary Disease (COPD). *Respiration*, Vol.68, No.1, (Januar 2001), pp. 4–19, ISSN 0025–7931

World Health Organization. (2003). *Adherence to long-term therapies: Evidence for action*, World Health Organization, Retrieved from: http://www.who.int/chp/knowledge/publications/adherence_full_report.pdf

Würtemberger, G. & Hütter, B.O. (2000). Health-related quality of life, psychological adjustment and compliance to treatment in patients on domiciliary liquid oxygen. *Monaldi Archives Chest Disease*, Vol.55, No.3, (June 2000), pp. 216–224, ISSN 1122–0643

Yeo, J.; Karimova, G. & Bansal, S. (2006). Co-morbidity in older patients with COPD – Its impact on health service utilisation and quality of life, a community study. *Age and Ageing*, Vol.35, No.1, (January 2006), pp. 33–37, ISSN 0002–0729

3

Noninvasive Positive-Pressure Ventilation Therapy in Patients with COPD

Zeynep Zeren Ucar
The Department of Pulmonary Disease and Sleep Disorders,
Dr Suat Seren Chest Diseases and Surgery
Training and Research Hospital, Izmir
Turkey

1. Introduction

Noninvasive positive pressure ventilation (NPPV) refers to the administration of ventilatory support without using an invasive artificial airway (endotracheal tube or tracheostomy tube). The use of NPPV has markedly increased over the past two decades. Rudimentary devices that provided continuous positive airway pressure were described in the 1930s, but the negative-pressure ventilators were the predominant method of ventilatory support until the polio epidemics overwhelmed their capacity in the 1950s. In the 1980s, increasing experience with positive-pressure ventilation delivered through a mask in patients with obstructive sleep apnea led to this type of ventilatory support, initially in patients with neuromuscular respiratory failure. Success led to its adoption in other conditions, and NPPV became especially promising in the treatment of patients with exacerbations of chronic obstructive pulmonary disease (COPD).

NPPV is defined as ventilatory support delivered by a non-invasive interface such as mask or similar device, acting as an alternative to intubation or tracheostomy. Consequently, by avoiding tracheal intubation, NPPV presents several potential advantages, such as reduction in pulmonary infections, barotrauma and need for sedation (British Thoracic Society Standards of Care Committee 2002). As a result, NPPV should be considered a standard of care to treat COPD exacerbation in selected patients, since it markedly reduces the need for intubation and improves outcome by lowering complication and mortality rates, and shortening hospital stay (Brochard et al. 1995; Kramer et al. 1995; Celikel et al. 1998; Martin et al. 2000; Conti et al. 2002; Squadrone et al. 2004; Lightowler et al. 2003; Nava, Navalesi, & Conti 2006). Weaker evidence indicates that NPPV could allow earlier extubation, avoid re-intubation in patients who fail extubation, and assist do-not-intubate patients, and thus could be beneficial for COPD patients who are suffering respiratory failure precipitated by superimposed pneumonia or postoperative complications, and COPD patients with severe stable disease who have substantial daytime hypercapnia and superimposed nocturnal hypoventilation.

This chapter will examine the evidence pertaining to the use of NPPV for various applications in COPD and make recommendation on patient, ventilation mode and interface selection as well as technical aspects of NPPV application in COPD. The literature review and consensus processes used to reach the recommendations presented here are the American College of Chest Physicians [ACCP] consensus report on clinical indications for NPPV in CRF due to restrictive lung disease, COPD and nocturnal hypoventilation published in 1999, the British Thoracic Society guidelines published in 2002, the Indian Society of Critical Care Medicine guidelines published in 2006, the guidelines from 12 German Medical Societies published in 2008 and the most recent guideline published in 2011 from Canadian Critical Care Trials Group/Canadian Critical Care Society Noninvasive Ventilation Guidelines Group.

2. Physiologic mechanism of NPPV effect in patients with COPD

Severe COPD places the respiratory muscles at a mechanical disadvantage (Rochester, Braun, & Arora 1979). During COPD exacerbation, this situation becomes catastrophic. Exacerbations of COPD increase the respiratory load in these patients, exceeding their ability to adequately ventilate through a variety of mechanisms, including increasing hyperinflation with decreased diaphragmatic excursion and strength, increasing intrinsic positive end-expiratory pressure (PEEP), changes in respiratory patterns and increased respiratory frequency leading to ineffective or inadequate tidal volume generation. NPPV effectively unloads the respiratory muscles by increasing tidal volume, decreasing the respiratory rate, and decreasing the diaphragmatic work of breathing, which translates into an improvement in oxygenation, a reduction in hypercapnia, and an improvement in dyspnea. NPPV treatment counterbalances auto-PEEP, assists inspiration, reduces transdiaphragmatic pressure, lowers respiratory rate, rests the accessory muscles, increases functional residual capacity, decreases respiratory load and work of breathing and leads to favorable changes in the ventilation/perfusion ratio as well as the respiratory center and the sensivity of chemoreceptors (Mansfield & Naughton 1999; de Miguel et al. 2002). Expiration positive airway pressure (EPAP) counterbalances intrinsic PEEP. Inspiration positive airway pressure (IPAP) is capable of increasing tidal volume and subsequently decreasing the elevated levels of PC02.

3. Indications of NPPV in patients with COPD

3.1 Acute respiratory failure/Exacerbation of COPD

Based upon the overwhelming evidence that NPPV reduces the need for intubation, reduces mortality and complications rates, and shortens the length of stay in both the intensive care unit (ICU) and hospital (Kramer et al. 1995; Brochard et al. 1995; Celikel et al. 1998; Martin et al. 2000; Carlucci et al. 2001; Mehta & Hill 2001) , NPPV should be considered as a standard of care in acute respiratory failure (ARF) due to COPD exacerbations (Keenan et al. 2011). Brochard et al. were the first to show that pressure-support ventilation administered via face mask significantly reduced the need for intubation, duration of mechanical ventilation, and ICU stay in patients with COPD exacerbations (Brochard et al. 1990). The patients with relatively mild COPD exacerbations are not likely to benefit from NPPV, which suggests that NPPV should be applied to selected patients who have moderate-to-severe COPD exacerbations. Though, patients with milder exacerbations appear to demonstrate a more rapid improvement in their level of dyspnea with NPPV treatment, the addition of NPPV to standard therapy for patients with milder exacerbations of COPD is not well tolerated (Keenan, Powers, & McCormack 2005). NPPV should be the first option for ventilatory support in patients with either a severe exacerbation of COPD or cardiogenic pulmonary edema(Keenan et al. 2011). Furthermore, consensus groups of experts advocate the routine use of NPPV for selected patients with COPD exacerbations (British Thoracic Society Standards of Care Committee 2002). High quality studies have shown that NPPV is an effective treatment for moderate to severe COPD exacerbation (Kramer et al. 1995; Celikel et al. 1998; Martin et al. 2000). In patients with mild to moderate ARF, characterized by pH levels between 7.25 and 7.35, the rate of NPPV failure was ranging from 15% to 20% (Elliott 2002; Lightowler et al. 2003). In more severely ill patients (pH<7.25), the rate of NPPV failure was inversely related to the severity of respiratory acidosis, rising up to 52%-62% (Conti et al. 2002; Squadrone et al. 2004). In patients with "mild" exacerbations, not complicated by respiratory acidosis, the use of NPPV was investigated in few studies, including patients in large majority with pH>7.35, which failed to demonstrate a better effectiveness of NPPV than standard medical therapy in preventing the occurrence of ARF (Bardi et al. 2000; Keenan, Powers, & McCormack 2005). Guidelines recommend the use of NPPV in addition to usual care in patients who have a severe exacerbation of COPD (pH<7.35 and relative hypercarbia) (grade 1A recommendation) (Keenan et al. 2011). Based on that evidence, the authors of the meta-analyses and the participants in the consensus groups recommended that NPPV should be used early in the course of a COPD exacerbation, in addition to the standard medical care (Lightowler et al. 2003; Keenan et al. 2003; British Thoracic Society Standards of Care Committee 2002) . NPPV is not appropriate for all COPD patients with ARF and the selection of candidates is important. Most of the indications and contraindications for NPPV in ARF are listed in Table 1 (Brochard et al. 1995). There are no absolute contraindications to NPPV although a number have been suggested (Ambrosino et al. 1995; Soo Hoo, Santiago, & Williams 1994). In part, these contraindications have been determined by the fact that they were exclusion criteria for the controlled trials. It is therefore accurate to state that NPPV is not proven in these circumstances rather than stating that it is contraindicated.

3.2 Severe community-acquired pneumonia in patients with COPD

The presence of pneumonia has been associated with poor outcome in patients treated with NPPV (Ambrosino et al. 1995). However COPD exacerbation is still an appropriate indication for NPPV even when complicated by community-acquired pneumonia (Confalonieri et al. 1999). In one randomized trial with patients suffering severe community-acquired pneumonia, NPPV reduced the need for intubation, and reduced mortality among the COPD subgroup of patients 2 months after hospital discharge (Confalonieri et al. 1999). But it is not clear whether NPPV should be used for severe community-acquired pneumonia in non-COPD patients.

3.3 Adjunct to early liberation

Patients with COPD can be considered for a trial of early extubation to NPPV in centres with extensive experience in the use of NPPV (Keenan et al. 2011). Guidelines suggest that NPPV be used to facilitate early liberation from mechanical ventilation in patients who have COPD, but only in centres that have expertise in this therapy (Grade 2B recommendation) (Keenan et al. 2011). Recent randomized controlled trials (RCTs) suggested benefit from NPPV after extubation in patients who had high risk of deterioration (Ferrer et al. 2006; Ferrer et al. 2009; Nava et al. 2005; Luo, Cheng, & Zhou 2001). The results of the RCTs of

Indications
• Increased dyspnea-moderate to severe • Tachypnea (>25 breaths per minute) • Signs of increased work of breathing, accessory muscle use, pursed lips breathing and abdominal paradox • Acute or chronic ventilatory failure (best indication), PaCO2 >45 mmHg, pH <7.35 • Hypoxaemia (use caution), PaO2/FiO2 ratio < 200
Contraindications
Absolute • Cardiac or respiratory arrest • Severe encephalopathy • Unable to fit mask Relative • Severe haemodynamic instability with or without cardiac ischemia or arrhythmia • Severe gastrointestinal bleeding • Agitated, uncooperative state • Upper airway obstruction • Inability to protect the airway and/or high risk of aspiration • Inability to clear secretions • Multiple organ failure • Recent facial, upper airway or upper gastrointestinal surgery

[NPPV= non-invasive positive pressure ventilation; PaCO2: arterial partial pressure of carbon dioxide; PaO2: arterial partial pressure of oxygen; FiO2: fraction of inspired oxygen]   ·

Table 1. Indications and contraindications for NPPV in ARF

early extubation in COPD patients with NPPV are controversial, some showing significant benefit and the other showing no important benefit, but no attributable harm in either (Girault et al. 1999; Ferrer et al. 2003). Intubated COPD patients are appropriate candidates for early extubation by NPPV, but clinicians are advised to be cautious when selecting patients. The inability to sustain 5–10 min of unassisted breathing, a prior difficult intubation, multiple co-morbidities, copious secretions, a weakened cough, or the need for high levels of pressure support prior to extubation (>20 cm H2O) should exclude patients from consideration for early extubation (Hill 2004).

3.4 After planned extubation

Extubation failure occurs after 5-20% of planned (Epstein, Ciubotaru, and Wong 1997) and 40-50% of unplanned extubation (Chevron et al. 1998) NPPV may prevent the need for reintubation if applied immediately after planned extubation. NPPV is recommended to be used after planned extubation in patients who are considered to be at high risk of recurrent respiratory failure, but only in centres that have expertise in this type of therapy (Grade 2B recommendation) (Keenan et al. 2011). We should be careful to avoid delays in intubation in the face of deterioration and to select the patients for extubation.

3.5 Postoperative patients

It has been shown that NPPV in post-lung-resection patients with acute respiratory failure results in significantly less need for intubation, shorter ICU stay, and lower mortality rate than conventionally treated controls (Auriant et al. 2001) . The use of NPPV in selected postoperative patients (especially COPD patients) could maintain improved gas exchange and avoid reintubation and its complications.

3.6 Do-not-intubate patients

In the studies of patients in whom endotracheal intubation was contraindicated or postponed, COPD subgroup were supported with NPPV and weaned more successfully than the pneumonia or cancer subgroup of patients (Benhamou et al. 1992; Meduri et al. 1994). Thus, NPPV is indicated in do-not-intubate patients with acutely reversible processes that are known to respond well, including COPD exacerbations. However, if NPPV is to be used in a do-not-intubate patient, the patient and/or the family should be informed that NPPV is being used as a form of life support that may be uncomfortable and can be removed at any time (Hill 2004).

3.7 Overlap syndrome

The term "overlap syndrome" was introduced by Flenly to describe the association of obstructive sleep apnea syndrome (OSAS) and COPD (Flenley 1985). Even by chance alone, a patient with one of the disorders has a greater than 10% probability of also having the other disorder. Thus, when seeing a patient with either OSAS or COPD, it is reasonable to screen for the lower and longer nocturnal oxyhemoglobin desaturations, which produces more severe pulmonary hemodynamic complications (Chaouat et al. 1995; Bednarek et al. 2005). Concomitant COPD in patients with severe OSAS so called critical care syndrome is frequently associated with diurnal hypercapnia and acute ventilatory failure (Fletcher et al. 1991). There is an increase in the morbidity and mortality and risk of developing pulmonary hypertension and hypercapnic respiratory failure in patients with overlap syndrome than patients with OSAS alone and patients with usual COPD (Chaouat et al. 1995; Chaouat et al. 1999). NPPV with or without supplemental oxygen is now the treatment of choice for the patients with overlap syndrome (Mayos et al. 2001).

Improvement in daytime hypercapnia and gas exchange has been reported in overlap syndrome with continuous positive airway pressure (CPAP) treatment (Owens & Malhotra. 2010). Mild bronchodilatory effect due to amelioration of chronic irritation and responsiveness of the upper airway and reduction of the chronic airway has also been suggested as the possible mechanisms for the benefits of CPAP. Bilevel positive airway pressure (BPAP) may be preferred if the patient experiences difficulty in exhaling against a fixed pressure or has persistent intermittent hypoxemia despite adequate airflow (Kushida et al. 2006). Supplemental oxygen can be added to NPPV to eliminate persistent intermittent nocturnal hypoxemia (Kakkar & Berry 2007). In a cohort of overlap syndrome patients, CPAP added to long term oxygen treatment as compared to long term oxygen treatment resulted in a survival benefit with 5 years-survival rates of 71% and 26%, respectively (Machado et al. 2010). In another study including COPD and overlap syndrome patients, CPAP therapy eliminated the additional risk of mortality due to OSA in overlap syndrome patients as compared to COPD- only patients (Marin et al. 2010) . One RCT and another study using a historical cohort showed reduction of mortality in overlap syndrome with NPPV (McEvoy et al. 2009; Windisch et al. 2009). In the study by Windisch et al., intensive pressure settings (average inspiratory pressure 28 cm H2O, average expiratory pressure 5 cm H2O and a high respiratory rate of about 21 breaths/min) were used with inhospital acclimatization and improvement in spirometry and arterial blood gas were reported (Windisch et al. 2009) . Finally, BPAP may be more comfortable and effective than CPAP in lowering CO2 and increasing tidal volume for patients with overlap syndrome, COPD component of which is much more related to moderate to severe hypercapnia and more prominent than the OSAS component.

3.8 Severe stable COPD/Chronic respiratory failure in patients with COPD

Despite the reported benefits of NPPV application in COPD patients with ARF, the role of NPPV in chronic respiratory failure (CRF) remains controversial. COPD patients with both increased hypercapnia and sleep-disordered breathing may be the ones, who are most likely to benefit from NPPV (Hill 2004). However the evidence to support the use of NPPV in CRF in the setting of severe stable COPD has been less consistent. COPD treatment guidelines does not recommend NPPV treatment routinely in end stage stable hypercapnic COPD in addition to conventional treatment (Global Initiative for Chronic Obstructive Lung Disease [GOLD] 2010).

Once hypercapnia develops, 2-year mortality is approximately 30-40% (Foucher et al. 1998). The reported studies show some physiological benefits for the use of NPPV in stable COPD, but clear survival benefit has not yet been demonstrated (Leger et al. 1994; Jones et al. 1998; Tuggey, Plant, & Elliott 2003). All of these and most other studies used a moderately aggressive ventilation to treat stable hypercapnic COPD patients and so an impressive reduction in hypercapnia was not achieved. In contrast, more aggressive form of ventilation with mean IPAP of up to 30 cmH20 or even higher was used in recent studies by Windish et al. and a remarkable reduction of PC02 was achieved (Windisch et al. 2002; Windisch et al. 2005; Windisch et al. 2006). Another RCT also has shown an improvement in survival with the application of nocturnal NPPV in end stage chronic hypercapnic COPD. The authors reported that the use of higher IPAP levels sufficient to be cardioprotective (but not to awake central respiratory drive) may result in greater treatment benefits (McEvoy et al. 2009). High intensity NPPV therefore offers a new and promising therapeutic option in the treatment of patients with CRF. High intensity NPPV is better tolerated in patients with severe chronic hypecapnic COPD and has been shown to be superior to the conventional and widely used form of low intensity NPPV in controlling nocturnal hypoventilation (Dreher et al. 2010). Nevertheless, higher leak volume, side effects and impairments in sleep quality are the main disadvantages of this modality.

NPPV might rest the chronically fatigued muscles and increase the muscle strength during daytime, could improve sleep time and efficiency, and sleep disordered breathing with episodes of hypoventilation. NPPV use in a select proportion of patients with severe stable COPD can improve gas exchange, exercise tolerance, dyspnea, work of breathing, frequency of hospitalisation, health-related quality of life and functional status (Kolodziej et al. 2007). Inconsistency in the effectiveness of all assessed outcomes may be due to the variability in degree of lung hyperinflation and NPPV levels and duration of use. As yet, no study has provided convincing evidence that survival in COPD is prolonged by NPPV. Further work is also required to evaluate the effect of NPPV on reducing frequency and severity of COPD exacerbation. The general consensus, however, is that there is insufficient evidence to recommend NPPV for routine use in stable hypercapnic COPD (Kolodziej et al. 2007; Wijkstra et al. 2003). Despite the insufficient evidence, the ACCP consensus group opined that a trial of NPPV was justified with a symptomatic but stable and optimally treated patient who has daytime PaCO2 > 55 mm Hg, if OSA had been excluded. For PaCO2 between 50 and 54 mm Hg, , the ACCP consensus group suggested that there should be evidence of worsening hypoventilation during sleep, as suggested by a sustained (> 5 min) desaturation during use of the usual oxygen supplementation. In addition, the need for repeated hospitalizations was deemed a justification for a trial of NPPV (ACCP consensus conference 1999).

The other limitation of NPPV use in patients with stable hypercapnic COPD is poor compliance to NPPV in this group of patients. Criner et al., found that only 50% of COPD patients were still using NPPV after 6 months, compared to 80% for neuromuscular patients (Criner et al. 1999). Reasons for poor adherence are unclear, but probably include the advanced age of COPD patients, frequent occurrence of co morbidities and cognitive defects, lack of motivation and appropriate/inefficient setting of NPPV. Close follow-up is probably helpful to optimize compliance rates.

3.9 Sleep related hypoventilation/Hypoxemia due to COPD

The latest edition of The International Classification of Sleep Disorders: Diagnostic and Coding Manual (ICSD-2) subsumes a broad range of disorders under the heading "Sleep Related Hypoventilation/hypoxemic Syndromes." (American Academy of Sleep Medicine. 2005). Some are quite common, such as COPD with worsening gas exchange during sleep; while some are exceedingly rare, such as congenital central hypoventilation syndrome. The ICSD-2 manual recommended the use of NPPV in addition to optimal treatment of the underlying disorder in selected subgroups of the patients (Casey, Cantillo, & Brown 2007).

In normal subjects, minute ventilation changes little, whereas minute ventilation in COPD patients falls approximately 16% from wakefulness to non REM sleep and almost 32% during REM sleep, compared to wakefulness, largely as a result of decreased tidal volumes. The greater drop in minute ventilation in subjects with COPD may reflect increased dependence on accessory muscles that become hypotonic during sleep, particularly in REM sleep leading to Sleep Related Hypoventilation/hypoxemic Syndrome due to COPD.

NPPV devices are used during sleep to treat patients with Sleep Related Hypoventilation/ hypoxemic syndromes. Compelling evidence exists to support the use of NPPV during sleep in the management of selected Sleep Related Hypoventilation/ hypoxemic syndromes. NPPV has been used in Sleep Related Hypoventilation/ hypoxemic due to central respiratory control disturbances, restrictive thoracic cage disorders, neuromuscular diseases and the obesity hypoventilation syndrome. A select subgroup of COPD patients also appears to have improved sleep after treatment with NPPV but specific characteristics that describe this subgroup well remain to be elucidated. It is unclear whether exclusively nocturnal hypoxemia in these patients will be deleterious and therefore whether isolated sleep-related hypoxemia should be treated. COPD patients with clear evidence of hypoventilation while awake as evidenced by daytime hypercapnia are a reasonable starting target group. Those COPD patients who also show continued sleep disruption or worsening hypercapnia and nocturnal hypoventilation despite oxygen therapy should be further investigated probably with polysomnography to rule out other sleep related breathing disorders. Finally we need to define optimal NPPV and interface design and settings in hopes of improving compliance of long-term therapy for all types of appropriate patients, who are likely to benefit from NPPV.

3.10 Adjunct to exercise training in pulmonary rehabilitation programs

Another potential application of NPPV in patients with severe stable COPD is to enhance exercise training during rehabilitation. It has been shown that when delivered during cycle ergometry, CPAP, pressure-support ventilation, and proportional-assist ventilation all reduce inspiratory effort and dyspnea in hypercapnic COPD patients (Petrof, Calderini, & Gottfried 1990; Bianchi et al. 1998). Recent studies in patients with severe COPD in a 6-week exercise training program has reported that, NPPV alone was more effective than supplemental oxygen alone as adjunct to physical exercise in improving submaximal exercise tolerance and health related quality of life (HRQOL) (Borghi-Silva et al. 2010). These studies demonstrated that NPPV can be used to increase or prolong the intensity of exercise training sessions in patients with severe COPD.

4. Where to administer NPPV?

Any patient on NPPV is classified as receiving Critical Care Level 2 care, defined as "Patients requiring more detailed observation or intervention including support for a single failed organ system". This suggest NPPV should be administered in an intensive care unit (ICU) or high dependency unit (HDU) setting, but it has been widely recognised that NPPV can be successfully used outside the ICU and HDU with dedicated NPPV team able to provide 24/7 care. This is however only feasible in large units with many trained staff (Manuel, Russell, & Jones. 2010). NPPV is more frequently used outside the ICU, in HDU, respiratory wards and emergency departments (EDs) (Brochard, Mancebo, & Elliott 2002; Hill 2004). It has been suggested that each hospital should have a specific designed area with experienced staff, where patients requiring NPPV can be transferred with the minimum delay (British Thoracic Society Standards of Care Committee 2002).

5. Selection of optimal ventilator and mode of NPPV

NPPV is broadly classified into volume preset and pressure preset devices, early studies of long-term domiciliary NPPV mainly concern patients on volume preset ventilators, whereas in the last 5-10 years pressure preset machines, particularly bilevel pressure support equipment has become more prominent.

Volume preset machines gives the adjusted tidal volume regardless of mechanics of respiratory system (i.e. compliance, resistance and active inspiration) and if there is a leak from mask or mouth, patient cannot deliver the adjusted tidal volume.

On the contrary **pressure preset** machines gives the adjusted pressure according to respiratory system mechanics by changing the flow and compensates the mask leaks. However pressure preset machines may not to be sufficient in patients who need high inspiratory pressure. Pressure support ventilators on a first line basis, especially with pressure support mode, is easier to adjust and to synchronise with the patient. CPAP and BPAP are the pressure support ventilators. CPAP as the name implies, requires the airway pressure not to change between inspiration and expiration. However BPAP therapy was originally conceived with the idea of varying the administered pressure between the inspiratory and expiratory cycles. BPAP is the commonly used pressure preset method. BPAP devices deliver separately adjustable inspiratory positive airway pressure (IPAP) and expiratory positive airway pressure (EPAP). The IPAP and EPAP levels are adjusted to maintain upper airway patency, and the pressure support (PS=IPAP-EPAP), which augments ventilation.

Three modes of NPPV were also defined according to principles of cycling of inspiration. NPPV devices can be used in the 1) **spontaneous mode** (the patient cycles the device from EPAP to IPAP), 2) the **spontaneous timed (ST)**/assisted-controlled (AC) mode (a backup rate is available to deliver IPAP for the set inspiratory time if the patient does not trigger an IPAP/EPAP cycle within a set time window otherwise patient the device from EPAP to IPAP), 3) the **timed (T)** /pressure controlled (PC) mode (patient cannot trigger and cycle the inspiration- inspiratory time and respiratory rate are fixed).

Volume assured pressure support / volume target BPAP (VT-BPAP) which is a hybrid mode of volume preset and pressure support ventilation was available by the end of the 1990s. Release of dual portable ventilators providing either pressure support ventilation or volume preset ventilation opened the way for new potent turbine pressure support ventilators able to deliver real volume ventilation with the average volume assured pressure support ventilation mode which represents a flexible way for managing the most difficult patients (Storre et al. 2006). Patient delivers the target tidal volume by the support of adjusted pressure support range. VT-BPAP has been developed in which the IPAP-EPAP difference is automatically adjusted to deliver a target tidal volume (Storre et al. 2006; Ambrogio et al. 2009; Janssens, Metzger, & Sforza 2009; Jaye et al. 2009)

Proportional Assist Ventilation is another mode still under investigation. It provides a level of ventilatory assistance which is proportional to the patient's respiratory effort throughout the respiratory cycle. Some studies reported better comfort and tolerance with proportional assist ventilation but found no differences in rates of mortality or intubation (Fernandez-Vivas et al. 2003; Gay, Hess, & Hill 2001). Guidelines make no recommendation about the use of proportional assist ventilation versus pressure support ventilation in patients who are receiving NPPV for ARF, due to lack of sufficient evidence.

6. Selection of interface

Interfaces connect the patient's airway to the NPPV tubing. The main six interfaces for NPPV are nasal mask, full face or oronasal mask, total face mask, helmet mask, nasal pillow or plugs and mouthpieces. Usually made of silicone, masks need to be carefully fitted to the individual to obtain optimum results. Variations include the bubble-type mask, and gel masks. Mask fit can be enhanced using mask cushions and seal/support rings which are supplied with the mask.

Nasal mask: Nasal mask covers nose and does not cover mouth so allows speaking, drinking and cough also reduces the risk of vomiting and asphyxia. Disadvantages of nasal masks are air leaks if mouth opens, possible nasal skin damage and the need for patent nasal passages.

Oronasal /Full face mask: Oronasal mask cover the nose and mouth and can prove valuable in patients with nasal airway blockage or acute confusional state. Oronasal mask is recommended rather than nasal mask in patients who have ARF. Although there was no difference in endotracheal intubation or mortality rates, the oronasal mask was better tolerated (Keenan et al. 2011). The use of an oronasal mask seem a logical solution to maximize the NPPV efficacy, presumably due to lower leakage with oronasal mask compared to nasal mask in dyspneic patients who are mostly mouth-breathers (Carrey, Gottfried, & Levy 1990). However during long-term use the face mask can be poorly tolerated, thus causing a premature NPPV interruption (Carlucci et al. 2001).

Total face mask: Total face mask covers mouth, nose and eyes. Advantages of this type of masks are minor air leaks, little cooperation required and easy fitting application. Risks of asphyxia, claustrophobia, speaking difficulty are the main disadvantages.

Helmet: Helmet mask covers whole head and all or part of the neck without a contact with face. Advantages of this type of masks are minor air leaks, little cooperation required and absence of nasal or facial skin damage. The risk of vomiting, worsening of CO_2 clearance due to rebreathing, asynchrony with pressure support ventilation and discomfort of axillae are the disadvantages of the helmet.

Nasal pillow or plugs: These masks are inserted into the nostrils. This type of the mask may be suitable for claustrophobic patients with chronic stable COPD who do not need high pressures. Nasal irritation is the main disadvantage.

Mouthpieces: They are placed between lips and held in place by lip seal. Mouthpieces can be applied with other interfaces. The risk of vomiting and salivation, possible air leaks, gastric distension and speaking difficulty are the disadvantages of the mouthpieces. Mouthpiece ventilation is mainly used in patients with neuromuscular disease.

7. Application, setting and adjustments of NPPV

The first hours of NPPV are associated with an increased workload for health care personnel that requires a specific management protocol, including monitoring mask ventilation and monitoring the patient (Nava and Hill 2009). Recommended application, setting and adjustments of NPPV in the ICU, HDU, respiratory wards and emergency departments (EDs) are summarised as in the following:

1. Explain technique to patient (if competent).
2. Choose correct interfaces and size.
3. Set pressure starting from low levels (minimum starting IPAP and EPAP should be 8 cm H_2O and 4 cm H_2O, respectively).
4. Place mask gently over face, holding it in place and start ventilation.
5. When patient is tolerant, tighten straps just enough to avoid major leaks, but not keep it too tight.
6. Set FiO_2 on ventilator or add low-flow oxygen into the circuit, aiming for $SO_2 > 90\%$.
7. Set alarms-low pressure alarm should be above PEEP level.
8. Be mindful of and try to optimise patient's comfort.
9. Reset pressures (pressure support increased to obtain inspired tidal volume 6mL/kg or higher, achieving a respiratory rate <25 breaths/min, $PaCO_2$ <45 mmHg and also raise EPAP to obtain SO_2 of 90% or higher). The recommended maximum IPAP should be 30 cm H_2O for patients $\geq$ 12 years. The recommended minimum and maximum levels of PS

are 4 cm H_2O and 20 cm H_2O, respectively. PS should be increased in order to optimize CO_2 removal and control of auto-positive end expiratory pressure (PEEP), according to the patient's tolerance. A backup rate (ST mode) should be used in all patients with low respiratory rate, in patients who unreliably trigger IPAP/EPAP cycle due to muscle weakness and in patients who do not achieve adequate ventilation or respiratory muscle rest with the maximum tolerated PS in the spontaneous mode. The inspiratory duration should be as short as possible.

10. Protect site of skin pressure from the interface.
11. Consider use of mild sedation if the patient is agitated.
12. Monitor comfort, respiratory rate, oxygen saturation and dyspnea every 30 minute for 6-12 hours and then hourly.
13. Measure arterial blood gases at baseline and within 1 hour from the start.
14. Humidification is advised for longer application.

Predictors of NPPV failure are no improvement or a fall in pH and PCO_2, no change or a rise in breathing frequency after 1-2 hours and lack of cooperation. Delays in intubation of these patients run the risk of unanticipated respiratory or cardiac arrest with attended morbidity and mortality. NPPV failure occurs more frequently in the first hours of ventilation, and was reported to be predicted by the following clinical factors: severe acidosis, high severity score, severe impairment of consciousness, presence of co-morbidities and lack of improvement of arterial blood gases after 1-2 hours of initial ventilation (Ambrosino et al. 1995; Elliott 2002; Nava & Ceriana 2004)

8. Complications of NPPV

Complications of NPPV therapy are minor and preventable. Major complications of NPPV such as pneumothorax and pneumocephalus are so rare (Grunstein 2005). The most common complications effecting almost half of the patients who are administered NPPV are due to mask leak and/or mask pressure injury (Pepin et al. 1999; Hoffstein et al. 1992; Abisheganaden et al. 1998; Lojander, Brander, & Ammala 1999; Sanders, Gruendl, & Rogers 1986). The main complications of NPPV therapy are listed in Table 2.

Due to Mask	Due to Device
Facial and nasal pressure injury/ ulcerations / pain	Rhinitis, Rhinorrhea
Mask allergy	Sinusitis
Conjunctivitis	Tinnitus
Dermatitis	Otitis /ear pain
Claustrophobia	Epistaxis
General	Gastric distension
Anxiety	Dry mucous membranes and thick secretions
Insomnia	Aspiration of gastric contents
Chest pain	Barotrauma (pneumothorax, pneumocephalus)
Headache	Central Sleep Apnea
Periodic Legs Movement Syndrome	Hypotension related to positive intrathoracic pressure

Table 2. Complications of NPPV Therapy

9. Conclusion

For COPD exacerbations NPPV should now be considered as a standard of care in properly selected patients, used in preference to invasive mechanical ventilation. Available evidence and experience have indicated that NPPV has an important role in managing COPD exacerbations, markedly by reducing the need for intubation and improving outcomes, including lowering complication and mortality rates, as well as shortening the hospital stay. NPPV can also be used in certain other situations in COPD patients: in respiratory failure precipitated by a superimposed pneumonia, in postoperative respiratory failure, in intubated patients to facilitate extubation with the aim of reducing the complications of prolonged intubation, in patients with postextubation failure to avoid reintubation, and in do-not-intubate patients; although the evidence to support these applications is not as strong as for NPPV in typical COPD exacerbations. For patients with severe stable COPD, currently available evidence suggests that NPPV can improve daytime and nocturnal gas exchange, prolong sleep duration, improve quality-of-life scores, and possibly reduce the need for hospitalization. However, the findings among studies have not been consistent on these benefits, partly related to numerous methodological shortcomings in most studies performed to date. Despite the weakness of the evidence base, however, some of the consensus and guidelines agree that COPD patients with substantial daytime carbon dioxide retention and evidence of superimposed nocturnal hypoventilation are the ones most likely to benefit (ACCP consensus conference 1999). Achieving desired NPPV adherence by COPD patients will remain still a challenge. Identification of eligible patients, establishment of the appropriate settings and close monitoring of the patients with trained staff are the key points of success of NPPV therapy. Technological improvement of NPPV devices and masks besides new guidelines on the selection of patient, ventilation mode and interface may achieve better NPPV adherence in patients with COPD in the future.

10. References

Abisheganaden, J., Chan C. C., Chee C. B., Yap J. C., Poh S. C., Wang Y. T., & Cheong T. H. (1998). The obstructive sleep apnoea syndrome--experience of a referral centre. Singapore Med J 39 (8):341-6.

Ambrogio, C., Lowman X., Kuo M., Malo J., Prasad A. R., & S. Parthasarathy. (2009). Sleep and non-invasive ventilation in patients with chronic respiratory insufficiency. Intensive Care Med 35 (2):306-13.

Ambrosino, N., Foglio K., Rubini F., Clini E., Nava S., & Vitacca M. (1995). Non-invasive mechanical ventilation in acute respiratory failure due to chronic obstructive pulmonary disease: correlates for success. Thorax 50 (7):755-7.

American Academy of Sleep Medicine. International classification of sleep disorders. Diagnostic and coding manual (ICSD-2), 2nd ed. American Academy of Sleep Medicine: Westchester, IL, 2005.

American College of Chest Physician Consensus Conference. Clinical indications for noninvasive positive pressure ventilation in chronic respiratory failure due to restrictive lung disease, COPD, & nocturnal hypoventilation--a consensus conference report. (1999). Chest 116 (2):521-34.

Auriant I., Jallot A., Hervé P., Cerrina J., Le Roy Ladurie F., Fournier J.L., Lescot B., & Parquin F. (2001). Noninvasive ventilation reduces mortality in acute respiratory failure following lung resection. Am J Respir Crit Care Med 164 (7):1231-5.

Bardi G., Pierotello R., Desideri M., Valdisserri L., Bottai M., & Palla A. (2000). Nasal ventilation in COPD exacerbations: early and late results of a prospective, controlled study. Eur Respir J 15 (1):98-104.

Bednarek, M., Plywaczewski R., Jonczak L., & Zielinski J. (2005). There is no relationship between chronic obstructive pulmonary disease and obstructive sleep apnea syndrome: a population study. Respiration 72 (2):142-9.

Benhamou, D., Girault C., Faure C., Portier F., & Muir J. F. (1992). Nasal mask ventilation in acute respiratory failure. Experience in elderly patients. Chest 102 (3):912-7.

Bianchi, L., Foglio K., Pagani M., Vitacca M., Rossi A., & Ambrosino N. (1998). Effects of proportional assist ventilation on exercise tolerance in COPD patients with chronic hypercapnia. Eur Respir J 11 (2):422-7.

Borghi-Silva, A., Mendes R. G., Toledo A. C., Malosa Sampaio L. M., da Silva T. P., Kunikushita L. N., Dutra de Souza H. C., Salvini T. F., & Costa D. Adjuncts to physical training of patients with severe COPD: oxygen or noninvasive ventilation? (2010). Respir Care 55 (7):885-94.

British Thoracic Society Standards of Care Committee. BTS Guideline: Non-invasive ventilation in acute respiratory failure. (2002). Thorax 57 (3):192-211.

Brochard L., Isabey D., Piquet J., Amaro P., Mancebo J., Messadi A.A., Brun-Buisson C., Rauss A., Lemaire F., & Harf A. (1990). Reversal of acute exacerbations of chronic obstructive lung disease by inspiratory assistance with a face mask. N Engl J Med 323 (22):1523-30.

Brochard L., Mancebo J., Elliott M.W. (2002). Noninvasive ventilation for acute respiratory failure. Eur Respir J 19 (4):712-21.

Brochard L., Mancebo J., Wysocki M., Lofaso F., Conti G., Rauss A., Simonneau G., Benito S., Gasparetto A., Lemaire F., Isabey D., & Harf A. (1995. Noninvasive ventilation for acute exacerbations of chronic obstructive pulmonary disease. N Engl J Med 333 (13):817-22.

Carlucci A., Richard J.C., Wysocki M., Lepage E., & Brochard L; SRLF Collaborative Group on Mechanical Ventilation. (2001). Noninvasive versus conventional mechanical ventilation. An epidemiologic survey. Am J Respir Crit Care Med 163 (4):874-80.

Carrey, Z., Gottfried S. B., & Levy R. D. (1990). Ventilatory muscle support in respiratory failure with nasal positive pressure ventilation. Chest 97 (1):150-8.

Casey, K. R., Cantillo K. O., & Brown L. K. (2007). Sleep-related hypoventilation/hypoxemic syndromes. Chest 131 (6):1936-48.

Celikel, T., Sungur M., Ceyhan B., & Karakurt S. (1998). Comparison of noninvasive positive pressure ventilation with standard medical therapy in hypercapnic acute respiratory failure. Chest 114 (6):1636-42.

Chaouat, A., Weitzenblum E., Krieger J., Ifoundza T., Oswald M., & Kessler R. (1995). Association of chronic obstructive pulmonary disease and sleep apnea syndrome. Am J Respir Crit Care Med 151 (1):82-6.

Chaouat, A., Weitzenblum E., Krieger J., Sforza E., Hammad H., Oswald M., & Kessler R. (1999). Prognostic value of lung function and pulmonary haemodynamics in OSA patients treated with CPAP. Eur Respir J 13 (5):1091-6.

Chevron, V., Menard J. F., Richard J. C., Girault C., Leroy J., & Bonmarchand G. (1998). Unplanned extubation: risk factors of development and predictive criteria for reintubation. Crit Care Med 26 (6):1049-53.

Clinical indications for noninvasive positive pressure ventilation in chronic respiratory
    failure due to restrictive lung disease, COPD, and nocturnal hypoventilation--a
    consensus conference report. Chest. 1999 Aug;116(2):521-34.

Confalonieri, M., Potena A., Carbone G., Porta R. D., Tolley E. A., & Umberto Meduri G.
    (1999). Acute respiratory failure in patients with severe community-acquired
    pneumonia. A prospective randomized evaluation of noninvasive ventilation. Am J
    Respir Crit Care Med 160 (5 Pt 1):1585-91.

Conti, G., Antonelli M., Navalesi P., Rocco M., Bufi M., Spadetta G., & Meduri G. U. (2002).
    Noninvasive vs. conventional mechanical ventilation in patients with chronic
    obstructive pulmonary disease after failure of medical treatment in the ward: a
    randomized trial. Intensive Care Med 28 (12):1701-7.

Criner, G. J., Brennan K., Travaline J. M., & Kreimer D. (1999). Efficacy and compliance with
    noninvasive positive pressure ventilation in patients with chronic respiratory
    failure. Chest 116 (3):667-75.

de Miguel, J., Cabello J., Sanchez-Alarcos J. M., Alvarez-Sala R., Espinos D., & Alvarez-Sala J.
    L. (2002). Long-term effects of treatment with nasal continuous positive airway
    pressure on lung function in patients with overlap syndrome. Sleep Breath 6 (1):3-10.

Dreher, M., Storre J. H., Schmoor C., & Windisch W. High-intensity versus low-intensity
    non-invasive ventilation in patients with stable hypercapnic COPD: a randomised
    crossover trial. (2010). Thorax 65 (4):303-8.

Elliott, M. W. (2002). Non-invasive ventilation in acute exacerbations of chronic obstructive
    pulmonary disease: a new gold standard? Intensive Care Med 28 (12):1691-4.

Epstein, S. K., Ciubotaru R. L., & Wong J. B. (1997). Effect of failed extubation on the
    outcome of mechanical ventilation. Chest 112 (1):186-92.

Fernandez-Vivas, M., Caturla-Such J., Gonzalez de la Rosa J., Acosta-Escribano J., Alvarez-
    Sanchez B., & Canovas-Robles J. (2003). Noninvasive pressure support versus
    proportional assist ventilation in acute respiratory failure. Intensive Care Med 29
    (7):1126-33.

Ferrer, M., Esquinas A., Leon M., Gonzalez G., Alarcon A., & Torres A. (2003). Noninvasive
    ventilation in severe hypoxemic respiratory failure: a randomized clinical trial. Am
    J Respir Crit Care Med 168 (12):1438-44.

Ferrer, M., Valencia M., Nicolas J. M., Bernadich O., Badia J. R., & Torres A. (2006). Early
    noninvasive ventilation averts extubation failure in patients at risk: a randomized
    trial. Am J Respir Crit Care Med 173 (2):164-70.

Ferrer, M., Sellares J., Valencia M., Carrillo A., Gonzalez G., Badia J. R., Nicolas J. M., &
    Torres A. (2009). Non-invasive ventilation after extubation in hypercapnic patients
    with chronic respiratory disorders: randomised controlled trial. Lancet 374
    (9695):1082-8.

Flenley, D. C. (1985). Sleep in chronic obstructive lung disease. Clin Chest Med 6 (4):651-61.

Fletcher, E. C., Shah A., Qian W., & Miller C. C., 3rd. (1991). "Near miss" death in obstructive
    sleep apnea: a critical care syndrome. Crit Care Med 19 (9):1158-64.

Foucher, P., Baudouin N., Merati M., Pitard A., Bonniaud P., Reybet-Degat O., & Jeannin L.
    (1998). Relative survival analysis of 252 patients with COPD receiving long-term
    oxygen therapy. Chest 113 (6):1580-7.

Gay, P. C., Hess D. R., & Hill N. S. (200)1. Noninvasive proportional assist ventilation for acute respiratory insufficiency. Comparison with pressure support ventilation. Am J Respir Crit Care Med 164 (9):1606-11.

Girault, C., Daudenthun I., Chevron V., Tamion F., Leroy J., & Bonmarchand G. (1999). Noninvasive ventilation as a systematic extubation and weaning technique in acute-on-chronic respiratory failure: a prospective, randomized controlled study. Am J Respir Crit Care Med 160 (1):86-92.

[GOLD] Global Initiative for Chronic Obstructive Lung Disease (updated 2010). [online]. URL: www.goldcopd.com

Grunstein, R. (2005). Continuous positive airway pressure treatment for obstructive sleep apnea-hypopnea syndrome. In Principles and practice of sleep medicine, edited by M. H. Kryger, Roth, T., Dement, W.C. Philadelphia: Elsevier Saunders.

Hill, N. S. (2004). Noninvasive ventilation for chronic obstructive pulmonary disease. Respir Care 49 (1):72-87; discussion 87-9.

Hoffstein, V., Viner S., Mateika S., & Conway J. (1992). Treatment of obstructive sleep apnea with nasal continuous positive airway pressure. Patient compliance, perception of benefits, & side effects. Am Rev Respir Dis 145 (4 Pt 1):841-5.

Janssens, J. P., Metzger M., & Sforza E. (2009). Impact of volume targeting on efficacy of bi-level non-invasive ventilation and sleep in obesity-hypoventilation. Respir Med 103 (2):165-72.

Jaye, J., Chatwin M., Dayer M., Morrell M. J., & Simonds A. K. (2009). Autotitrating versus standard noninvasive ventilation: a randomised crossover trial. Eur Respir J 33 (3):566-71.

Jones, S. E., Packham S., Hebden M., & Smith A. P. (1998). Domiciliary nocturnal intermittent positive pressure ventilation in patients with respiratory failure due to severe COPD: long-term follow up and effect on survival. Thorax 53 (6):495-8.

Kakkar, R. K., & Berry R. B. (2007). Positive airway pressure treatment for obstructive sleep apnea. Chest 132 (3):1057-72.

Keenan, S. P., Sinuff T., Cook D. J., & Hill N. S. (2003). Which patients with acute exacerbation of chronic obstructive pulmonary disease benefit from noninvasive positive-pressure ventilation? A systematic review of the literature. Ann Intern Med 138 (11):861-70.

Keenan, S. P., Powers C. E., & McCormack D. G. (2005). Noninvasive positive-pressure ventilation in patients with milder chronic obstructive pulmonary disease exacerbations: a randomized controlled trial. Respir Care 50 (5):610-6.

Keenan, S.P., Sinuff T., Burns K.E., Muscedere J., Kutsogiannis J., Mehta S., Cook D.J., Ayas N., Adhikari N.K., Hand L., Scales D.C., Pagnotta R., Lazosky L., Rocker G., Dial S., Laupland K., Sanders K., & Dodek P.; Canadian Critical Care Trials Group/Canadian Critical Care Society Noninvasive Ventilation Guidelines Group. (2011). Clinical practice guidelines for the use of noninvasive positive-pressure ventilation and noninvasive continuous positive airway pressure in the acute care setting. CMAJ 183 (3):E195-214.

Kolodziej, M. A., Jensen L., Rowe B., & Sin D. (2007). Systematic review of noninvasive positive pressure ventilation in severe stable COPD. Eur Respir J 30 (2):293-306.

Kramer, N., Meyer T. J., Meharg J., Cece R. D., & Hill N. S. (1995). Randomized, prospective trial of noninvasive positive pressure ventilation in acute respiratory failure. Am J Respir Crit Care Med 151 (6):1799-806.

Kushida, C.A., Littner M.R., Hirshkowitz M., Morgenthaler T.I., Alessi C.A., Bailey D., Boehlecke B., Brown T.M., Coleman J. Jr, Friedman L., Kapen S., Kapur V.K., Kramer M., Lee-Chiong T., Owens J., Pancer J.P., Swick T.J., & Wise M.S.; American Academy of Sleep Medicine. (2006). Practice parameters for the use of continuous and bilevel positive airway pressure devices to treat adult patients with sleep-related breathing disorders. Sleep 29 (3):375-80.

Leger, P., Bedicam J. M., Cornette A., Reybet-Degat O., Langevin B., Polu J. M., Jeannin L., & Robert D. (1994). Nasal intermittent positive pressure ventilation. Long-term follow-up in patients with severe chronic respiratory insufficiency. Chest 105 (1):100-5.

Lightowler, J. V., Wedzicha J. A., Elliott M. W., & Ram F. S. (2003). Non-invasive positive pressure ventilation to treat respiratory failure resulting from exacerbations of chronic obstructive pulmonary disease: Cochrane systematic review and meta-analysis. BMJ 326 (7382):185.

Lojander, J., Brander P. E., & Ammala K. (1999). Nasopharyngeal symptoms and nasal continuous positive airway pressure therapy in obstructive sleep apnoea syndrome. Acta Otolaryngol 119 (4):497-502.

Luo, H., Cheng P., & Zhou R. (2001). [Sequential BiPAP following invasive mechanical ventilation in COPD patients with hypercapnic respiratory failure]. Hunan Yi Ke Da Xue Xue Bao 26 (6):563-5.

Machado, M. C., Vollmer W. M., Togeiro S. M., Bilderback A. L., Oliveira M. V., Leitao F. S., Queiroga F. Jr., Lorenzi-Filho G., & Krishnan J. A. (2010). CPAP and survival in moderate-to-severe obstructive sleep apnoea syndrome and hypoxaemic COPD. (2010). Eur Respir J 35 (1):132-7.

Mansfield, D., & Naughton M. T. (1999). Effects of continuous positive airway pressure on lung function in patients with chronic obstructive pulmonary disease and sleep disordered breathing. Respirology 4 (4):365-70.

Manuel, A., Russell R. E., & Jones Q. (2010). Noninvasive ventilation: has Pandora's box been opened? Int J Chron Obstruct Pulmon Dis 5:55-6.

Marin, J. M., Soriano J. B., Carrizo S. J., Boldova A., & Celli B. R. Outcomes in patients with chronic obstructive pulmonary disease and obstructive sleep apnea: the overlap syndrome. (2010). Am J Respir Crit Care Med 182 (3):325-31.

Martin, T. J., Hovis J. D., Costantino J. P., Bierman M. I., Donahoe M. P., Rogers R. M., Kreit J. W., Sciurba F. C., Stiller R. A., & Sanders M. H. (2000). A randomized, prospective evaluation of noninvasive ventilation for acute respiratory failure. Am J Respir Crit Care Med 161 (3 Pt 1):807-13.

Mayos, M., Hernandez Plaza L., Farre A., Mota S., & Sanchis J. (2001). [The effect of nocturnal oxygen therapy in patients with sleep apnea syndrome and chronic airflow limitation]. Arch Bronconeumol 37 (2):65-8.

McEvoy, R. D., Pierce R. J., Hillman D., Esterman A., Ellis E. E., Catcheside P. G., O'Donoghue F. J., Barnes D. J., & Grunstein R. R. Australian trial of non-invasive Ventilation in Chronic Airflow Limitation (AVCAL) Study Group. (2009).

Nocturnal non-invasive nasal ventilation in stable hypercapnic COPD: a randomised controlled trial. Thorax 64 (7):561-6.

Meduri, G. U., Fox R. C., Abou-Shala N., Leeper K. V., & Wunderink R. G. (1994). Noninvasive mechanical ventilation via face mask in patients with acute respiratory failure who refused endotracheal intubation. Crit Care Med 22 (10):1584-90.

Mehta, S., & Hill N. S. (2001). Noninvasive ventilation. Am J Respir Crit Care Med 163 (2):540-77.

Nava, S., & Ceriana P. (2004). Causes of failure of noninvasive mechanical ventilation. Respir Care 49 (3):295-303.

Nava, S., Gregoretti C., Fanfulla F., Squadrone E., Grassi M., Carlucci A., Beltrame F., & Navalesi P. (2005). Noninvasive ventilation to prevent respiratory failure after extubation in high-risk patients. Crit Care Med 33 (11):2465-70.

Nava, S., Navalesi P., & Conti G. (2006). Time of non-invasive ventilation. Intensive Care Med 32 (3):361-70.

Nava, S., & Hill N. (2009). Non-invasive ventilation in acute respiratory failure. Lancet 374 (9685):250-9.

Owens, R. L., & Malhotra A. (2010). Sleep-disordered breathing and COPD: the overlap syndrome. Respir Care 55 (10):1333-44; discussion 1344-6.

Pepin, J. L., Krieger J., Rodenstein D., Cornette A., Sforza E., Delguste P., Deschaux C., Grillier V., & Levy P. (1999). Effective compliance during the first 3 months of continuous positive airway pressure. A European prospective study of 121 patients. Am J Respir Crit Care Med 160 (4):1124-9.

Petrof, B. J., Calderini E., & Gottfried S. B. (1990). Effect of CPAP on respiratory effort and dyspnea during exercise in severe COPD. J Appl Physiol 69 (1):179-88.

Rochester, D. F., Braun N. M., & Arora N. S. (1979). Respiratory muscle strength in chronic obstructive pulmonary disease. Am Rev Respir Dis 119 (2 Pt 2):151-4.

Sanders, M. H., Gruendl C. A., & Rogers R. M. (1986). Patient compliance with nasal CPAP therapy for sleep apnea. Chest 90 (3):330-3.

Soo Hoo, G. W., Santiago S., & Williams A. J. (1994). Nasal mechanical ventilation for hypercapnic respiratory failure in chronic obstructive pulmonary disease: determinants of success and failure. Crit Care Med 22 (8):1253-61.

Squadrone, E., Frigerio P., Fogliati C., Gregoretti C., Conti G., Antonelli M., Costa R., Baiardi P., & Navalesi P. (2004). Noninvasive vs invasive ventilation in COPD patients with severe acute respiratory failure deemed to require ventilatory assistance. Intensive Care Med 30 (7):1303-10.

Storre, J. H., Seuthe B., Fiechter R., Milioglou S., Dreher M., Sorichter S., & Windisch W. (2006). Average volume-assured pressure support in obesity hypoventilation: A randomized crossover trial. Chest 130 (3):815-21.

Tuggey, J. M., Plant P. K., & Elliott M. W. (2003). Domiciliary non-invasive ventilation for recurrent acidotic exacerbations of COPD: an economic analysis. Thorax 58 (10):867-71.

Wijkstra, P. J., Lacasse Y., Guyatt G. H., Casanova C., Gay P. C., Meecham Jones J., & Goldstein R. S. (2003). A meta-analysis of nocturnal noninvasive positive pressure ventilation in patients with stable COPD. Chest 124 (1):337-43.

Windisch, W., Vogel M., Sorichter S., Hennings E., Bremer H., Hamm H., Matthys H., & Virchow J. C., Jr. (2002). Normocapnia during nIPPV in chronic hypercapnic COPD reduces subsequent spontaneous PaCO2. Respir Med 96 (8):572-9.

Windisch, W., S. Kostic, M. Dreher, J. C. Virchow, Jr., & S. Sorichter. (2005). Outcome of patients with stable COPD receiving controlled noninvasive positive pressure ventilation aimed at a maximal reduction of Pa(CO2). Chest 128 (2):657-62.

Windisch, W., Dreher M., Storre J. H., & Sorichter S. (2006). Nocturnal non-invasive positive pressure ventilation: physiological effects on spontaneous breathing. Respir Physiol Neurobiol 150 (2-3):251-60.

Windisch, W., Haenel M., Storre J. H., & Dreher M. (2009). High-intensity non-invasive positive pressure ventilation for stable hypercapnic COPD. Int J Med Sci 6 (2):72-6.

4

Novel Concept in Pulmonary Delivery

Maria Carafa[1], Carlotta Marianecci[1],
Paolino Donatella[2], Luisa Di Marzio[3],
Christian Celia[4], Massimo Fresta[4] and Franco Alhaique[1]
*[1]Department of Drug Chemistry and Technologies,
"Sapienza", University of Rome, Rome
[2]Department of Experimental and Clinical Medicine,
Faculty of Medicine, University "Magna Graecia" Catanzaro
[3]Department of Drug Science,
University of Chieti "G. D'Annunzio", Chieti
[4]Department of Pharmacobiological Sciences,
Faculty of Pharmacy, University "Magna Graecia" Catanzaro
Italy*

1. Introduction

This chapter deals with recent advances in the nanovector approach to the pulmonary delivery of therapeutic substances; it also describes briefly the physiology of the lungs and the main factors affecting pulmonary delivery (Figure 1).

The development of an innovative nanocarrier, able to deliver the drug to the desired site of action, is highly dependent on the nature of the active substance and on its desired mode of action.

A delivery technology can thus be used to:

- reduce systemic exposure and improve drug targeting;
- circumvent the parenteral route or reduce the number of injections;
- achieve sustained plasma levels of the drug;
- reduce side – effects;
- modulate the effect of the drug, specifically in the case of vaccines, where the delivery system can modify the ratio of humoral and cellular response;
- increase patient compliance;
- reduce the price of the therapy;
- increase patent life and/or circumvent patents of competitors.

Numerous approaches involving non - parenteral routes, such as intestinal, nasal, buccal, transdermal and rectal, have been examined, but most of them are inadequate for a satisfactory therapeutic response. On the other hand, the pulmonary route represents a great promise for the systemic delivery and bioavailability of peptides and proteins, since lungs are highly permeable and accessible by normal inhalation methods. Actually, the pulmonary

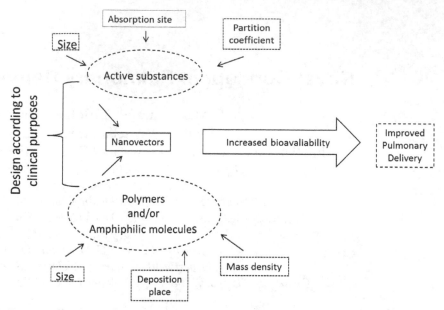

Fig. 1. Factors affecting pulmonary delivery

route typically shows from 10 to 200 times greater bioavailability with respect to other non - invasive routes (Patton & Byron, 2007). Thus, various pharmaceutical techniques have been introduced to take advantage of this route. These include formulations using specific and innovative excipients, chemical modifications of drugs, polymeric and/or amphiphilic Drug Delivery Systems (DDSs), particle engineering, inhalation devices.

In particular, over the past decade, the use of DDSs involving micro or nanocarriers and particle engineering techniques were remarkably developed and the resulting pharmaceutical techniques have been eagerly applied to the pulmonary delivery of drugs.

Inhalation is also a proven means of systemic delivery for drugs that have limited bioavailability by other routes or would benefit from rapid onset of action and a variety of products are being developed for this purpose (Gonda, 2006; Patton & Byron, 2007).

At the same time, in recent decades, advances in device design and formulation science have addressed the need for more efficient inhalers that are capable of delivering larger doses to the lung with low extrathoracic deposition. Once deposited in the lungs, drug disposition (dissolution, absorption, distribution, metabolism and elimination) and the influence of pulmonary pharmacokinetics (PK) are the critical determinants of clinical outcomes in terms of drug efficacy and safety. Pulmonary disposition remains poorly understood despite modern capabilities in imaging, analytical and biological science which make measurement of drug disposition and mode of action more accessible. For these reasons the development of new inhaled medicines capable to allow improvements in current therapy is a promising challenge in the development new DDSs.

A number of benefits result from inhalation of drugs and a continuously increasing number of inhaled drugs and nanomedicines are becoming available for the treatment various diseases. Inhalation of drugs is convenient and extremely efficient to treat diseased airways. It allows a targeted therapy with high drug concentrations in the tissue of interest and low systemic drug exposure (and thereby reduced side effects). Inhalation aerosols have also been developed for systemic drug administration. The large absorptive surface area, the very thin diffusion path to the bloodstream and the elevated blood flow make the lung a port of entry to the systemic circulation and proteins are absorbed more efficiently from the lungs than from any other non-invasive route of drug administration.

Only one inhaled therapeutic protein is currently available on the market. It is recombinant human deoxyribonuclease I (Dornase alfa) indicated for the treatment of cystic fibrosis (CF) and marketed since 1994.

Recombinant human deoxyribonuclease I is a glycoprotein of 37 kDa, which selectively cleaves DNA. In CF patients, retention of viscous purulent secretions in the airways contributes both to reduced pulmonary function and to exacerbation of infection. Purulent pulmonary secretions contain very high concentrations of extracellular DNA released by degenerating leukocytes. Dornase alfa is delivered to CF patients by inhalation of an aerosol mist produced by a pneumatic nebulizer. It hydrolyses the DNA in airway secretions and reduces their viscoelasticity.

Inhalation can represent the most favourable non-invasive route of administration for insulin (5.8 kDa) because insulin bioavailability can reach 37% following inhalation while it reaches at most 1% following oral, sublingual, nasal or transdermal administration without chemical enhancers (Cefalu, 2004; Illum, 2002). The first inhaled insulin product, Exubera®, was approved in January 2006 but withdrawn from the market already in October 2007 due to disappointing sales.

Another inhaled insulin product, AFREZZA™, is currently under review by the FDA for the treatment of type 1 and type 2 diabetes (Neumiller & Campbell 2010; Rossiter et al., 2010).

AFREZZA™ is an ultra rapid acting insulin comprising Technosphere® insulin powder in unit dose cartridges for administration with the inhaler. The Technosphere® powder formulation is prepared by precipitating insulin from solution onto preformed diketopiperazine particles, which readily dissolve once in the lung environment. AFREZZA™ appears to overcome several limitations of Exubera®. Technosphere® insulin is both rapidly absorbed and eliminated and its pharmacokinetic profile mimics more closely normal physiologic insulin release than injection of regular human insulin as well as of rapid-acting analogues.

A few small-scale clinical trials have been conducted on inhalation of other systemically-acting therapeutic proteins, including interferon alpha-2b (19.3 kDa), human growth hormone (22 kDa) (Walvoord et al., 2009), an erythropoietin-Fc fusion protein (112 kDa) (Dumont et al., 2005). Inhalation of growth hormone is a potential alternative to growth hormone injection, which could offer improved patient adherence especially in pediatric patients. The bioavailability of inhaled growth hormone was 3.5% relative to subcutaneous injection in children, while it reached 7.6% in adults (Walvoord et al., 2009). The hypothesis behind this difference is that children have smaller oropharynx and larynx, which results in different deposition patterns as compared to adults. Although children preferred the inhalation route of therapy, ongoing development of growth hormone inhalation has been delayed due to its low bioavailability. An erythropoietin-Fc fusion protein was absorbed in the bloodstream following delivery to the central lung regions in humans, with a dose-dependent concentrations in the serum, suggesting that large therapeutic molecules can be delivered to humans via the lungs using the FcRn-mediated transport pathway (Dumont et al., 2005).

2. Practical issues in the pulmonary delivery

2.1 Physiological features of the lungs

The lung resembles an inverted tree, where the trachea or trunk subdivides into two main bronchi and these latter successively branch into more and more narrow and short bronchioles. In total, the trachea undergoes 23 bifurcations before it reaches the alveolar sacs. The first 16 generations compose the conducting region where air is filtered, warmed, humidified and conducted to the respiratory region. Gas exchange between airspaces and blood capillaries occurs in the respiratory region, which includes the respiratory bronchioles, the alveolar ducts and the alveolar sacs.

Two different epithelia line the conducting and respiratory regions. A pseudo stratified columnar epithelium lines the proximal conducting airways and is composed of ciliated columnar cells, goblet or mucus secreting cells and basal or progenitor cells (Parkes, 1994). It is progressively replaced by a simple cuboidal cell layer in the more distal airways and by a very thin epithelial lining in the alveoli. Squamous type I pneumocytes cover 95% of the alveolar surface, owing to their large apical surface and thinness (0.05 µm). Cuboidal type II pneumocytes produce the lung surfactant and are progenitor for type I cells. Type II pneumocytes are located in the corners of the alveoli. The surface area of the alveolar epithelium reaches 100 m², which is enormous as compared to the 0.25m² surface area of the airways (Crapo et al.,1982; Mercer et al., 1994).

Mucociliary clearance is one of the most important defense mechanisms to eliminate dust and microorganisms in the lungs (Van der Schans, 2007).

The mucus is produced by goblet cells and sub-mucosa glands. It covers the entire airway surface and its thickness ranges from 5 µm to 55 µm (Clunes & Boucher, 2007; Lai et al., 2009). It consists of an upper gel phase made of 95% water, 2% mucin, a highly glycosylated and entangled polymer, as well as salts, proteins and lipids (Bansil & Turner, 2006). A periciliary liquid layer underlies the mucus gel and its low viscosity allows effective cilia beating. The mucus is transported by the coordinated beating of the cilia and by expiratory airflow towards the oropharynx at an average flow rate of 5 mm per minute. Mucus, cells and debris coming from the nasal cavities and from the lung meet in the pharynx, are mixed with saliva and are swallowed.

Pulmonary surfactant is responsible for biophysical stabilizing activities and innate defense mechanisms. It lines the alveolar epithelial surfaces and overflows into the conductive airways so that the surfactant film is continuous between alveoli and central airways (Bernhard et al., 2004). Pulmonary surfactant is composed of 80% phospholipids (half of which being dipalmitoylphosphatidylcholine), 5–10% neutral lipids (mainly cholesterol), 5–6% specific surfactant proteins and 3–4% non-specific proteins (Perez-Gil, 2008).

The phospholipids are mainly responsible for forming the surface active film at the respiratory air–liquid interface. In water, phospholipids self-organize in the form of bilayers.

Bilayers are also the structural form in which surfactant is assembled and stored by pneumocytes in lamellar bodies. At the air–liquid interface, phospholipids form oriented monolayers, with the hydrophilic headgroups oriented towards the aqueous phase and the hydrophobic acyl chains pointing towards the air. The higher the concentration of phopholipid molecules at the interface, the lower the surface tension, the lower the energy required to enlarge the alveolar surface during inspiration.

Specific surfactant proteins include SP-A, SP-B, SP-C and SP-D. SP-A and SP-D are hydrophilic while SP-B and SP-C are hydrophobic. SP-A is able to bind multiple ligands, including sugars, Ca^{2+} and phospholipids. This property allows SP-A to bind to the surface of pathogens, contributing to their elimination from the airways. Recognition of SP-A by specific receptors on alveolar macrophages stimulates phagocytosis of the pathogens. SP-B is strictly required for the biogenesis of pulmonary surfactant and its packing into lamellar bodies. Both, SP-B and SP-C promote rapid transfer of phospholipids from bilayers stores into air– liquid interfaces.

Luminal airway and alveolar macrophages are at the forefront of lung defence and their primary role is to participate in innate immune responses, that is, chemotaxis, phagocytosis, and microbial killing (Geiser, 2010). They also downregulate adaptive immune responses and protect the lung from T-cell-mediated inflammation (Holt et al., 2008). Macrophages are tightly applied on the surface of respiratory epithelia. They are immersed in the lung lining fluid beneath the surfactant film.

Although they occupy only 1% of the alveolar surface, they are capable to clean particles from the entire alveolar surface due to amoeboid movements (Geiser, 2010). In contrast to surface macrophages, interstitial macrophages are primarily involved in adaptive immunity by interfacing with lymphocytes via antigen presentation and production of cytokines (Geiser, 2010).

The lung presents a lower level of metabolism than the gastrointestinal tract and liver. Yet, various peptidases are distributed on the surface of different cell types in the lung, including bronchial and alveolar epithelial cells, submucosal glands, smooth muscles, endothelial cells, connective tissue. Proteases are largely present in lysosomes (Buhling et al., 2004). Proteases that degrade the extracellular matrix are secreted by different structural cells or are membrane bound (Stamenkovic, 2003).

Proteases play an essential role in cell and tissue growth, differentiation, repair, remodelling, cell migration and peptide-mediated inflammation (van der Velden & Hulsmann, 1999). Proteases can also be released in the airspaces by activated macrophages and neutrophils in case of inflammatory reactions in the respiratory tract (Buhling et al., 2006; Tetley, 2002). Blood supply to the lungs is divided among the pulmonary and systemic circulations (Altiere & Thompson, 1996). The pulmonary circulation consists of the pulmonary artery that leaves the right heart, branches into a dense pulmonary capillary bed that surrounds the alveoli and finally coalesces into the pulmonary vein that drains into the left heart. One hundred percent of the cardiac output flows through the pulmonary circulation. Its principal functions are gas exchange with air in the alveoli and nutrients supply to terminal respiratory units. The lungs receive a second blood supply via the systemic circulation, commonly referred to as the bronchial circulation. The bronchial circulation originates from the aorta and provides oxygenated blood and nutrients to all structures of the tracheobronchial tree. Lymphatic vessels exist in close proximity of major blood vessels and of the airways (El-Chemaly et al., 2009). The lungs have unique physiological features and provide many conditions that favour the absorption of peptides and proteins.

2.2 Barriers to the pulmonary delivery of active substances

2.2.1 Deposition of nanocarriers through the respiratory tract

As pointed out in the section on lung physiology, the structure of the lung tissue largely varies according to airway generation and the fate of nanomedicines will similarly vary depending on the structures on which they deposit. The site of deposition of an inhaled formulation within the respiratory tract depends on the aerodynamic diameter of the aerosol particles. The aerodynamic diameter of a particle, d_{aer}, is equivalent to the diameter of a unit density (ρ_0) sphere that has the same terminal velocity in still air as the particle:

$$d_{aer} = d\sqrt{\frac{\rho}{\rho_0 X}} \qquad (1)$$

where d is the geometric diameter of the particle, ρ is the particle density and χ is the particle dynamic shape factor denoting deviation of shape from sphericity (Hinds, 1999).

Filtering of large particles (d_{aer} >5 µm) occurs in upper airways (mouth, trachea and main bronchi) by inertial impaction. One to 5 µm d_{aer} particles deposit by gravitational settling in the central and distal tract. Particles with d_{aer} <1 µm remain suspended in the air and are mostly exhaled. Ultrafine particles (<100 nm) can largely deposit in the respiratory tract by random Brownian motion: particles <100 nm reach the alveolar region while particles <10 nm already deposit in the tracheo-bronchial region due to their high diffusion coefficients (Heyder at al., 1986).

Drug delivery inhalers, that include nebulizers, metered-dose inhalers and dry powder inhalers, generate particles with a d_{aer} in the micron-size range for deposition in the tracheo-bronchial tree (3–10 µm) in order to treat the airways (e.g., β2 mimetics) or in the alveolar region (1–3 µm) for systemic drug absorption (e.g., insulin) (Figure 2).

Therapeutic proteins can be delivered to the lungs by any medical inhaler. Yet, medical inhalers are not designed to produce ultrafine particles. Ultrafines require enormous energy for their creation, that is, for the atomization of the solution into nano-sized liquid droplets or for the complete de-agglomeration of nanosized dry powder particles. Therefore, drug formulations based on nanoparticles are most often delivered to the respiratory tract by nebulization of colloidal suspensions (Dailey et al., 2003). Developments of the preparation of dry powder microparticles as nanoparticles carriers for pulmonary drug delivery were also reported quite recently (Tsapis et al., 2002). It should be noted, ultrafines are generated in abundance in our environment by the most significant pollution sources, which are those related to combustion processes (Morawska et al., 2005). Epidemiologic studies have provided evidence that an increase in atmospheric ultrafines is associated with adverse pulmonary and cardiovascular effects in susceptible parts of the population. Therefore, significant research has focused on the fate of inhaled ultrafines in the body and ultrafines have been frequently produced in laboratories using spark generators (Geiser et àl., 2008).

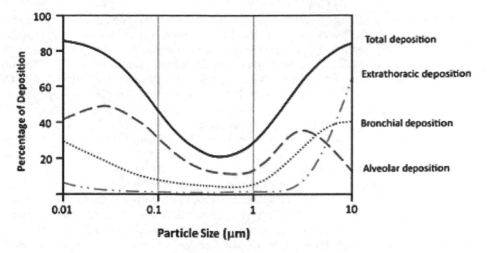

Fig. 2. Deposition of nanocarriers in human respiratory tract as a function of size

Data from several of these studies have been included in this review as the pulmonary fate of atmospheric ultrafines has likely similarities with the pulmonary fate of nanomedicines (Geiser et al., 2008; Furuyama et al., 2009).

2.2.2 Clearance mechanisms

Various elimination pathways for nanoparticles exist in the lungs, including coughing, dissolution, mucociliarly escalator, translocation from the airways to other sites, phagocytosis by macrophages and neuronal uptake (Figure 3); but the quantitative relationship among these pathways has not yet been established (Muhlfeld et al., 2008).

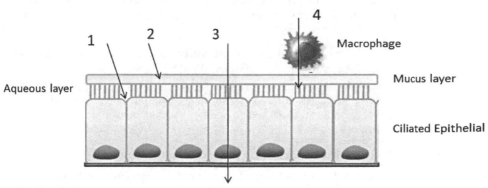

1 = dissolution
2 = mucociliary clearance
3 = translocation
4 = phagocytosis

Fig. 3. Pathways involved in nanocarriers absorption

When a nanoparticle has landed on the airways, it first encounters the surfactant on the top of the airway lining fluid. The surfactant will enhance particle wetting thus helping it to sink into the fluid, passing first through the gel phase and then to the sol phase. Compared with sulphur colloidal particles (220 nm), human serum albumin molecules (HSA, 66 kDa) were cleared 3 times more slowly from the bronchi of dogs. This difference was attributed to the possibility that sulphur nanoparticles resided on the gel phase (i.e. the top layer of the periciliary fluid) whereas HSA dissolved and partitioned into the sol (i.e. bottom layer) which may be transported less effectively by mucociliary clearance (MCC). If extrapolated to inhaled drugs, the more soluble ones will behave like HSA and should be hence less susceptible to MCC (Edsbacker et al., 2008), but more likely absorbed through the epithelium. For nanoparticle agglomerates, it is likely that the particles will first reside on the gel phase. Depending on the aqueous dispersibility and solubility in the airway fluid, the agglomerates may remain in the gel phase behaving like the microsized particles, or they may then disperse into nanoparticles followed by dissolution and absorption. Nanoparticles delivered within a liquid droplet (e.g. from a nebulizer) might be different from dry particles, as the droplet liquid may interact with the gel layer making the nanoparticles easier to wet and partition into the sol layer, i.e. potentially more readily to escape the MCC (Zhang et al., 2011).

2.2.2.1 Dissolution

Dissolution depends on the site of deposition, which determines the volume of airway fluids available for dissolution and, hence, whether the dissolution occurs in sink or non-sink conditions, as well as on the solubility and dose of the drugs. Freely water soluble drugs include organic salts (e.g., salbutamol sulphate, terbutaline sulphate and disodium cromoglycate) and polar compounds (e.g. mannitol). These drugs will dissolve readily in the airway fluid followed by absorption or elimination by the mucociliarly escalator. Sparingly soluble drugs include the inhaled corticosteroids, which have aqueous solubility ranging from 140 to below 0.1 µg/mL (Edsbacker et al., 2008). Once dissolved, the drug molecules are diluted in the airway fluid where they can bind to proteins, opsonins, or other constituents and be metabolized and/or absorbed into the blood and lymph (Schmid et al., 2010).

Absorption of the drugs depends on the site such as alveolar or conducting airways (which affects the barrier thickness and surface area) and the drug molecule itself (which impacts on passive diffusion and active uptake by the epithelium. It must be pointed out that absorption of most drugs from the lungs is rapid: as an example, it has been reported that following inhalation of formoterol fumarate (4.5 nmol/L) and budesonide (136 pmol/L, the peak plasma concentrations occurred at 20 and 10 min, respectively.

2.2.2.2 Mucociliary clearance (MCC)

MCC operates in the ciliated airways where the movement of the cilia transports the mucus carrying the drug nanoparticles or dissolved drug (not yet absorbed) on the epithelial surface towards the pharynx/larynx. The drug-containing mucus will then be swallowed to the GI tract. The average transport velocity in the human trachea has been estimated at 3–10 mm/min, but the value varies widely among subjects. Using well-developed techniques of depositing radiolabelled sulfur colloids in the central airways, Daviskas and her colleagues reported a MCC rate remarkably reduced in patients with bronchiectasis, asthma, and CF, with respect to healthy individuals. Actually, MCC and dissolution occur simultaneously and their relative importance should depend on the elimination rate from each of these contributions. While insoluble particles of 6 µm are practically all cleared from the bronchial airways by MCC in 24 h, smaller particles are retained for a longer period showing almost an inverse relationship between the 24 h airway retention and the geometric particle size. Nanoparticles with enhanced mobility may partition through the mucus into the periciliary spaces, where they can be taken up by the airway macrophages and bronchial epithelial cells, causing a reduction of MCC (Schmid et al., 2009).

2.2.2.3 Macrophage uptake

Alveolar macrophages are responsible for clearance of nanoparticles deposited in the alveolar region, in which MCC is absent. In response to the deposited nanoparticles, alveolar macrophages will migrate to the particles and phagocytize them via chemotaxis involving opsonisation. Macrophage uptake is believed to complete within 6–12 h after deposition of the particles in the alveoli (Oberdörster, 2007). nce internalized in the macrophages, the particles will be either disintegrated (e.g. by enzymes in lysosomes) or accumulated in the lymphatic system (Schmid et al., 2009) draining both airways and alveoli and finally terminating in the mediastinal and hilar lymph nodes (Geiser & Kreyling, 2010). A minor fraction of the particle-carrying macrophages will migrate to the ciliated airways where they are removed by MCC (Schmid et al., 2009). However, with a retention half-time of up to 700 days in humans (Oberdörster, 2007), clearance of solid particles by alveolar macrophages is a relatively slow mechanism. Phagocytosis of particles below 100 nm is not effective (Oberdörster, 2007), most probably because of a less effective recognition (~20%) of nanoparticles by the macrophages (Schmid et al., 2009). The reduced recognition is possibly due to more scattered and diluted chemotactic signals as a result of i) higher number concentration of nanoparticles (compared with micron-sized particles at the same dose) and ii) fewer opsonin molecules available per particle. Conversely, since nanoparticles are more readily taken up by epithelial cells, they become less available to be phagocytized by macrophages (Madl & Pinkerton, 2009). Macrophages are also present in the ciliated airway but their role in nanoparticle clearance is probably less important compared with MCC.

2.2.2.4 Translocation into cells, blood and lymph

This process involves transcytosis of the particles into the epithelial cells and/or across the epithelia of the respiratory tract into the interstitium and then to blood and lymph. As described earlier, translocation to the lymphatic system can be facilitated by macrophage uptake. The transport may be protein-mediated, requiring binding of certain proteins on the nanoparticle surface for recognition by the receptors (Schmid et al., 2009). The transport may also be receptor-mediated transcytosis via caveolae (Oberdörster, 2007), which have a diameter of 50–100 nm. Surface coating of the particles by albumin and lecithin may facilitate cellular uptake by pneumocytes and transcytosis across capillaries (Yang et al., 2008). Once internalized, nanoparticles can bind to mitochondria and even DNA in the nucleus (Muhlfeld et al., 2008; Oberdörster, 2007).

When translocated to the systemic circulation, nanoparticles could cause unwanted effects on the blood (e.g. accumulation in platelets) and other organs in the body (Oberdörster, 2007). Some biological effects may include inflammation, oxidative stress, cytotoxicity, fibrosis, and immunologic responses (Madl & Pinkerton, 2009; Unfried et al., 2007).

Surface area has been proposed as the single most important particle dose parameter for the toxicity of nanoparticles (Schmid et al., 2009). This is particularly relevant for inflammatory and oxidative stress reactions, such as surface area of a catalyst (i.e. nanoparticles), that determines the oxidative reaction rate. However, oxidative stress involves the formation of reactive oxygen species (ROS) from the particles containing reactants such as transition metals or polyaromatic hydrocarbons (which induce the expression of the CYP1A1 protein). Drug nanoparticles, which do not contain such reactants, are therefore less likely to cause oxidative stress in the lungs. Biodegradabile nanoparticles indeed showed significantly lower inflammatory response in-vitro (Sung et al., 2007). Interestingly, translocation in the reverse direction with particles re-entrained from the lung capillaries or interstitium to the luminal side of the epithelium have been shown in animal models using rabbits and rats. Such back-translocation was suggested to be macrophage-mediated.

2.2.2.5 Neuronal uptake

Translocation into afferent vagal nerves in the tracheobronchial airways has been proposed but still not well studied (Oberdorster et al., 2005). Nanoparticles deposited in the nasal cavity have been reported to be taken up by the olfactory lobe and translocated to the central nervous system (Oberdorster et al., 2005). However, such a neuronal uptake pathway is relevant only if the drug nanoparticles are inhaled nasally. Existing data from epidemiologic and toxicological studies showed longer retention of inhaled nanoparticles in the lungs, but the applicability of these findings on nanoparticles is under investigation. In theory, inhaled nanodrug particles have the potential to be retained longer in the lungs followed by cellular uptake and translocation into the systemic circulation thus causing nanotoxicity. It can be speculated that the fate of the nanoparticles in the lungs, regarding the elimination pathways, will depend on the properties of both the particle and the drug molecule. Micron-sized aggregates of nanoparticles will deposit by sedimentation in the tracheobronchial (TB) region where MCC will operate to eliminate both the dissolved and undissolved drugs. Even discrete nanoparticles can deposit by diffusion in the TB region. Drug nanoparticles deposited in the alveolar region will dissolve in the airway fluid and be absorbed. This is likely to be the case even for hydrophobic drugs with low aqueous solubility like inhaled corticosteroids due to the relatively low doses that are used. As a result of the low persistence of drug nanoparticles, dissolution and mucociliary escalator will likely be the major clearance pathways responsible for these particles before macrophage phagocytosis and other translocation pathways would start to play a significant role.

3. Nanocarriers for lung delivery

Nanomedicine can be defined as the application of nanotechnology to medicine. Nanotechnology involves the understanding and control of matter at dimensions of 1 to 100-200 nm, where unique phenomena enable novel applications. Artificial nanostructures are of the same size as biological entities and can readily interact with biomolecules on both the cell surface and within the cell (Figure 4). Here our attention is focused on the fate of nanomedicines delivered to the lung, in particular an innovative glucocorticoid delivery system will be considered.

The understanding the fate of nanomedicines in the lungs is important because fate and therapeutic activity are closely related. Interaction of nanomedicines with cells of the

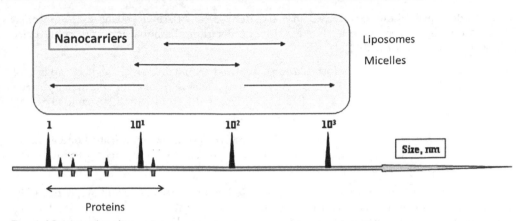

Fig. 4. Nanocarrier size

respiratory system will determine the pharmacodynamic response. For instance, the rapid uptake of particles by alveolar macrophages can be a way of targeting anti-tuberculosis drugs to this type of cells (Nimje et al., 2009). Conversely, macrophages uptake represents a clearance pathway for drugs acting on other cells within the lungs (e.g., β_2 mimetics).

Nowadays, biopharmaceuticals and conventional drugs are frequently engineered or incorporated in carriers in order to direct their fate in preferential pathways (Schmidt, 2009; Veronese & Pasut, 2005). Nano-size drug carriers can incorporate various therapeutics (e.g.,poorly water soluble drugs) and present several advantages for drug delivery to the lung including controlled release, protection from metabolism and degradation, decreased drug toxicity and targeting capabilities. Moreover, the successful integration of novel drugs with devices capable of delivering defined doses to the respiratory tract has resulted in a proven track record for inhalation as a route of administration that limits systemic exposure and provides localized topical delivery. Thus, a number of orally inhaled products have been successfully developed over the last 50 years, providing symptomatic relief to millions of patients with asthma and chronic obstructive pulmonary disease (COPD).

There are numerous types of nanoparticle systems now being explored for drug delivery to lungs, especially in cancer treatment (Haley & Frenkel, 2008).

The types of nanoparticle used at present in research for cancer therapeutic applications include polymeric nanoparticles, protein nanoparticles, ceramic nanoparticles, viral nanoparticles and metallic nanoparticles (Balak et al., 2010).

Liposomes are the most extensively investigated system for controlled drug delivery to the lungs (Mansour et al., 2009). A few liposome-encapsulated antibiotics have been delivered to the lungs in phase II clinical trials. These include amikacin (Weers et al., 2009) and ciprofloxacin (Bruinenberg et al., 2010) Multiple treatment cycles with ARIKACE™ (liposomal amikacin for inhalation) showed sustained improvement in lung function with significant reduction in bacterial density in CF patients who have chronic Pseudomonas lung infections (Okusanya et al., 2009).

A nanoscale liposomal formulation of amikacin has been shown to slowly release the drug in rat lungs and to penetrate Pseudomonas biofilms and CF sputum in vitro (Meers et al., 2008).

Mitsopoulos and Suntres reported that the delivery of N-acetylcysteine as a liposomal formulation improves its effectiveness in counteracting Paraquat-induced cytotoxicity (Mitsopoulos & Suntres, 2011).

Liposomal drug dry powder formulations, realized to obtain novel devices capable of delivering defined doses of drugs, represent promising tools for pulmonary drug administration, such as selective localization of drug, reduced local and systemic toxicities, increased patient compliance and high dose loading.

In liposomal dry powder formulations, drug encapsulating liposomes are homogenized, dispersed into the carrier and converted into dry powder by using freeze drying, spray drying or supercritical fluid technologies.

The most commonly used liposomes are composed of lung surfactants and synthetic lipids. Liposomal formulation have been proposed to delivery anticancer drugs, corticosteroids, immunosuppressants, antimicotic drugs, antibiotics for local pulmonary infections and CF and opioid analgesics for pain management using. Many of them have reached the stage of clinical trials for the treatment of several pulmonary diseases (Misra et al., 2009).

A promising application of nanocarriers to lung targeting is related to gene delivery. Gene therapy is currently being developed for a wide range of acute and chronic lung diseases, incuding CF, cancer and asthma (Griesenbach & Alton, 2009; Lam et al., 2011). Nguyen et al (2009) developed a highly efficient nanocomposite aerosol for pulmonary gene delivery, consisting of a biodegradable polymer core.

Respiratory diseases have attracted particular attention as targets of siRNA - mediated therapeutics, due to the lethality and prevalence of certain illnesses and the lung's accessibility to therapeutic agents via both local and systemic delivery routes. However, one of the major challenges to realize the RNAi therapeutic potential in lung diseases is to deliver the siRNAs to the lung tissue, in particular, to the target cells with high efficiency and high specificity (Yuan et al., 2011).

Several clinical trials have been conducted in order to assess the efficacy and safety of pulmonary DNA delivery using viral and non-viral vectors, especially in the case of CF. Yet, none of these formulations have been pursued due to low transfection efficiency, transient gene expression or immune elimination of the gene vector. Identifying the barriers to cell transfection might help to improve gene transfer efficiency of non-viral vectors (Griesenbach & Alton, 2009). An efficient and safe cationic lipid, 6-lauroxyhexyl lysinate (LHLN), was proposed to prepare cationic liposomes. *In vitro* tests showed that, compared with Lipofectamine2000, the new cationic liposome formulation using LHLN exhibited lower cytotoxicity and similar transfection efficiency in A549 and HepG2 lung cancer cells (Peng et al., 2011).

Ishitsuka et al. (2011) developed a multifunctional envelope-type nano device (MEND), in which plasmid DNA is condensed using a polycation to form a core particle that is encapsulated in a lipid envelope, modified with the IRQ peptide (IRQRRRR) to enhance transgene expression in lungs. (Ishitsuka et al., 2011).

Clinical applications of liposomes and nanoparticles for drug delivery to the respiratory tract are still in early stages. The key to future innovation may lie at the interface between biology and particle engineering. Improved understanding of biological processes including particle clearance, cellular targeting, intracellular trafficking, and drug absorption are needed to better design formulations that deliver to the "target" with the optimal balance of pharmacodynamic, pharmacokinetic, and safety profiles. More specifically, continued advances are needed in the development of: (1) controlled release formulations; (2) formulations with improved regional targeting within the lungs (e.g., airway versus alveoli and vice versa); (3) formulations containing active targeting moieties; (4) formulation strategies for improving the systemic bioavailability of inhaled macromolecules; (5) formulation strategies for delivering macromolecules, including siRNA and DNA, into cells; and (6) formulations with improved dose consistency. It is likely that such innovation will require the development of novel excipients and particle engineering strategies. Future innovation must also take into account the changing marketplace and the diverse set of customers (patient, healthcare professional, heath authorities, payers, and politicians) who must be satisfied. The pharmacoeconomics of new delivery systems will be closely scrutinized, so it is imperative that cost factors should be taken into account. Otherwise, the new technology option may overshoot the evolving inhalation marketplace.

4. Toxicity of nanoparticles to the lung

Epidemiological studies have confirmed a positive correlation between levels of particulate pollution and increased morbidity and mortality rates among general populations (Gwinn & Vallyathan, 2006; Stone et al., 2007).

The adverse health effects seem to be dominated by pulmonary symptoms. For instance, many reports have addressed that occupational exposure of inhaled rigid nanoparticles (NPs) can lead to respiratory diseases such as pneumoconiosis (pulmonary fibrosis) and bronchitis (Byrne & Baugh, 2008; Lkhasuren et al., 2007).

Increasing inhalation of ambient ultrafine particles has been linked with exacerbation of respiratory symptoms and mortality among COPD sufferers (Xia et al., 2009). It has also been documented that NPs can instigate oxidative stress and cellular toxicity in various types of cells (Huang et al., 2009).

It was also reported that chronic exposure to NPs can potentially predispose humans to lung inflammation and increase the risk of COPD.

A concentration range of NPs within the level found in ambience and in nanotechnology industries (Klaine et al., 2008) can promote mucin aggregation.

The second safety aspect of deep lung deposition is the interaction of nanoparticles with the alveolar environment. The alveolar space is covered with a thin surfactant film. This film has important physiological functions e.g. to accelerate gas exchange and to lower the surface tension in the alveolar space. Compromising these functions by inhalable nanoparticles might cause life threatening consequences. Therefore, the compatibility of a delivery system with the alveolar environment must be considered (Azarmi et al., 2008).

For these reasons vesicular nanocarriers, composed of lung surfactants and/or synthetic amphiphiles, provide an efficient delivery system for the treatment of pulmonary disorders due to their biocompatibility, biodegradability and non-toxic nature (Taylor & Newton, 2004).

5. Chronic obstructive pulmonary disease (COPD)

COPD is the fourth leading cause of death in the United States and Europe, with COPD mortality more than doubling in the last two decades (Mannino et al., 2002). COPD can be defined as a preventable and treatable disease state characterized by airflow limitation that is not fully reversible. The airflow limitation is usually progressive and is associated with an abnormal inflammatory response of the lungs to noxious particles or gases, primarily caused by cigarette smoking. Although COPD affects the lungs, it also produces significant systemic consequences (Celli & MacNee, 2004). It is interesting to point out how the definition of COPD has evolved including the systemic consequences of the disease. The natural history of the disease reveals numerous extrapulmonary manifestations and comorbidity factors that complicate the evolution of COPD, thereby altering the prognosis and quality of life of patients (Barnes & Celli, 2009; Agusti & Soriano, 2008). Many extrapulmonary effects of COPD have been described over the last two decades, including renal and hormonal abnormalities, muscle wasting (Remels et al., 2007), osteoporosis, anemia and reduction in circulating bone marrow progenitors (Palange et al., 2006). Although these systemic manifestations have been described for years in COPD patients, it is still unclear whether they represent consequences of the pulmonary disorder, or whether COPD should be considered as a systemic disease. The importance of establishing the distinction between a respiratory disease with extrapulmonary manifestations and a systemic inflammatory state with multiple compromised organs is justified by different therapeutic options: in the first definition, therapy is primarily centred on the lungs, whereas in the second, therapy could aim at the systemic inflammatory state. Both submucosal gland hypertrophy and airway surface goblet cell metaplasia are prominent features of the chronic bronchitis that occurs in most COPD patients. While cough and chronic expectoration helps to remove excess mucus from the large airways, impaired mucociliary function in COPD causes ineffective mucus clearance from small airways (≤ 2 mm diameter) which are not well cleared by cough. Like asthma and CF, COPD is strongly associated with the accumulation of inflammatory mucous exudates in the lumens of small airways (Hogg et al., 2004). Accordingly, declining lung function, respiratory infections, hospital admission, and mortality are significantly associated with chronic expectoration.

Among the numerous extrapulmonary effects of COPD, systemic inflammation has been widely studied and considered as an important key between the pulmonary disease and the related systemic manifestations. Many studies reported changes in various inflammatory cells and mediators, including neutrophils, lymphocytes, acute-phase reactants, and cytokines. Recently it was shown that systemic inflammation is present during COPD exacerbations and stable phases of the disease: increased numbers of leukocytes, levels of acute-phase response proteins (C-reactive protein and fibrinogen), cytokines such as interleukin (IL)-6, and tumor necrosis factor (TNF)-α are present in the peripheral blood of COPD patients (Gan et al., 2004). Systemic inflammation has been implicated in the pathogenesis of the majority of COPD systemic effects, including weight loss (Wouters, 2002), skeletal muscle dysfunction, cardiovascular diseases (Sin & Man, 2003), and osteoporosis, although it is still controversial whether this so called low-grade systemic inflammation represents the consequence of pulmonary inflammation into the systemic vascular bed (Agusti` et al. 2003), or whether it is a systemic inflammation. Although inflammation is certainly one of the major features of COPD, we still need to understand whether the local inflammation is sufficient to induce systemic effects, or whether a second pathogenetic event is required (Evans & Koo, 2009; Huertas & Palange 2011).

Over the years it was evidenced that mucus hypersecretion is an important manifestation of COPD. In the classical phenotype of chronic bronchitis, mucus hypersecretion is the key presenting symptom that appears independent of airflow obstruction. A more recent work demonstrated that obstruction of the small airways by inflammatory exudates containing mucus is predictive of early death after volume reduction surgery in patients with advanced COPD (Hogg et al., 2007). It was suggested that such occlusion enhanced the probability of infection in the lower respiratory tract. In addition, several epidemiological studies showed an association between mucus hypersecretion and outcomes in patients with COPD. Mucus hypersecretion is not an innocent disorder. However, despite these observations, until now few studies have focused on the effects of mucolytic drugs in patients with COPD, even though some of these mucolytic drugs also appear to have antioxidant properties (Dekhuijzen, 2004; Rahman et al., 1997; Rahman & Kilty 2006; Decramer & Janssens, 2010).

Histopathological findings from surgical specimens clearly show that increased goblet cell numbers and increased MUC5AC and MUC5B production and secretion are found in the lumen of small airways in COPD patients (Caramori et al., 2004). These findings are inversely associated with pre-surgical Forced Expiratory Volume in the 1st second (FEV1). Thus, patients with higher FEV1 have less goblet cell metaplasia than patients with lower FEV1, suggesting that the presence of mucin-producing cells in the airways is related to increased airflow obstruction. The presence of a prominent goblet cell phenotype also negatively correlates with FEV1 improvement following lung volume reduction surgery (Kim et al., 2005). Collectively, these results show that mucus secretion may be significant enough to result in physiologically and clinically measurable mechanical obstruction of small airways, and it may significantly impact disease pathogenesis and prognosis. The main cause of COPD in humans is cigarette smoking. In mice, chronic cigarette smoke exposure causes strain dependent mucous metaplasia. Cigarette smoke itself has also been shown to promote mucin synthesis directly in vitro by activation of the EGFR cascade (Shao et al., 2004). Inhalation, of one of the many potential toxicants present in cigarette smoke, acrolein (acrylic aldehyde), induces mucous metaplasia and MUC5AC production in animals. Acrolein also induces MUC5AC production in human airway epithelial cell lines, and it is found at significantly elevated levels in the induced sputum and exhaled breath condensates of COPD patients, (Deshmukh et al., 2008).

It has been suggested that mucus can also serve as a suitable medium for adherence and growth of some bacterial pathogens, such as non-typeable H. influenzae. Gram positive and gram negative bacteria products up-regulate MUC5AC and MUC2 gene expression and mucin secretion in human respiratory epithelial cell lines in vitro, and the same effect can be seen in some animal models in vivo. Viral infections are also closely associated with COPD exacerbations in humans (Wedzicha & Donaldson, 2003; Beckham et al., 2005). Surgical specimens from smokers with COPD show increased goblet cell numbers in the epithelium of peripheral airways compared to non-smokers. This is accompanied by increased macrophages and CD8 positive T-lymphocytes, both of which are indicative of viral. Roles for IL-6 and virus-induced mucin overproduction have been suggested. In vivo, IL-6 production is enhanced during the early phase of bacterial or viral-induced inflammation.

Accordingly, IL-6 levels are increased in COPD patients (Bucchioni et al., 2003), and during experimental respiratory viral infections in humans and mice (Decramer & Janssens, 2010).

5.1 Mucus rheological properties

Mucus rheology plays a critical role in maintaining respiratory health. Mucins are large, highly glycosylated proteins. The polyanionic nature of mucin stems primarily from sialic acid, sulfate, and carboxyl groups present in these linked oligosaccharides. Beside physical entanglement, cationic calcium ions can act as crosslinkers that condense the mucin matrices inside mucin granules before exocytosis. Upon release, phase transition mainly driven by the Donnan effect triggers the massive decondensation of mucin networks. Hydrogen bonding, hydrophilic and hydrophobic interactions have also been proposed to contribute to the gel properties of mucin The gel characteristics and rheological properties of mucin are critical for the maintainance the integrity of epithelia by trapping bacteria and viruses and for mucociliary clearance (Bansil & Stanley, 1995; Verdugo, 1990).

Mucus is mainly composed of large and heavily glycosylated glycoproteins called mucins. The gel-forming mucins rapidly hydrate after exocytosis and, due to their tangle network properties, anneal with other mucins to form a protective barrier at the airway-surface liquid layer. The mucin gel layer lines the epithelial surface of various organs such as the vaginal tract, eyes, gastric wall and pulmonary lumen. Mucus in the airway of lungs serves as an innate immune defense against inhaled particulates, bacteria and viruses. Maintenance of the airway protection mechanism stems from the delicate balance between normal mucus production, transport and clearance. The mucin polymer network of mucus has a characteristic tangled topology. Since the rheological properties of mucus are governed mainly by the tangle density of mucin polymers, which decreases with the square of the volume of the mucin matrix, the mucin network hydration (degree of swelling) is the most critical factor in determining the rheological properties of mucus. The diffusivity of mucin matrices, which is closely related to mucin viscosity, can be calculated from polymer swelling kinetics. Based on the polymer network theory, polymer diffusivity is inversely proportional to its viscosity (Lodge, 1999). Thus, lower rate of mucin diffusivity is associated with higher viscosity, less dispersed and less transportable mucins that appear to characterize the clinical symptoms of thick mucus accumulation and obstruction commonly found in asthma, COPD and CF 44. (Rogers, 2007).

The clinical manifestation of major respiratory diseases (Rogers & Barnes, 2006; Quinton, 2008) are related to thick mucus.

The relationship between mucin dehydration and defective mucus clearance has been well established (Mall et al., 2004). As a result, the poorly hydrated, highly viscous and less transportable mucus appears to accumulate within airway passages (Randell et al., 2006). Obstruction of airway lumen with viscous mucus is usually accompanied by chronic bacterial infection, inflammation and impaired mucociliary transport.

6. Case studies

Although the use of liposomes for aerosol formulations is certainly encouraging, liposome nebulization still presents some problems, i.e. storage stability (mainly related to oxidation processes) and leakage of encapsulated drugs. In addition, it should be also considered that synthetic phospholipids are usually expensive and, on the other side, natural phospholipids show a variable degree of purity (Desai & Finlay, 2002).

An alternative approach to the liposomal approach is the use of liposome-like vesicles made up of non-ionic surfactants, the so-called niosomes. These carriers were proposed for both topical (Carafa et al., 2000; Carafa et al., 2004; Paolino et al., 2007; Paolino et al., 2008) and systemic administration (Cosco et al., 2009).

Here we report the evaluation of the possible advantages of a new type of non-phospholipid vesicle system for pulmonary drug delivery that can lead to an improved mucus permeation. Vesicles consisting of one or more surfactant bilayers enclosing aqueous spaces (non ionic surfactant vesicles NSVs), are of particular interest because they offer several advantages with regard to chemical stability, lower cost and availability of materials compared to conventional liposomes

In the formulation of inhaled drugs for the treatment of asthma and COPD, considerable attention has been devoted to new aerosol morphologies which can either enhance the local effect and/or increase the penetration through the mucus, secreted in bronchial inflammatory diseases. In diseases characterized by bronchial hypersecretion, lipophilic substances, such as corticosteroids, can be remarkably impeded in reaching their receptors, which are localized within the cytoplasm of bronchial epithelial cells.

In particular, alveolar macrophages are important target cells for the therapeutic action of glucocorticoids, because these cells are the major source of both proinflammatory and antiinflammatory cytokines. The action of glucocorticoids is mediated by an intracellular receptor belonging to the steroid thyroid/retinoic acid receptor superfamily (Oakley et al., 1999).

With the purpose of carrying out research leading to an innovative formulation for lung delivery capable of permeating the mucous layer and of an efficient delivery to alveolar macrophages, beclomethasone dipropionate (BDP), clinically used for the treatment of asthma and COPD, was entrapped in non-phospholipid vesicles.

BDP, as a reference model drug, was encapsulated in vesicular structures obtained with polysorbate 20. The aim of the study was to evaluate *in vitro* the effectiveness of such delivery system that should enhance permeation through mucosal barriers because of the presence of vesicles formed with a remarkably hydrophilic non-ionic surfactant usually considered as unsuitable for the formation of vesicular structures because of its high HLB value (HLB 16.7) (Santucci et al., 1996).

The intracellular availability of BDP and the safety of the delivery system are the two main issues to be addressed to propose these innovative non-ionic surfactant vesicles as carriers for the pulmonary delivery of this drug to be effectively used for the treatment of pulmonary inflammatory diseases. Therefore, the aim of this investigation was the evaluation of the interaction between our innovative non-ionic surfactant vesicles and human lung fibroblast (HLF) cells, the carrier tolerability, the vesicle localization within the cells and the amount of BDP actually internalized by the cells.

Unilamellar vesicles were obtained from a non-ionic surfactant/BDP aqueous dispersion (Hepes pH 7.4) by means of the "film" method as previously reported (Santucci et al., 1996), according to the compositions reported in Table 1.

Sample	Polysorbate 20	Cholesterol	BDP
1	1.84	0.58	0.5
2	1.84	0.58	1.0
3	1.84	0.58	3.0
4	1.84	0.58	5.0
5	3.68	1.16	0.5
6	3.68	1.16	1.0
7	3.68	1.16	3.0
8	3.68	1.16	5.0

Table 1. Sample composition (expressed as % w/v)

All compositions are able to form nanovesicles with different size and zeta potential (ζ-potential) according to the various formulations (Table 1). The size and the polydispersity index (PDI) obtained by dynamic light scattering measurements indicated those formulations with the smallest size and the most homogeneous nanovesicles population that can be obtained: samples 2 and 8, chosen to perform further experiments.

Size measurement experiments indicate that BDP-loaded vesicles are slightly larger than empty ones as reported in Table 2 for samples 2 and 8 of Table 1, there is an increase in diameter between 10 and 20%, and this expected effect can be related to drug partition between the bilayer and the aqueous core of the vesicles. Accordingly, the presence of BDP in the formulation may affects the ζ-potential values; as it is possible to observe from Table 2, the corresponding samples 2 and 8 show a significant decrease in ζ-potential that approaches the value obtained with BDP alone. This effect can be related to the chemical steroidic structure of the drug that is somehow similar to that of cholesterol, thus allowing it to fit well within the vesicular structure.

Sample	Dimensions (nm)	ζ-potential (mV)
2	163±0.03	-32±0.2
8	174±0.02	-34±0.3
Empty vesicles	146±0.05	-40±0.2
BDP solution 0.05% w/v	=	-30±0.1

Table 2. Vesicle dimensions (nm) and ζ- potential (mV) of analyzed samples (n=3; ±SD)

Furthermore, it should be pointed out that electron microscopy carried out on numerous samples (10) indicated that nebulization does not influence drug-loaded vesicle dimensions (Figure 5A and B).

Analyzed samples showed a good stability in terms of possible changes in vesicle dimensions after aggregation.

Size measurement experiments indicated that after 1 month at 25 °C, no appreciable vesicle dimension variations could be detected.

The best entrapment efficiency (e.e.) was obtained for sample 8 and the calculated drug e.e. indicated that only about 20% of the overall amount of BDP is actually enclosed within the vesicles. This result is in agreement with the data reported by previous authors (Montenegro

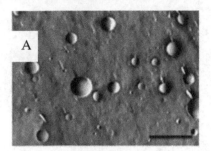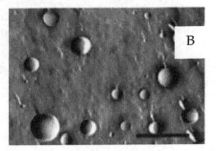

Fig. 5. Trasmission electron micrographs of BDP-loaded vesicles after freeze-fracture, before (A) and after (B) nebulization. The scale bar represents 0.5 μm.

et al., 1996; Darwis et al., 2001). For this reason, for permeation and nebulization experiments the formulation corresponding to sample 8 of Table 1 was used.

The possibility to use the novel vesicular dispersion in a conventional jet nebulizer, widely used in clinical applications, was also evaluated. For this purpose, samples were characterized also by means of rheological measurements and the aerodynamic diameter was determined (Table 3) as well as the nebulizer mass output (Figure 6) after completion of nebulization. Evaluation of Mass Median Aerodynamic Diameter (2.0±0.2 μm) and of geometric standard deviation (GSD) were also carried out; the GSD value (1.5) demonstrates the polydisperse nature of the distribution of the aerosolized droplets that, on the other side, contained a monodisperse vesicular system.

Aerodynamic diameter	Percentage
<10	100
<5	99.5
<2	65

Table 3. Percentage of particles with aerodynamic diameter <10, < 5, <2 μm, containing non-ionic surfactant vesicles, delivered by a jet nebulizer

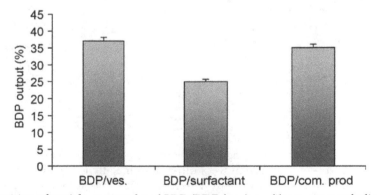

Fig. 6. Deposition of vesicle-encapsulated BDP (BDP/ves) on filters upon nebulization, compared to a BDP/surfactant solution and to a BDP commercial product (n=3, ±SD).

Furthermore, in all conditions of nebulization (TurboBoy nebulizer and Clenny nebulizer), the dispersion BDP/vesicles releases a greater amount of drug, dosed by HPLC, with respect to commercial formulations.

An important aspect to be taken into account for an actual application of these non-ionic surfactant vesicles as possible carriers to be aerosolized for the pulmonary delivery of drugs is their colloidal and storage stability.

In fact, the occurrence of aggregation phenomena can lead to a significant worsening of the biopharmaceutical features of nanosized colloidal suspensions, such as NSVs. Therefore, the colloidal stability of BDP-loaded NSVs was evaluated using the Turbiscan Lab® Expert (Celia et al., 2009) i.e. the optical transmission and the photon backscattering profiles of various samples were recorded. Any variation of the vesicle volume fraction (migration) or mean size (coalescence) triggers the variation of backscattering (BS) and transmission (T) signals, which are graphically reported as positive (backscattering/transmission increase) or negative (backscattering/transmission decrease) peaks. It can be assumed that no variation of particle size occurs when the ΔBS and ΔT profiles are within an interval of ±2% while variations greater than 10% either as a positive or a negative value are representative of an instable formulation.

Two different BDP concentrations, i.e. 50 mg/ml (sample BDP-50) and 0.4 mg/ml (BDP-0.4), were used in this stability investigations. The first concentration led to the maximum possible amount of drug entrapment within the NSVs, while the second concentration led to an amount of entrapped drug similar to that actually present in the most common commercial products.

The ΔBS and ΔT profiles of BDP -loaded and unloaded non-ionic surfactant vesicles are shown in Figure 7.

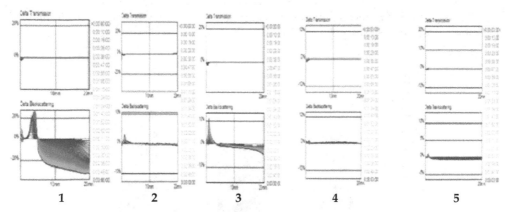

1   2   3   4   5

Fig. 7. Transmission and backscattering profiles of niosomes by using Turbiscan Lab® Expert. The image represents the analysis of different formulations: (1) unpurified BDP-50-niosomes; (2) purified BDP-50-niosomes; (3) unpurified BDP-0.4-niosomes; (4) purified BDP-0.4-niosomes; (5) unloaded niosomes. Data are reported as a function of time (0–3 h) and sample height (from 2 to 20 mm).

The transmission signal remained close to the base line value and ΔT profiles close to 0% were observed for all the investigated NSV formulations during the entire time of analysis.

Therefore, NSVs suspensions maintained a constant opalescent aspect along the height of various samples. At the same time, positive or negative variations of the backscattering profiles of the different formulations (Figure 7) were not correlated to destabilization processes under the sample height of 2 mm and over that of 20 mm, the values having been determined by enclosed air in the bottom and/or on the top of the cylindrical glass tube, respectively. Different NSVs formulations showed that backscattering emerged as the prevalent signal in the different measurements (Figure 7). ΔBS signals are close to ~1% during the time of analysis for the entire height of the samples of both purified BDP-loaded and unloaded non-ionic surfactant vesicles (Figure 7 panels B, D and F). It was interesting to observe that the different amounts of the entrapped drug do not influence the colloidal stability of non-ionic surfactant vesicles both in terms of vesicle migration and coalescence. Different stability behaviors, as shown by ΔBS profiles (Figure 7 panels A and C), were observed in the case of not purified BDP loaded non-ionic surfactant vesicles (i.e. before gel exclusion chromatography).

In particular, vesicles prepared in the presence of the highest drug concentration (50 mg/ml) showed a high colloidal instability just after the beginning of the analysis. A moderate stability (ΔBS profile within the 10% during the 3 h of analysis) was observed for unpurified non-ionic surfactant vesicles prepared in the presence of 0.4 mg/ml of the drug, while an elevated stability (equal to purified formulations) was observed for unpurified unloaded vesicles (Figure 7 panel E). These findings can be due to the presence of high amount of free drug, that with time leads to the formation of aggregates. Therefore, the purification procedure is essential to achieve a stable vesicular colloidal carrier for the delivery of BDP. The stability findings by Turbiscan Lab® Expert measurement were also supported by light scattering size analysis during a storage period of 3 months, which showed no appreciable vesicle size variation for purified BDP-loaded non-ionic surfactant vesicles.

According to the aim of this research, the capability of ensuring a better penetration through the mucus layer of vesicular formulation was tested.

In Figure 8, the permeation rate of BDP from the vesicular dispersion is reported and compared with that obtained using a BDP/polysorbate 20 (at the same concentration used for vesicle preparation) suspension as well as with that of the commercial preparation. The vesicular formulation (BDP-0.4) was used in its unpurified form, thus with the drug partitioned inside and outside the vesicular structure.

This situation allows an appropriate comparison with the other preparations used in permeation experiments: since both micellar surfactant solutions and the commercial one contained free BDP and BDP included within aggregated structures (micelles). As it can be observed, the presence of NSVs in the formulation remarkably increases the permeation rate through the model mucosal barrier with respect to the other tested preparation thus indicating that the novel BDP formulation can be proposed for a better targeting of corticosteroids in the treatment of COPD.

An important aspect to evaluate an innovative drug delivery system is its safety. This aspect is much more relevant in the case of pulmonary delivery, since several side effects may

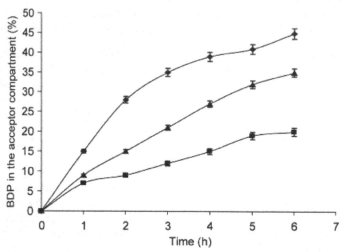

Fig. 8. Comparison of the permeation patterns through a gel-like mucin solution (0.1%w/v), expressed as percentage of permeated drug as a function of time (n=3, ±SD) (■BDP/surfactant ▲BDP/commercial product ◆BDP/vesicles).

result from an unsafe material, i.e. fibrosis, pulmonary oedema, inflammation, as reported in section 4.

Safety of empty non-ionic surfactant vesicles was evaluated in vitro on HLF cells by using the trypan blue dye exclusion assay (cell mortality) and MTT viability test. Purified and unpurified empty NSVs were assayed in vitro at different surfactant concentrations (from 0.01 to 10 μM) and incubation-times (24, 48 and 72 h).

Purified non-ionic surfactant vesicles did not show a significant cytotoxic activity on HLF cells at all incubation times for concentrations ranging from 0.01 to 1 μM, i.e. the mortality values ranged from 1.2 to 5.81%, respectively. Only at the highest investigated concentration (10 μM) and after 48 h of incubation a slight cytotoxic effect was observed (mortality value of 16%).

It is interesting to point out that unpurified vesicles showed a significant (P<0.001) increase of cytotoxicity with respect to purified vesicles at all the investigated conditions (exposition times and surfactant concentrations). In this sense it was also observed that the increase of the cytotoxic effect was dependent on surfactant concentration but not on the exposition time. This finding was due to the fact that the cytotoxic action of unpurified NSVs was determined by the presence of the free molecules of surfactants, which were able to exert immediately their cytotoxic action during the incubation period by noticeably perturbing the cellular membranes (Dimitrijevic et al., 2000; Lin et al., 2007) and hence causing the cellular death. This hypothesis was strongly supported by the evidence that HLF cells treated with the free surfactants showed a greater (P<0.001) cytotoxic insult than those treated with unpurified non-ionic surfactant vesicles. Therefore, the assembling of surfactant into non-ionic surfactant vesicles determined a drastic reduction of cytotoxicity, due to a concomitant reduction of the free surfactant molecules in solution and/or surfactant micelles, which are able to alter the cellular permeability and homeostasis.

Another important feature of an innovative drug delivery system is to increase the amount of active compound in the target district, thus improving the therapeutic effect of the drug. Therefore, to evaluate the delivery ability and the mechanisms of interaction of fluorescein-labelled non-ionic surfactant vesicles with HLF cells, CLSM experiments were carried out.

Figure 9 shows how the fluorescein-labelled vesicles interacted with HLF cells at different incubation times. A green fluorescence distribution was observed in the cells just after 1 h incubation. After 3 h incubation the fluorescence of the cellular membrane and the cytoplasm became more intense and increased slightly up to 24 h of incubation. These findings prompted us to suppose that the main mechanism involved in the NSVs/cell interaction was the endocytosis of the carrier (Di Marzio et al., 2008), which enabled a rapid internalization in the cytoplasm. It is worthy of note that at all incubation times the localization of fluorescence was in the cytoplasm compartment and these results represent an important aspect because the glucocorticoid receptor is localized in the cytoplasm.

No fluorescence was detected in the untreated HLF cell line (control) and hence there was no interfering auto-fluorescence phenomenon (Figure 9 panel 6).

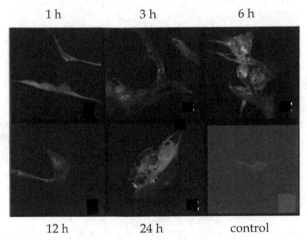

Fig. 9. CLSM micrographs of the interaction of fluoresceine-labelled NSVs with primary HLF cells as a function of the incubation times,. The reflectance CLSM micrographs of untreated cells were used as controls and no significant cellular fluorescence was observed

As a consequence, the improved interaction of NSVs with primary HLF cells should lead to a greater intracellular delivery of the entrapped drug.

For this reason the intracellular uptake of BDP prompted by the various formulations was investigated as a function of time (Figure 10).

Considering that surfactant molecules and unloaded non-ionic surfactant vesicles may act as drug cellular penetration enhancers and to evaluate the effective role of the vesicles in the promotion of the intracellular uptake of BDP, a mixture surfactant/BDP and a mixture empty vesicles/BDP was also assayed. As reported in Figure 10, BDP loaded non-ionic surfactant vesicles (BDP-0.4) showed a significant improvement of the intracellular uptake of the drug with respect to a mixture surfactant/BDP, a mixture empty non-ionic surfactant

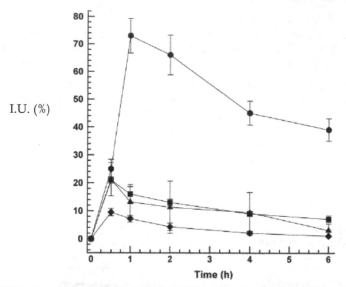

Fig. 10. HLF intracellular uptake (I.U. at 37 °C) of beclomethasone dipropionate (expressed as percentage of the applied dose) as a function of time by different formulations: BDP loaded NSVs (BDP-0.4), •; surfactant/BDP mixture, ▲; empty non-ionic surfactant vesicle/BDP mixture, ■; free drug, ♦.

vesicle/BDP and a free drug solution. This result was correlated to the ability of NSVs to easily penetrate across cell membranes of primary HLF cells (in full agreement with CSLM experiments), thus achieving a noticeable cytoplasm accumulation of BDP. These results clearly evidenced that the improvement of the drug intracellular uptake was mainly mediated by the vesicular carrier and no positive influence was exerted by the surfactant molecules and/or empty vesicles, i.e. the drug has to be entrapped within the carrier. In fact, the mixtures surfactant/drug and empty vesicle/drug showed only a slight improvement of the intracellular uptake of BDP. The profiles of BDP intracellular uptake as a function of time showed (Figure 10) a Tmax (time at which the maximum drug concentration was reached) value of 1 h followed by a gradual reduction of the intracellular drug accumulation up to 6 h in the case of the drug-loaded non-ionic surfactant vesicles. On the other side, all other tested formulations showed Tmax values of 30 min.

The rapid internalization of BDP formulated in niosomes was not considered as a critical parameter.

The evidence of the improved intracellular entrance of NSVs and the noticeable increase of the intracellular uptake of BDP mediated by the vesicular carrier should match an improved pharmacological activity of the delivered drug. For this reason the anti-inflammatory activity of BDP-loaded non-ionic surfactant vesicles was evaluated in comparison with the free drug, as the capacity to inhibit the secretion of NGF.

NGF is an important inflammatory mediator, which contributes to the development of airway hyper-responsiveness (de Vries et al., 1999). The NGF production is stimulated by the presence of pro-inflammatory cytokines and asthma-associated cytokines, i.e. IL-1β, and inhibited by anti-inflammatory glucocorticoids. Therefore, the in vitro determination of the levels of NGF secreted by HLF cells is a direct evidence of the pro- or anti-inflammatory effect of a substance.

As shown in Figure 11, the stimulation of HLF cells with IL-1β led to an over-secretion of NGF up to 210% of basal values (control). The treatment with the free BDP (1 μM) significantly reduced both the constitutive and the IL-1β-stimulated secretion of NGF by 18.7% and 61.23%, respectively. BDP-loaded non-ionic surfactant vesicles (BDP-0.4) were much more effective than the free drug, i.e. a reduction of 68% and 85% with respect to the constitutive and IL-1β-stimulated NGF secretion were respectively observed. These findings are in agreement with both CLSM and intracellular uptake experiments.

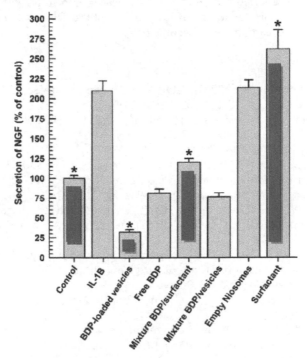

Fig. 11. Anti-inflammatory activity of various formulations containing BDP (1 μM) evaluated as inhibition of NGF secretion in primary HLF cells treated with IL-1β (as pro-inflammatory stimulating agent). Control was untreated HLF cells, which secrete the basal level of NGF.

The use of NSV formulations was investigated not only to increase intracellular uptake of BDP in HLF cells and to improve diffusion through mucus layer but also to design an innovative system able to increase therapeutic efficacy of BDP in pulmonary diseases thus reducing the dosage and potential side effects of this drug.

7. Conclusions

Despite the many promising proof - of - concepts of various delivery technologies, there is still a long way ahead that must be covered. This means there are still many challenges that are being faced, which, in turn, mean there are still many chances for the academic and industrial scientist to make a decisive impact.

Further research efforts are needed to ensure the safety of long-term in vivo applications. There is an urgent requirement for cautiously designed toxicology and toxicokinetic studies for each nanocarrier type; the protocols should be customized for an appropriate clinical use. Furthermore, it should be pointed out that scale up from laboratory to industry is still poorly investigated in this specific area, despite its obvious importance in the ultimate goal of the development a product that can reach the market and actually give benefits to the patients.

In spite of the above reported difficulties and challenges; hopefully, within a few years, the safety and large - scale production at affordable costs of the delivery technologies described in this book will be a dream that will become true.

8. References

Augustí, A.G. & Soriano, J.B. (2008). COPD as a systemic disease. *COPD*, Vol. 5, No. 2, (January 2008), pp. 133-138, ISSN 1541-2555.

Augustí, A.G., Noguera, A., Sauleda, J., Sala, E., Pons, J. & Busquets, X. (2003). Systemic effects of chronic obstructive pulmonary disease. *Eur Respir J*, Vol. 21, No. 2, (February 2003), pp. 347-360, ISSN 0903-1936.

Altiere, R.J. & Thompson, D.C. (1996). Pulmonary physiology and pharmacology of the airways, In: *Inhalation Aerosols: Physical and Biological Basis for Therapy*, Antony J. Hickey, pp. 96–99, Informa, ISBN: 0849341604, New York.

Azarmi, S., Roa , W. H. & Löbenberg, R. (2008). Targeted delivery of nanoparticles for the treatment of lung diseases. *Adv Drug Deliv Rev*, Vol. 60, No. 8, (May 2008), pp. 863–875, ISSN 0169-409X.

Bansil, R. & Turner, B.S. (2006). Mucin structure, aggregation, physiological functions and biomedical applications. *Curr. Opin. Colloid Interface Sci.*, Vol. 11, No. 2-3, (June 2006), pp. 164–170, ISSN 1359-0294.

Bansil, R., Stanley, E. & LaMont, J.T. (1995). Mucin Biophysics. *Ann Rev Physiol*, Vol. 57, (March 1995), pp. 635–657, ISSN 0066-4278.

Barnes, P.J. & Celli, B.R. (2009). Systemic manifestations and comorbidities of COPD. *Eur Respir J*, Vol. 33, No. 5, (May 2009), pp 1165-1185, ISSN 0903-1936.

Beckham, J.D., Cadena, A., Lin, J, Piedra, P.A., Glezen,W.P., Greenberg, S.B. & Atmar, R.L. (2005). Respiratory viral infections in patients with chronic, obstructive pulmonary disease. *J Infect*, Vol. 50, No. 4, (May 2005), pp. 322–330, ISSN 0163-4453.

Bernhard, W., Haslam, P.L. & Floros, J. (2004). From birds to humans: new concepts on airways relative to alveolar surfactant. *Am J Respir Cell Mol Biol*, Vol. 30, No. 1, (January 2004), pp. 6–11, ISSN 1044-1549.

Bruinenberg, P., Serisier, D., Cipolla, D. & Blanchard, J. (2010). Safety, tolerability and pharmacokinetics of novel liposomal ciprofloxacin formulations for inhalation in healthy volunteers and non-cystic bronchiectasis patients. *Am J Respir Crit Care Med*, Vol. 181, B49 Meeting Abstract, (May 2010), A3192, ISSN 1073-449X.

Bucchioni, E., Kharitonov, S.A., Allegra, L. & Barnes, P.J. (2003). High levels of interleukin-6 in the exhaled breath condensate of patients with COPD. *Respir Med,* Vol. 97, No. 12, (December 2003), pp. 1299–1302, ISSN 0020-1324.

Buhling, F., Groneberg, D. & Welte, T. (2006). Proteases and their role in chronic inflammatory lung diseases. *Curr Drug Targets,* Vol. 7, No. 6, (June 2006), pp. 751–759, ISSN 1389-4501.

Buhling, F., Waldburg, N., Reisenauer, A., Heimburg, A., Golpon, H. & Welte, T. (2004). Lysosomal cysteine proteases in the lung: role in protein processing and immunoregulation. *Eur Respir J,* Vol. 23, No. 4, (April 2004), pp. 620–628, ISSN 0903-1936.

Byrne, J.D. & Baugh, J.A. (2008), The significance of nanoparticles in particle-induced pulmonary fibrosis. *Mcgill J Med,* Vol. 11, No. 1, (January 2008), pp. 43–50, ISSN 1201-026X.

Carafa, M., Marianecci, C., Lucania, G., Marchei, E. & Santucci, E. (2004). New vesicular ampicillin-loaded delivery systems for topical application : characterization, in vitro permeation experiments and antimicrobial activity. *J Control Release,* Vol. 95, No. 1, (February 2004), pp. 67–74, ISSN 0168-3659.

Carafa, M., Santucci, E. & Lucania, G. (2002). Lidocaine-loaded non-ionic surfactant vesicles: characterization and in vitro permeation studies, *Int J Pharm,* Vol. 231, No. 1, (January 2002), pp. 221–232, ISSN 0378-5173.

Caramori, G., Di Gregorio, C., Carlstedt, I., Casolari, P., Guzzinati, I. & Adcock, I.M. (2004). Mucin expression in peripheral airways of patients with chronic obstructive pulmonary disease. *Histopathology,* Vol. 45, No. 5, (November 2004), pp. 477–484, ISSN 1365-2559.

Cefalu, WT. (2004). Concept, strategies, and feasibility of noninvasive insulin delivery. *Diabetes Care,* Vol. 27, No. 1, (January 2004), pp. 239–46, ISSN 0149-5992.

Celia, C., Trapasso, E., Cosco, D., Paolino., D. & Fresta, M. (2009). Turbiscan Lab® Expert analysis of the stability of ethosomes® and ultradeformable liposomes containing a bilayer fluidizing agent. *Colloids Surf. B Biointerface,* Vol. 72, No. 1, (August 2009), pp. 155–160 ISSN 0927-7765.

Celli, B.R. & MacNee, W. (2004). Standards for the diagnosis and treatment of patients with COPD: A summary of the ATS/ ERS position paper. *Eur Respir J,* Vol.23, No. 6, (June 2004), pp. 932–946, ISSN 0903-1936.

Clunes, M.T. & Boucher, R.C. (2007). Cystic fibrosis: the mechanisms of pathogenesis of an inherited lung disorder. *Drug Discov Today Dis Mech,* Vol. 4, No. 2, (June 2007), pp. 63–72, ISSN 1740-6765.

Cosco, D., Paolino, D., Muzzalupo, R., Celia, C., Citraro, R., Caponio, D., Picci, N. & Fresta, M. (2009) Novel PEG-coated niosomes based on bola-surfactant as drug carriers for 5-fluorouracil. *Biomed. Microdevices,* Vol. 11, No. 5 ,(October 2009), pp. 1115–1125, ISSN 1387-2176.

Crapo, J.D., Barry, B.E., Gehr, P., Bachofen, M. & Weibel, E.R. (1982). Cell number and cell characteristics of the normal human lung. *Am Rev Respir Dis,* Vol. 126, No. 3, (August 1982), pp. 332–337, ISSN 0003-0805.

Dailey, L.A., Schmehl, T., Gessler, T., Wittmar, M., Grimminger, F., Seeger, W., & Kissel, T. (2003). Nebulization of biodegradable nanoparticles: impact of nebulizer technology and nanoparticle characteristics on aerosol features. *J Control Release,* Vol. 86, No. 1, (January 2003), pp.131–44, ISSN: 0168-3659.

Darwis, Y. & Kellaway, I.W. (2001). Nebulization of rehydrated freeze-dried beclomethasone dipropionate liposomes. *Int J Pharm,* Vol. 215, No. 1-2, (March 2001), pp. 113–121. ISSN 0378-5173.

Daviskas, E., Anderson, S.D., Shaw, J., Eberl, S., Seale, J.P., Yang, I.A. & Young, I.H. (2005). Mucociliary clearance in patients with chronic asthma: effects of beta agonists. *Respirology,* Vol. 10, No. 4, (September 2005), pp. 426–435, ISSN: 1440-1843.

de Vries, A., Dessing, M.C., Engels, F., Henricks, P.A.J. & Nijkamp, F.P. (1999). Nerve growth factor induces a neurokinin-1 receptor-mediated airway hyperresponsiveness in guinea pigs. *Am J Respir Crit Care Med,* Vol. 159, No. 5, (May 1999), pp. 1541–1544, ISSN 1073-449X.

Decramer, M. & Janssens, J. (2010). Mucoactive therapy in COPD. *Eur Respir Rev,* Vol. 19, No. 116, (June 2010), 134–140, ISSN 0905-9180.

Dekhuijzen, P.N. (2004). Antioxidant properties of N-acetylcysteine: their relevance in relation to chronic obstructive pulmonary disease. *Eur Respir J,* Vol. 23, No. 4, (April 2004), pp. 629–636, ISSN 0903-1936.

Desai, T.R. & Finlay, W.H. (2002). Nebulization of niosomal all-trans-retinoic acid : an inexpensive alternative to conventional liposomes. *Int J Pharm,* Vol. 241, No. 2 (July 2002), pp. 311–317, ISSN 0378-5173.

Deshmukh, H. S., Shaver, C., Case, L.M., Dietsch, M., Wesselkamper, S. C. & Hardie,W. D. (2008). Acrolein-activated matrix metalloproteinase 9 contributes to persistent mucin production. *Am J Respir Cell Mol Biol,* Vol. 38, No. 4, (April 2008), pp. 446–454, ISSN 1044-1549.

Di Marzio, L., Marianecci, C., Cinque, B., Nazzarri, M., Cimini, A.M., Cristiano., L., Cifone, M.G., Alhaique, F. & Carafa, M. (2008). pH-sensitive non-phospholipid vesicle and macrophage-like cells: binding, uptake and endocytotic pathway. *Biochim Biophys Acta,* Vol. 1778, No. 12, (December 2008), pp. 2749–2756 ISSN 0005-2736.

Dimitrijevic, D., Shaw, A.J. & Florence, A.T. (2000). Effects of some non-ionic surfactants on transepithelial permeability in Caco-2 cells. *J Pharm Pharmacol,* Vol. 52, No. 2, (February 2000), pp. 157–162 ISSN 0022-3573

Dumont, J.A., Bitonti, A.J., Clark, D., Evans, S., Pickford, M. & Newman, S.P. (2005). Delivery of an erythropoietin-Fc fusion protein by inhalation in humans through an immunoglobulin transport pathway. *J Aerosol Med,* Vol. 18, No. 3, (September 2005), pp. 294–303, ISSN 0894-2684.

Edsbäcker, S, Wollmer, P., Selroos, O., Borgstroem, L., Olsson, B. & Ingelf J. (2008). Do airway clearance mechanisms influence the local and systemic effects of inhaled corticosteroids? *Pulm Pharmacol Ther,* Vol. 21, No. 2, (April 2008), pp. 247–258, ISSN 1094-553.

El-Chemaly, S., Pacheco-Rodriguez, G., Ikeda, Y., Malide, D. & Moss, J. (2009). Lymphatics in idiopathic pulmonary fibrosis: new insights into an old disease. *Lymphat Res Biol,* Vol. 7, No. 4, (December 2009),pp. 197–203, ISSN 1539-6851

Evans, C.M. & Koo, J.S. (2009). Airway mucus: the good, the bad, the sticky. *Pharmacol Ther,* Vol. 121, No. 3, (March 2009), pp. 332-348, ISSN 0163-7258.

Furuyama, A., Kanno., S., Kobayashi, T. & Hirano., S. (2009). Extrapulmonary translocation of intratracheally instilled fine and ultrafine particles via direct and alveolar macrophage-associated routes. *Arch Toxicol*, Vol. 83, No. 5, (May 2009), pp. 429–437, ISSN 0340-5761.

Gan, W.Q., Man, S.F., Senthilselvan, A. & Sin, D.D. (2004). Association between chronic obstructive pulmonary disease and systemic inflammation: a systematic review and a meta-analysis. *Thorax*, Vol. 59, No. 6, (June 2004) pp. 574-580, ISSN 1468-3296.

Geiser M. & Kreyling, W.G. (2010). Deposition and biokinetics of inhaled naNo.particles. *Part. Fibre Toxicol*, Vol. 7, No. 2, (January 2010), pp. 1-17, ISSN 1743-8977.

Geiser, M. (2010). Update on macrophage clearance of inhaled micro- and nanoparticles. *J Aerosol Med Pulm Drug Deliv*, Vol. 23, No. 4, (August 2010), pp. 207–17, ISSN 1941-2711.

Geiser, M., Casaulta, M., Kupferschmid, B., Schulz, H., Semmler-Behnke, M. & Kreyling, W. (2008). The role of macrophages in the clearance of inhaled ultrafine titanium dioxide particles. *Am J Respir Cell Mol Biol*, Vol. 38, No. 3, (March 2008), pp. 371–376, ISSN: 1044-1549.

Gonda, I. (2006). Systemic delivery of drugs to humans via inhalation. *J Aerosol Med*, Vol. 19, No. 1, (March 2006), pp. 47–53, ISSN 0894-2684.

Griesenbach, U. & Alton, E.W. (2009). Gene transfer to the lung: lessons learned from more than 2 decades of CF gene therapy. *Adv Drug Deliv Rev*, Vol. 61, No. 2, (February 2009), pp. 128–139, ISSN 0169-409X.

Haley, B. & Frenkel, E. (2008). Nanoparticles for drug delivery in cancer treatment. *Urol Oncol*, Vol. 26, No. 1, (January-February 2008), pp. 57-64, ISSN 1078-1439.

Heyder, J., Gebhart, J., Rudolf, G., Schiller, C.F. & Stahlhofen, W. (1985). Deposition of particles in the human respiratory tract in the size range 0.005–15 μm. *J Aerosol Sci*, Vol. 17, No. 5, (May 1985), pp. 811–25, ISSN 0021-8502.

Hinds, W.C. (1999). Uniform Particle Motion. In: *Aerosol Technology: Properties, Behavior and Measurement of Airborne Particles Second ed.*, William C. Hinds, pp. 53–55, Wiley, ISBN 978-0-471-19410-1, New York.

Hogg, J. C., Chu, F., Utokaparch, S., Woods, R., Elliott, W. M. & Buzatu, L. (2004). The nature of small-airway obstruction in chronic obstructive pulmonary disease. *N Engl J Med*, Vol. 350, No. 26, (June 2004), pp. 2645–2653, ISSN 0028-4793.

Hogg, J.C., Chu, F.S. & Tan, W.C. (2007). Survival after lung volume reduction in chronic obstructive pulmonary disease: insights from small airway pathology. *Am J Respir Crit Care Med*, Vol. 176, No. 4, (August 2007), pp. 454–459, ISSN 1044-1549.

Holt, P.G., Strickland, D.H., Wikstrom, M.E. & Jahnsen, F.L. (2008). Regulation of immunological homeostasis in the respiratory tract. *Nat Rev Immunol*, Vol. 8, No. 2, (February 2008), pp. 142–52, ISSN 1474-1733.

Huang, C.C., Aronstam, R.S., Chen, D.R. & Huang, Y.W. (2010). Oxidative stress, calcium homeostasis, and altered gene expression in human lung epithelial cells exposed to ZnO nanoparticles. *Toxicol In Vitro*, Vol. 24, No. 1, (February 2010), pp. 45–55, ISSN 0887-2333.

Huertas, A. & Palange, P. (2011). COPD: a multifactorial systemic disease. *Ther Adv Respir Dis*, Vol. 5, No. 3, (March 2011), pp. 217-224, ISSN 1753-4658.

Illum L. (2002). Nasal drug delivery: new developments and strategies. *Drug Discov Today*, Vol. 7, No. 23, (December 2002), pp. 1184–1189, ISSN 1359-6446.

Ishitsuka, T, Akita, H. & Harashima, H. (2011). Functional improvement of an IRQ-PEG-MEND for delivering genes to the lung. *J Control Release*, Vol. 154, No. 1, pp. 77-83, ISSN 0168-3659.

Kim, V, Criner, G.J., Abdallah, H.Y., Gaughan, J.P., Furukawa, S. & Solomides, C.C. (2005). Small airway morphometry and improvement in pulmonary function afterlung volume reduction surgery. *Am J Respir Crit Care Med*, Vol. 171, No. 1, (January 2005), pp. 40–47, ISSN 1044-1549.

Klaine, S.J., Alvarez, P.J.J., Batley, G.E., Fernandes, T.F. & Handy, R.D. (2008). Nanomaterials in the environment: Behavior, fate, bioavailability, and effects. *Environ Toxicol Chem*, Vol. 27, No. 9, (September 2008), pp. 1825–1851, ISSN 0730-7268.

Kurmi, B.D., Kayat, J., Gajbhiye, V., Tekade, R.K. & Jain, N.K. (2010). Micro- and nanocarrier-mediated lung targeting. *Expert Opin Drug Deliv*, Vol. 7, No. 7, (July 2010), pp. 781-794, ISSN 1742-5247.

Lai, S.K., Wang, Y.Y. & Hanes, J. (2009). Mucus-penetrating nanoparticles for drug and gene delivery to mucosal tissues. *Adv Drug Deliv Rev*, Vol. 61, No. 2, (February 2009), pp. 158–171, ISSN 0169-409X.

Lam, J.K., Liang, W. & Chan, H.K. (2011). Pulmonary delivery of therapeutic siRNA. *Adv Drug Deliv Rev*, Article in Press, ISSN 0169-409X.

Li, P., Liu, D., Sun, X., Liu, C., Liu, Y. & Zhang, N. (2011). A novel cationic liposome formulation for efficient gene delivery via a pulmonary route. *Nanotechnology*, Vol. 22, No. 24, (June 2011), art. No. 245104 (11 pages), ISSN 1361-6528.

Lin, H., Gebhardt, M., Bian, S., Kwon, K.A., Shim, C.K., Chung, S.J. & Kim D.D (2007). Enhancing effect of surfactants on fexofenadine HCl transport across the human nasal epithelial cell monolayer, *Int J Pharm*, Vol. 330, No. 1-2, (February 2007), pp. 23–31, ISSN 0378-5173.

Lkhasuren, O., Takahashi, K. & Dash-Onolt, L (2007). Occupational lung diseases and the mining industry in Mongolia. *Int J Occup Environ Health*, Vol. 13, No. 2, (April 2007), pp. 195–201, ISSN 1077-3525.

Lodge, T.P. (1999). Reconciliation of the molecular weight dependence of diffusion and viscosity in entangled polymers. *Phys Rev Lett*, Vol. 83, No. 16, (October 1999), pp. 3218-3221, ISSN 0031-9007.

Madl, A.K. & Pinkerton, K.E. (2009). Health effects of inhaled engineered and incidental nanoparticles. *Crit Rev Toxicol*, Vol. 39, No. 8, (September 2009), pp. 629–658, ISSN 1040-8444.

Mall, M., Grubb, B.R., Harkema, J.R., O'Neal, W.K. & Boucher, R.C. (2004). Increased airway epithelial Na+ absorption produces cystic fibrosis-like lung disease in mice. *Nat Med*, Vol. 10, No. 4, (April 2004), pp. 487–493, ISSN 1078-8956.

Mannino, D.M., Homa, D.M., Akinbami, L.J., Ford, E.S., & Redd, S.C. (2002). Chronic obstructive pulmonary disease surveillance—United States, 1971–2000. *Respir Care*, Vol. 47, No. 10, (October 2002), pp.1184–1199, ISSN 0020-1324.

Mansour, H.M., Rhee, Y.S. & Wu, X. (2009). Nanomedicine in pulmonary delivery. *Int J Nanomedicine*, Vol. 4, (December 2009), pp. 299–319, ISSN 1176-9114.

Meers, P., Neville, M., Malinin, V., Scotto, A.W., Sardaryan, G., Kurumunda, Mackinson, R., James, G., Fisher, S. & Perkins, W.R. (2008). Biofilm penetration, triggered release and in vivo activity of inhaled liposomal amikacin in chronic Pseudomonas aeruginosa lung infections. *J Antimicrob Chemother*, Vol. 61, No. 4, (April 2008), pp. 859–868, ISSN 0305-7453.

Mercer, R.R., Russell, M.L., Roggli, V.L. & Crapo, J.D. (1994). Cell number and distribution in human and rat airways. *Am J Respir Cell Mol Biol*, Vol. 10, No. 6, (June 1994), pp. 613–624, ISSN 1044-1549.

Misra, A., Jinturkar, K., Patel, D., Lalani, J. & Chougule, M. (2009). Recent advances in liposomal dry powder formulations: preparation and evaluation. *Expert Opin Drug Deliv*, Vol. 6, No. 1, (January 2009), pp. 71-89, ISSN 1742-5247.

Mitsopoulos, P. & Suntres, Z. E (2011). Protective effects of liposomal N-acetylcysteine against paraquat-induced cytotoxicity and gene expression. *J Toxicol*, Vol. 2011, Article ID 808967 (14 pages), ISSN 1687-8205.

Montenegro, L., Panico, A.M. & Bonina, F. (1996). Quantitative determination of hydrophobic compound entrapment in DPPC liposomes by DSC. *Int J Pharm*, Vol. 138, No. 2, (July 1996), pp.191-197, ISSN 0378-5173.

Morawska, L., Hofmann, W., Hitchins-Loveday, J., Swanson, C. & Mengersen, K. (2005). Experimental study of the deposition of combustion aerosols in the human respiratory tract. *J Aerosol Sci*, Vol. 36, No. 8, (August 2005), pp. 939–957, ISSN 0021-8502.

Muhlfeld, C., Gehr, P. & Rothen-Rutishauser, B. (2008). Translocation and cellular entering mechanisms of nanoparticles in the respiratory tract. *Swiss Med Wkly*, Vol. 138, No. 27-28, (July 2008), pp. 387–391, ISSN 1424-7860.

Muhlfeld, C., Rothen-Rutishauser, B., Blank, F., Vanhecke, D., Ochs, M. & Gehr, P. (2008). Interactions of nanoparticles with pulmonary structures and cellular responses. *Am J Physiol Lung Cell Mol Physiol*, Vol. 294, No. 5, (May 2008), pp. 817–829, ISSN 1040-0605.

Neumiller, J.J. & Campbell, R.K. (2010). Technosphere insulin: an inhaled prandial insulin product. *BioDrugs*, Vol. 24, No. 3, (June 2010), pp. 165–172, ISSN 1173-8804.

Nguyen, J., Reul, R., Betz, T., Dayyoub, E., Schmehl, T., Gessler, T., Bakowsky, U., Seeger, W. & Kissel, T. (2009). Nanocomposites of lung surfactant and biodegradable cationic nanoparticles improve transfection efficiency to lung cells. *J Control Release*, Vol. 140, No. 1, (November 2009), pp. 47-54, ISSN 0168-3659.

Nimje, N., Agarwal, A., Saraogi, G.K., Lariya, N., Rai, G., Agrawal, H. & Agrawai, G.P. (2009). Mannosylated nanoparticulate carriers of rifabutin for alveolar targeting. *J Drug Target*, Vol. 17, No. 10, (December 2009), pp. 777–787, ISSN 1061-186X.

Oakley, R.H., Jewell, C.M., Yudt, M.R., Bofetiado, D.M. & Cidlowski, J.A. (1999). The dominant negative activity of the human glucocorticoid receptor beta isoform. Specificity and mechanisms of action. *J Biol Chem*, Vol. 274, No. 3, (Septmber 1999), pp. 27857–27866, ISSN 0021-9258.

Oberdörster, G. (2007). Biokinetics and effects of nanoparticles, In: *Nanotechnology – Toxicological Issues and environmental safety*, P.P. Simeonova, N. Opopol, M.I. Luster, pp. 15–51, Springer, ISBN 978-1-4020-6074-8, Netherlands.

Oberdorster, G., Oberdorster, E. & Oberdorster, J. (2005). Nanotoxicology: an emerging discipline evolving from studies of ultrafine particles. *Environ Health Persp*, Vol. 113, No. 7, (July 2005), pp. 823–839, ISSN 0091-6765.

Oberdorster, G., Stone, V. & Donaldson K. (2007). Toxicology of nanoparticles: a historical perspective. *Nanotoxicology*, Vol. 1, No. 1, (January 2007), pp. 2–25, ISSN 1743-5390.

Okusanya, O.O., Bhavnani, S.M., Hammel, J., Minic, P., Dupont, L.J., Forrest, A., Mulder, G.J, Mackinson, C., Ambrose, P.G., Gupta, R. (2009). Pharmacokinetic and pharmacodynamic evaluation of liposomal amikacin for inhalation in cystic fibrosis patients with chronic pseudomonal infection. *Antimicrob Agents Chemother*, Vol. 53, No. 9, (September 2009), pp. 3847–3854, ISSN 0066-4804.

Palange, P., Testa, U., Huertas, A., Calabro`, L., Antonucci, R. & Petrucci, E. (2006). Circulating haemopoietic and endothelial progenitor cells are decreased in COPD. *Eur Respir J.* Vol. 27, No. 3 (March 2006), pp. 529–541, ISSN 0903-1936.

Palko, H.A., Fung, J.Y. & Louie, A.Y. (2010). Positron emission tomography: a novel technique for investigating the biodistribution and transport of nanoparticles. *Inhal Toxicol,* Vol. 22, No. 8, (July 2010), pp. 657–688, ISSN 0895-8378.

Paolino, D., Cosco, D., Muzzalupo, R., Trapasso, E., Picci, N. & Fresta, M. (2008). Innovative bolasurfactant niosomes as topical delivery systems of 5-fluorouracil for the treatment of skin cancer. *Int J Pharm,* Vol. 353, No. 1-2, (April 2008), pp. 233–242, ISSN 0378-5173.

Paolino, D., Muzzalupo, R., Ricciardi, A., Celia, C., Picci, N. & Fresta, M. (2007). In vitro and in vivo evaluation of Bola-surfactant containing niosomes for transdermal delivery. *Biomed. Microdevices,* Vol. 9, No. 4 (August 2007), pp. 421–433, ISSN 1387-2176.

Parkes, W.R. (1994). Morphology of the respiratory tract, In: *Occupational lung disorders,* Butterworth-Heinemann, pp. 1-17, Butterworth-Heinemann Medical, ISBN 075061403X, Oxford, UK.

Patton, J.S. & Byron, P.R. (2007). Inhaling medicines: delivering drugs to the body through the lungs. *Nat Rev Drug Discov,* Vol. 6, No. 1, (January 2007), pp. 67 – 74, ISSN 1474-1776.

Perez-Gil, J. (2008). Structure of pulmonary surfactant membranes and films: the role of proteins and lipid–protein interactions. *BBA,* Vol. 1778, No. 7-8, (July-August 2008), pp. 1676–1695, ISSN 0005-2736.

Quinton, P.M. (2008). Cystic fibrosis: impaired bicarbonate secretion and mucoviscidosis. *Lancet,* Vol. 372, No. 9636 (August 2008), pp. 415–417, ISSN 0140-6736.

Rahman, I & Kilty, I. (2006). Antioxidant therapeutic targets in COPD. *Curr Drug Targets,* Vol. 7, No. 6 (June 2006), pp. 707–720, ISSN 1389-4501.

Rahman, I., Skwarska, E. & MacNee, W. (1997). Attenuation of oxidant/antioxidant imbalance during treatment of exacerbations of chronic obstructive pulmonary disease. *Thorax,* Vol. 52, No. 6, (June 1997), pp. 565–568, ISSN 1468-3296.

Randell, S.H. & Boucher, R.C. (2006). Effective mucus clearance is essential for respiratory health. *Am J Respir Cell Mol Biol,* Vol. 35, No. 1, (July 2006), pp. 20–28, ISSN 1044-1549.

Remels, A.H., Gosker, H.R., van der Velden, J., Langen, R.C. & Schols, A.M. (2007). Systemic inflammation and skeletal muscle dysfunction in chronic obstructive pulmonary disease: State of the art and novel insights in regulation of muscle plasticity. *Clin Chest Med,* Vol. 28, No. 3, (September 2007), pp. 537-552, ISSN 0272-5231.

Robinson, M., Eberl, S., Tomlinson, C., Daviskas, E., Regnis, J.A., Bailey, D.L., Torzillo, P.J., Menache, M. & Bye, P.T. (2000). Regional mucociliary clearance in patients with cystic fibrosis. *J. Aerosol Med.,* Vol. 13, No. 2, (June 2000), pp. 73–86, ISSN 0894-2684.

Rogers, D.F. & Barnes, P.J. (2006). Treatment of airway mucus hypersecretion. *Ann Med,* Vol. 38, No. 2, (January 2006), pp.116–125, ISSN 0785-3890.

Rogers, D.F. (2007). Physiology of airway mucus secretion and pathophysiology of hypersecretion. *Respir Care*, Vol. 52, No. 9, (September 2007), pp. 1134–1146, ISSN 0020-1324.

Rossiter, A., Howard, C.P., Amin, N., Costello, D.J. & Boss A.H. (2010). Technosphere® Insulin: Safety in Type 2 Diabetes Mellitus. *ADA Scientific Sessions*, Orlando Florida, June 2010.

Santucci, E., Carafa, M., Coviello, T., Murtas, E., Riccieri, F.M., Alhaique, F., Modesti, A. & Modica, A. (1996). Vesicles from polysorbate 20 and cholesterol. A simple preparation and a characterization. *STP Pharma Sci*, Vol. 6, No. 1, (January 1996), pp. 29–32, ISSN 1157-1489.

Schmid, O., Moller, W., Semmler-Behnke, M., Ferron, G.A., Karg, E., Lipka, J., Schulz, H., Kreyling, W.G. & Stoeger, T. (2009). Dosimetry and toxicology of inhaled ultrafine particles. *Biomarkers*, Vol. 14, No. 1, (July 2009), pp. 67–73, ISSN 1354-750X.

Schmidt, S.R. (2009). Fusion-proteins as biopharmaceuticals–applications and challenges. *Curr Opin Drug Discov Dev*, Vol. 12, No. 2, (March 2009), pp. 284–295, ISSN 1367-6733.

Shao, M.X., Nakanaga, T. & Nadel, J.A. (2004). Cigarette smoke induces MUC5AC mucin overproduction via tumor necrosis factor-alpha-converting enzyme in human airway epithelial (NCI-H292) cells. *Am J Physiol Lung Cell Mol Physiol*, Vol. 287, No. 2, (August 2004), pp. 420–427, ISSN 1040-0605.

Sin, D.D. & Man, S.F. (2003). Why are patients with chronic obstructive pulmonary disease at increased risk of cardiovascular diseases? The potential role of systemic inflammation in chronic obstructive pulmonary disease. *Circulation*, Vol. 107, No. 6, (June 2003), pp. 1514-1519, ISSN 0009-7322.

Stamenkovic, I. (2003). Extracellular matrix remodelling: the role of matrix metalloproteinases. *J Pathol*, Vol. 200, No. 4, (July 2003), pp. 448–464, ISSN 1096-9896.

Sung, J.C., Pulliam, B.L. & Edwards, D.A. (2007). Nanoparticles for drug delivery to the lungs. *Trends Biotechnol*, Vol. 25, No. 12, (December 2007), pp. 563–570, ISSN 0167-7799.

Tetley,T.D. (2002). Macrophages and the pathogenesis of COPD. *Chest*, Vol. 121, No. 1, (January 2002), pp. 156S–159S, ISSN 0012-3692.

Tsapis, N., Bennett, D., Jackson, B., Weitz, D.A. & Edwards, D.A. (2002). Trojan particles: large porous carriers of nanoparticles for drug delivery. *Proc Natl Acad Sci*, Vol. 99, No. 19, (September 2002), pp. 12001–12005, ISSN 0027-8424.

Unfried, K., Albrecht, C., Klotz, L.O., Von Mikecz, A., Grether-Beck, S., Schins, R.P.F. (2007). Cellular responses to nanoparticles: target structures and mechanisms. *Nanotoxicology*, Vol. 1, No. 1, (January 2007), pp. 51-71, ISSN 1743-5390.

Van der Schans, C.P. (2007). Bronchial mucus transport. *Respir Care*, Vol. 52, No. 9, (September 2007), pp. 1150–1156, ISSN 0020-1324.

van der Velden, V. & Hulsmann, A.R. (1999). Peptidases: structure, function and modulation of peptide-mediated effects in the human lung. *Clin Exp Allergy*, Vol. 29, No. 4, (April 1999), pp. 445–456, ISSN 1365-2222.

Verdugo, P. (1990). Goblet cells secretion and mucogenesis. *Ann Rev Physiol*, Vol. 52 (March 1990), pp.157–176, ISSN 0066-4278.

Veronese, F.M. & Pasut, G. (2005). PEGylation, successful approach to drug delivery. *Drug Discov Today*, Vol. 10, No. 21, (November 2005), pp. 1451–1458, ISSN 1359-6446.

Walvoord E.C., de la PAZ, Park, S., Silverman, B., Cuttler,L., Rose, S.R. (2009). Inhaled growth hormone (GH) compared with subcutaneous GH in children with GH deficiency: pharmacokinetics, pharmacodynamics, and safety. *J Clin Endocrinol Metab*, Vol. 94, No. 6, (March 2009), pp. 2052–2059, ISSN 0021-972X.

Wedzicha, J.A. & Donaldson, G.C. (2003). Exacerbations of chronic obstructive pulmonary disease. *Respir Care*, Vol. 48, No. 12, (December 2003), pp. 1204–1213, ISSN 0020-1324.

Weers, J., Metzheiser, B., Taylor, G., Warren, S., Meers, P. & Perkins, W.R. (2009). A gamma scintigraphy study to investigate lung deposition and clearance of inhaled amikacin-loaded liposomes in healthy male volunteers. *J Aerosol Med Pulm Drug Deliv*, Vol. 22, No. 2, (June 2009), pp. 131–138, ISSN 1941-2711.

Wouters, E.F. (2002). Systemic effects in COPD. *Chest*, Vol.121, No. 1, (January 2002), pp. 127S-130S, ISSN 0012-3692.

Xia, T., Li, N. & Nel, A.E. (2009). Potential health impact of nanoparticles. *Annu Rev Public Health*, Vol. 30, (April 2009), pp. 137–150, ISSN 0163-7525.

Yang W., Peters, J.I. & Williams, R.O. (2008). Inhaled nanoparticles – a current review. *Int. J. Pharm*, Vol. 356, No. 1-2, (May 2008), pp. 239–247, ISSN 0378-5173.

Yuan, X., Naguib, S., Yuan, X., Naguib, S. & Wu, Z (2011). Recent advances of siRNA delivery by nanoparticles. *Expert Opin Drug Deliv*, Vol. 8, No. 4, (April 2001), pp. 521-536, ISSN 1742-5247.

Zhang, J., Wu, L., Chan, H. & Watanabe, W. (2011). Formation, characterization, and fate of inhaled drug nanoparticles. *Adv Drug Deliv Rev*, Vol. 63, No.6, (May 2011), pp. 441–455, ISSN 0169-409X.

5

Types of Physical Exercise Training for COPD Patients

R. Martín-Valero, A. I. Cuesta-Vargas and M. T. Labajos-Manzanares

School of Nursing, Physiotherapy, Podiatry and Occupational Therapy
Psyquiatry and Physiotherapy Department
Málaga University
Spain

1. Introduction

Pulmonary diseases are increasingly important causes of morbidity and mortality in the modern world (Ries et al., 2007). Chronic obstructive pulmonary disease (COPD) is the most common chronic lung disease, and a major cause of lung-related death and disability (Fishman, 2008). COPD is characterized by chronic airflow limitation, progressive and largely irreversible, associated with an abnormal inflammatory reaction (Ancochea Bermúdez et al., 2009). COPD is very disabling and features extra-pulmonary manifestations, but it can be prevented and treated.

The disease is diagnosed by a clinical history based on the combination of history, physical examination and confirmation of the presence of airflow obstruction with the use of spirometry (Figure 1 Spirometry). Spirometric assessment is performed according to the guidelines of the American Thoracic Society (ATS) (Laszlo, 2006). The technician asks the subjects three exhaling exercises and the best is used for the analysis (Miller et al., 2005). If the Tiffenau rate (value of FEV_1/FVC) is less than seventy percent, COPD exists (Global initiative for chronic obstructive lung disease *[GOLD]*, 2010). Smoking is the major risk factor for the disease (Hilberink et al. 2011).

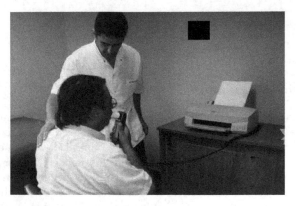

Fig. 1. Spirometry

The most common symptoms of COPD are breathlessness, chronic cough, wheezing, sputum production, recurrent respiratory infection may be associated with some of the following systematic effects such as undernourishment, weight loss, exercise limitation and muscle weakness (*GOLD, 2010*). Knowledge regarding the disturbance of muscle function that occurs in patients with COPD is continuously increasing. Initially muscular dysfunction was considered to be a self-limiting disease resulting from inactivity and lack of exercise. However, recent studies have shown that in addition to this factor, peripheral muscles such as the quadriceps seem to have some type of myopathy (Couillard & Prefaut, 2005). Although the presence of myopathy is still being debated, there is some evidence pointing to myopathy associated with oxidative stress (Rabinovich et al., 2001). Recent studies in COPD have highlighted the role of the ubiquitine proteasome system in the breakdown of skeletal muscle protein in COPD patients. Malfunction of the mitochondria has also recently been identified in these patients (Rabinovich & Vilaro, 2010).

COPD is a major cause of disability and mortality worldwide and the prevalence increases with age. COPD will increase by more than thirty percent in the next ten years, if the population does not cut down smoking (Ancochea Bermúdez et al., 2009). Actually, due to high prevalence, associated to high morbidity, economic and social cost COPD is a major health problem (Ramsey & Sullivan, 2003; Sullivan, Ramsey, & Lee, 2000). COPD is not curable, but treatments can help to control symptoms and improve quality of life of patients. It is necessary to reduce risk factors such as smoking and physical inactivity (*GOLD, 2010*).

Many people suffer from COPD for years and die prematurely of it or its complications. The goals of the Global Initiative for Chronic Obstructive Lung Disease (GOLD) (Rabe et al., 2007) are to improve prevention and management of COPD through a concerted worldwide effort of people involved in all facets of health care and health care policy, and to encourage an expanded level of research interest in this highly prevalent disease. The GOLD report separates COPD patients into the four different stages (figure 2) (*GOLD, 2010*).

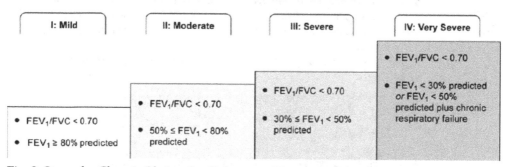

Fig. 2. Stages for Chronic Obstructive Pulmonary Disease

Pulmonary rehabilitation has emerged as a recommended standard of care for patients with chronic lung disease based on a growing body of scientific evidence. The American Thoracic Society and European Respiratory Society (ATS /ERS) published a document in 2006 defining respiratory rehabilitation as "a multidisciplinary and comprehensive intervention has proved effective from the perspective of evidence-based medicine for patients with chronic respiratory diseases who are symptomatic and often have decreased daily life activities. Integrated into individualized treatment of the patient, pulmonary rehabilitation is designed to reduce symptoms, optimize functional status, increase participation, and reduce health-care costs by stabilizing or reversing systemic manifestations of the disease" (Nici et al., 2006). This definition focuses on three aspects of successful rehabilitation: a multidisciplinary approach; an individualized program; tailored to the patient´s needs; and attention to physical psychological and social functioning (Ries, 2008). Not forgetting a primary goal of rehabilitation interventions for people with COPD is to optimize function (Nici et al., 2006).

The components of multidisciplinary respiratory rehabilitation programs include education of patients and their families, chest physiotherapy, muscle training, the emotional support, nutritional support, occupational therapy (Ries et al., 2007). Physiotherapy consists of various phases of treatment (exercise training, peripheral and respiratory muscle training, and breathing exercises) that are considered cornerstones of the physiotherapeutic intervention (Langer et al., 2009). Also consider patients that are incorporated into a respiratory rehabilitation program must have an optimal pharmacological treatment, although not analyzed in this chapter.

There is no consensus of opinion regarding the optimal duration of the pulmonary rehabilitation intervention (Ries et al., 2007). The duration depends on changes in the patient´s lifestyle. A number of external factors also influence program duration including health-care systems and reimbursement policies, access to programs, level of functional disability, health-care provider referral patterns, and the ability of individual patients to make progress toward treatment goals.

Few clinical trials have focused on the impact of program duration on rehabilitation outcomes, but existing data suggest that gains in exercise tolerance may be greater following longer programs (Berry et al., 2003; Foy, Rejeski, Berry, Zaccaro, & Woodard, 2001; Green, Singh, Williams, & Morgan, 2001; Troosters, Gosselink, & Decramer, 2000). Besides Verrill et al. (2005) demonstrated that patients achieved significant gains in exercise tolerance in the six minute walk distance, after twelve weeks of pulmonary rehabilitation. However, in an older trial Wijkstra et al. (1995) showed that there was no difference noted between groups in the magnitude of gains in the six minute walk distance for patients who underwent 18 months and three months of home-based rehabilitation.

Moreover, although some studies suggest that the duration of the pulmonary rehabilitation program has an impact on exercise tolerance improvement, it is not clear that other outcomes such as health status or dyspnea are similarly affected by program duration (Ries et al., 2007). Thus, given the variations found in types of rehabilitation programs and content as on duration (Clini et al., 2001). Besides the differences found in clinical study design, patient populations, health systems in different countries, program location, and program content.

The purpose of this literature review is to compare the effectiveness of various exercises training programmes in the rehabilitation of COPD patients. This study analyzes the different types of aerobic exercises that are carried out with different intensities, doses and frequencies.

2. Exploratory testing

The chronic symptoms of COPD (cough, expectoration, wheezing, dyspnea and exercise tolerance) are the major factors responsible for altering the relationship between health and quality of life. Studies of health-related quality of life (HRQoL) in patients with COPD with varying degrees of severity have consistently shown that patients have significant decrements in HRQoL (Okubadejo, Jones, & Wedzicha, 1996; Schrier, Dekker, Kaptein, & Dijkman, 1990). Therefore, HRQoL is an important clinical outcome in COPD. The Chronic Respiratory Disease Questionnaire (CRQ) (Guyatt, Berman, Townsend, Pugsley, & Chambers, 1987) and St George's Respirtory Questionnaire (SGRQ) (Jones, Quirk, Baveystock, & Littlejohns, 1992; Jones, 2001) are the main questionnaires used to measure the quality of life in COPD patients.

The evidence-based clinical practice guidelines document concluded that there was a strong level of type A evidence, that Pulmonary Rehabilitation Programmes (PRP) improve the symptom of dyspnea in patients with COPD with a strong level of type A evidence (Jones, 2002). Dyspnea is a sensation of respiratory discomfort and the evaluation of the degree of dyspnea provides an independent dimension that is not provided by pulmonary function tests or by measuring dyspnea in an exercise laboratory. So, dyspnea is a main symptom associated with exercise performance and, therefore, quality of life. One of the major goals of COPD treatment is a reduction in dyspnea. The severity of the disease can be determined by the intensity of dyspnea (Camargo & Pereira, 2010). The severity of COPD is habitually classified by forced expiratory volume in the first second (FEV_1) after bronchodilator use (Rabe et al., 2007). Various instruments are available to measure the degree of dyspnea during exercise; the modified Medical Research Council (mMRC) dyspnea scale is the most used (Barbera et al., 2001). The mMRC has five levels that increase with the level of activity in which dyspnea appears. It assesses common tasks the patient can develop without displaying dyspnea. Levels of Dyspnea are graded as follows. Grade 0: "I only get breathless with strenuous exercise"; grade 1: "I get short of breath when hurrying or walking up a slight hill"; grade 2: "I walk slower than people of the same age because of breathlessness or have to stop for breath when walking at my own pace"; grade 3: "I stop for breath after walking 100 yards or after a few minutes"; grade 4: "I am too breathless to leave the house".

The mMRC was unidimensional, to overcome this limitation; Mahler (Mahler, Mejia-Alfaro, Ward, & Baird, 2001) designed the index known as the Baseline Dyspnea Index (BDT), which was later supplemented with the Transitional Dyspnea Index (TDI). BDT analyzes dyspnea from a triple perspective; the difficulty of the task, magnitude of effort and functional impairment, each of the sections will be assessed from 0 (severe) to 4 (none), so total amount can range between 0 and 12 (Mahler, 2006). TDI assessed changes over time compared to baseline (BDI), the changes in each of the three sections are measured between -3 and +3. Therefore, the total score can be between +9 and -9. A score of 0 indicates no changes have occurred, while -9 is very negative result (Sobradillo et al., 1999). Both multidimensional scales, BDT and TDI, are clinical instruments that can be used during cardiopulmonary exercise testing for clinical and research purposes. Besides, Borg et al., (Borg, Borg, Larsson, Letzter, & Sundblad, 2010) described the matching of the increase in dyspnea related to ventilation and oxygen consumption in exercise.

In a review of application of dyspnea and quality of life scales in COPD, it was concluded that a unidimensional scale can be used if applied in conjunction with specific quality of life scales. Alternatively, a multidimensional scale, which correlates better with quality of life, can be used (Bausewein, Farquhar, Booth, Gysels, & Higginson, 2007). Consequently, multidimensional clinical instruments were developed in order to provide a more comprehensive assessment of the severity of dyspnea, combined with the Chronic Respiratory Disease Questionnaire (CRQ) incorporates five physical activities that are specific for individual patients (Guyatt et al., 1987). These instruments have been shown to be valid, reliable, and responsive (Reda, Kotz, Kocks, Wesseling, & van Schayck, 2010).

In 2004, Celli et al. created a mortality prediction index, known as the BODE index. It encompassed the body mass index (B), the degree of airflow obstruction as expressed by the FEV_1 (O), dyspnea with the modified medical research council (D), and exercise (E) measured with six-minute walk distance (Table 1 Variables and point value used for the computation of BODE index) data adapted from Celli et al. (2004). The cut-off values for the assignment of points are shown for each variable. *The FEV_1 categories were identified by the American Thoracic Society (1995).† Scored on the modified Medical Research Council (mMRC) dyspnea scale can range from 0 to 4, with a score of 4 indicating that the patient is too breathless to leave the house or becomes breathless when dressing or undressing.

BODE index

Variables	Points on BODE index			
	0	1	2	3
FEV_1% of predicted *	≥ 65	50–64	36–49	≤ 35
Six-minute walk distance (m)	≥ 350	250–349	150–249	≤ 149
MRC dyspnea score †	0–1	2	3	4
Body mass index (kg/m²)	>21	≤ 21		

Table 1. Variables and point value used for the computation of BODE index, adapted from Celli et al. (2004)

The BODE index is a multidimensional classification system that systemically determines the degree of mortality in individuals with COPD, that provides useful prognostic information in patients with COPD and might be able to measure health status. However, it is unknown whether the BODE index is a sensitive tool for predicting the impact of quality of life in such patients. Araujo (Araujo & Holanda, 2010) found correlations between the BODE index scores and all of the CRQ domains in COPD patients. Moreover, there are studies where patients who moved from moderate to high physical activity improved their SGRQ scores by 18.4 and their CRQ scores by 14.8 (Esteban et al., 2010).

Over recent decades, several organizations have championed pulmonary rehabilitation and developed comprehensive statements, practice guidelines, and evidence-based guidelines (Ries, 2008), however there are differences about how assessment of severity of disease. The 2010 NICE Guidelines defended that multidimensional assessment tool (BODE index) is a better predictor of mortality and exacerbation rate than FEV_1 alone (Gruffydd-Jones & Loveridge, 2011).

Exercise testing is frequently used in the clinical evaluation of patients with COPD to evaluate the functional impact of a treatment (American Thoracic Society & American College of Chest Physicians, 2003). Exercise testing is a useful evaluative tool, allowing standardized measurement of exertional dispnea and exercise tolerance (GOLD, 2010). There is, however, no consensus regarding which exercise testing protocol should be used for this application (Pepin, Saey, Whittom, LeBlanc, & Maltais, 2005). A research indicated that walking, as performed in the endurance shuttle walk, is sensitive to detect changes in exercise performance after bronchodilation (Pepin et al., 2005). Besides Pepin et al. (2007)

indicate that the response of the 6MWT test is not sensitive to change and may not be appropriate for an assessment tool. Another research also suggests that the endurance shuttle walk is more responsive to the effects of pulmonary rehabilitation than the 6MWT for detecting changes in exercise performance following broncholdilations (Eaton, Young, Nicol, & Kolbe, 2006). Together, these findings provide growing support for the use of the endurance shuttle walk as an evaluative tool to monitor response to treatment to COPD.

The six minute walk test (6MWT) is used in order to determine the six-minute walk distance (6MWD), which correlates with the performance of activities of daily living in patients with COPD (ATS Committee on Proficiency Standards for Clinical Pulmonary Function Laboratories, 2002; Brooks, Solway, & Gibbons, 2003). The 6MWT measures the global and integrated responses of all organ systems involved during exercise, has been shown to be an important parameter related to morbility and mortality in COPD (Casanova et al., 2007), and is also part of the BODE index (Celli et al., 2004). Although rehabilitation improves both exercise tolerance and quality of life in COPD, it is not known whether these improvements are related to each other. Several trials show the weak correlation between quality of life and the six minute walking distance in patients with COPD suggests that these parameters measure different aspects of health (Wijkstra et al., 1995).

Recently, the use of accelerometer has been incorporated as an objective measure to assess physical activity level of the patient performs daily (Troosters et al., 2010). It is necessary to analyze physical activity in daily life in patients across different disease stages according to GOLD. Other studies have shown that grip strength in the wrist is a strong independent predictor of mortality in COPD (Cortopassi, Divo, Pinto-Plata, & Celli, 2011). A significant relationship was found between hand grip strength and peripheral muscle strength (flexion of elbow and knee) and strong relationship ($r = - 0.75$, $p < 0.0001$) with the force respiratory muscles (maximum inspiratory muscles, inspiratory capacity, forced vital capacity and maximum volume ventilation).

There is no clinical trial review that has found a connection between rehabilitation respiratory programs and an increase in exercise tolerance. It is necessary to clarify the change in quality of life was related with a change in exercise tolerance in COPD patients. The difference between current studies and previous controlled studies (Sinclair, 1980; Vale, Reardon, & ZuWallack, 1993) are the use of the 12 minute walking distance which is probably more sensitive to change than the six minute walking distance (Wijkstra et al., 1995).

COPD is often associated with exacerbation of symptoms. An exacerbation of COPD is defined as "an event in the natural course for the disease characterized by a change in the patient´s baseline dyspnea, cough, and/or sputum that is beyond normal day-to-day variations, is acute in onset, and may warrant a change in regular medication in a patient with underlying COPD" (Burge & Wedzicha, 2003). The most common causes of an exacerbation are infection of the tracheobronchial tree and air pollution (White, Gompertz, & Stockley, 2003). Studies investigating effects on pulmonary function and oxigenation did not show benefits in either acute exacerbations of COPD (Newton & Bevans, 1978) or in chronic COPD (May & Munt, 1979). Assessment of the severity of an exacerbation is based on the patient´s medical history before the exacerbation, pre-existing comorbidities, symptoms, physical examination, arterial blood gas measurements, and other laboratory test. Physicians should obtain the results of previous evaluations, where possible, to compare with the current clinical data. Specific information is required on the frequency and severity of attacks of breathlessness and cough, sputum volume and color, and limitation of daily activities (Vilaró et al., 2007).

Other targets of rehabilitation are anxiety control, dyspnea reduction and improvement of the health-related quality of life (Lacasse et al., 2006). The illness evolution can be associated with extra-pulmonary components, such as muscle loss is related with reduction of physical activity. After exacerbation, symptoms of depression have been identified as an independent factor of mortality risk (Yohannes, Baldwin, & Connolly, 2005), as well as risk a factor for rehabilitation program drop-outs (Garrod, Marshall, Barley, & Jones, 2006). The skeletal muscle dysfunction and depressive symptoms are potencially amenable to rehabilitation with exercise training (Rodrigues, 2010). We have made the following figure 3 in order to collect intra-pulmonary components (airways obstruction and dyspnea) with extra-pulmonary factors (muscle wasting, reduce mobility, exercise limitation, depression and sedentary lifestyle).

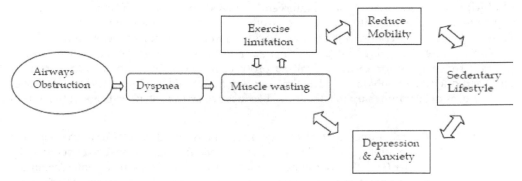

Fig. 3. Relation between intra-pulmonary components with extra-pulmonary factors.

3. Types of exercises

Physical activity is defined as any bodily movement produced by skeletal muscles that results in energy expenditure beyond resting energy expenditure (Thompson et al., 2003). Information on the importance of physical activity in COPD has grown, especially in the last few years, although major questions remain to be answered. The present chapter aims to provide an update on the most important studies of physical activity in COPD (Esteban, 2009).

Findings from meta-analysis of pulmonary rehabilitation strongly supports that exercise training as part of treatment of patients with COPD should last at least four weeks (Lacasse, Goldstein, Lasserson, & Martin, 2006). Exercise training should be available to people with COPD, because it improves breathlessness, quality of life, exercise tolerance and functional ability (Lacasse et al., 2006). Physical therapists are crucial to the delivery of rehabilitation because of their training in exercise and movement therapies (Garrod & Lasserson, 2007).

The primary goal of the rehabilitation programs is to restore the patient to the highest possible level of independent function (Ries et al., 2007). This goal is accomplished by helping patients become more physically active, and to learn more about their disease, treatment options, and how to cope. Within the program of rehabilitation, the physiotherapeutic intervention is responsible for various treatment phases (specifically physical exercise training, peripheral and respiratory muscle training, and breathing exercises) (Langer et al., 2009).

Aerobic exercise is the main non-pharmacological treatment better tolerated by patients with COPD (Martín-Valero, Cuesta-Vargas, & Labajos-Manzanares, 2010). Exercise training is one of the key components of pulmonary rehabilitation. The exercise prescription for the training program is guided by the following three parameters: intensity; frequency; and duration.

The standarized criterions on intervention period, dose, intensity of physical exercises in COPD patients is needed. Seven (Coppoolse et al., 1999; Kurabayashi et al., 2000; O'Shea, Taylor, & Paratz, 2004; Puente-Maestu, Sanz, Sanz, Cubillo et al., 2000; Puente-Maestu, Sanz, Sanz, Ruiz de Ona et al., 2000; Wadell, Sundelin, Henriksson-Larsen, & Lundgren, 2004; Wijkstra et al., 1995) agreed with the criteria of the American College of Sports Medicine (ACSM) (Garber et al., 2011) for the intervention period and number of sessions varied from eight weeks in the majority on trials to twelve weeks in two trials and from two to four sessions a weeks. Therefore, the number sessions a week were at least between two or four sessions a week. Only one trial (Wijkstra et al., 1995) took into account, that patients had to practise twice a day for an individualised protocol, for 0 to 5 hours the first three months and then once a day only for 0-5. The time of sessions is variable in these seven articles with a minimum of 20 minutes up to 60 minutes because two articles do not talk about the time of sessions.

According to the recommendations of the American Association of Cardiovascular and Pulmonary Rehabilitation (AACVPR), *high-intensity training targets* have been operationally defined to be at least 60 to 80% of the peak work rate achieved in an incremental maximum exercise test. The intensity of the training sessions in five articles (Coppoolse et al., 1999; Puente-Maestu, Sanz, Sanz, Cubillo et al., 2000; Puente-Maestu, Sanz, Sanz, Ruiz de Ona et al., 2000; Wadell, Sundelin, Henriksson-Larsen, & Lundgren, 2004; Wijkstra et al., 1995) showed that the goal is 60-90% of heart rate maximum (HR_{max}) set by the ACSM for improving aerobic fitness ("American college of sports medicine position stand. exercise and physical activity for older adults,"1998a; "American college of sports medicine position stand. The recommended quantity and quality of exercise for developing and maintaining cardiorespiratory and muscular fitness, and flexibility in healthy adults,"1998b)

Exercise training intervention can be adapted to the individual exercise limitations of the patient (Troosters, Gosselink, Langer, & Decramer, 2007). Troosters et al. review focused on different training types (endurance, interval and resistance training) (Troosters et al., 2007). In this chapter regarding types of exercise training intervention, it has been divided into aerobic and resistance training types. Aerobic exercise training for older people should have a target intensity of 50-85% of the oxygen uptake reserve – a range that includes both moderate exercise (minimum of 30 minute five days a week) or vigorous exercise (20 minutes three days each week)(Garber et al., 2011).

Resistance training is an ideal intervention for patients with peripheral muscle weakness and pronounced symptoms of dyspnea during exercise (O´Shea, Taylor, & Paratz, 2004).

There is not consensus on the optimal method of resistance training (callisthenics, resistance weight training, isometrics or isokinetic-type training) in patients with COPD. Each type produces strength gains highly specific to the type of training. There are no studies that compared different intensities of resistance training in patients with COPD. It is recommended to use (lower limb) resistance training according to ACSM (two or three times a week) ("ACSM", 1998a; "ACSM", 1998b; Garber et al., 2011). Exercises should be performed at 60-80% of the first repetition maximum (RM), resistance exercises should train 8-10 exercises involving the major muscle groups in bouts of 8-15 repetitions at least 30 minutes a day of moderate-intensity activity on two or three non-consecutive days each week (Nelson et al., 2007). Multiple sets of repetitions (2-5 sets) provide greater benefit (Langer et al., 2009). Resistance activities include a progressive-weight training program, done with therabands (wrist or ankle weights) or progressive weight.

Given that muscle weakness is a common problem in this population, progressive resistance exercise represents a beneficial treatment for improvements in muscle strength (O'Shea, Taylor, & Paratz, 2009). Moreover, improvements in muscle strength can be obtained when progressive resistance exercise is conducted alone or in combination with aerobic training, indicating that it can be successfully performed in conjunction with other training types during pulmonary rehabilitation (O'Shea, Taylor, & Paratz, 2009).

Careful consideration is also required when prescribing progressive resistance exercise programs for people with COPD who have comorbid health conditions (O'Shea, Taylor, & Paratz, 2004). Therefore, progresive resitance exercise may not be appropriate for all people with COPD attending pulmonary rehabilitation, and it is recommended that prescription be targeted to the individual (Storer, 2001).

It is essential to educate the patient about the importance of the training program begining with an initial phase: warming up and stretching (Table 2 Session outline). The central part consists in aerobic training (endurance or interval exercise), resistance training and breathing retraining. Finally, the sessions finish with stretching and relaxation exercises.

Initial phase	Central phase	Final phase
*Stretching *Warming up	*Aerobic training (Endurance or Interval) *Resistance training *Breathing retraining	*Stretching *Relaxation exercises

Table 2. Session outline

It is recommended to apply training strategies that enable patients to resume participation in a rehabilitation programme after an acute exacerbation as soon as possible (Puhan, Scharplatz, Troosters, Walters, & Steurer, 2009). Resistance training and interval training are best suited for early reactivation of patients. Moreover, arm exercises in patients with COPD were shown to increase arm muscle force (Epstein et al., 1997) and reduce symptoms of dyspnea and fatigue during arm activities (Bauldoff, Hoffman, Sciurba, & Zullo, 1996).

Patient education is included as an important recommendation in current clinical practice guidelines for COPD (GOLD, 2010; Celli, MacNee, & ATS/ERS Task Force, 2004) Education should be an integral component of pulmonary rehabilitation (Ries et al., 2007). Moreover, education should include information on collaborative self-management and prevention and treatment of exacerbation. So, patient education interventions are necessary to ensure long-term maintenance of treatment effects. Studies with successful results in chronically ill adults both used physical activity self-monitoring (pedometers or diaries) and applied behavioural strategies to increase patient's self efficacy and self-regulatory skills (Conn, Hafdahl, Brown, & Brown, 2008). It is necessary to initiate and maintain physical activity behaviour change during and after supervised physical exercise training programs. Rose et al., (Baraniak & Sheffield, 2011; Rose et al., 2002) evaluated psychosocial interventions to treat anxiety and panic in patients with COPD; however the data indicated that there were no changes in cognitive function. Overall, the educational intervention may have facilitated aspects of program adherence.

3.1 Continuous or incremental aerobic exercise

In this section different types of physical exercise training that can be applied to improve exercise performance in patients with COPD are presented. The authors have compared programmes with constant load training and incremental load training in COPD patients. There is high level evidence that aerobic training is effective for aerobic capacity and there is moderate evidence that interval training is effective for strength, endurance, functionality and psychosocial parameters (Normandin et al., 2002).

Endurance or continuous training

Supervised continuous training is recommended for patients in all stages of the disease who are able to perform continuous training of at least moderate intensity. Training frequency should be three times weekly in the first weeks of the exercise programme (Langer et al., 2009). Patients with severe symptoms of dyspnea during exercise are frequently not capable of performing high-intensity (70 to 80% of the peak work rate) continuous type training (Casaburi et al., 1997; Maltais et al., 1997). It seems that moderate intensity continuous training (50 to 60% of the peak work rate or 5-6 out of 10 according to the modified Borg Scale) is minimally required to achieve changes in physical fitness. Improvements in health-related quality of life after training at moderate intensities were comparable with those observed after high intensity training (Puente-Maestu, Sanz, Sanz, Cubillo et al., 2000).

Lower extremity exercise training at higher exercise intensity produces greater physiologic benefits than lower intensity training in patients with COPD. Moreover, both low-intensity and high-intensity exercise training produce clinical benefits for patients with COPD (Ries, 2008).

Two categories of tasks can be found during everyday activities, endurance and strength tasks. Endurance tasks require repetitive actions over an extended period of time (walking, cycling and swimming) as shown in figure 4. While strength tasks require explosive performance over short time periods (jumping, lifting weights, sprinting)(Ries et al., 2007). The addition of a strength-training component to a program of pulmonary rehabilitation increases muscle strength and muscle mass (Ries, 2008).

Interval training

Interval training is recommended as an alternative to continuous training in patients with severe symptoms of dyspnea due to the fact that they are unable to sustain continuous

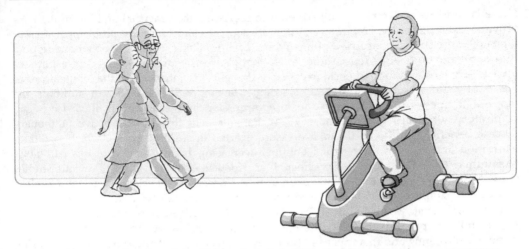

Fig. 4. Endurance tasks taken from "Manual de Rehabilitación Respiratoria para personas con EPOC".

training at the recommended intensities. Short high intensity (at least 70-80% of peak work rate) exercise bouts of 30-180 seconds are necessary during interval training. Recommended frequency of training is the same as with continuous training (Langer et al., 2009).

Only one article (Puente-Maestu, Sanz, Sanz, Cubillo et al., 2000) showed that patients responded to supervised training with incremented loads also changed their ventilatory pattern to deeper, slower breathing. Therefore, improved ventilation this type of incremental training also tended to be more efficient with an average decrease in dead space. Perhaps, the quality of life questionnaires are not sensitive tools to detect changes in the functional variables of disease progression. The changes produced by aerobic physical training in COPD do not have clinical relevance, but they are a success because it slows down disease progression.

Most patients with severe COPD are not able to sustain a continuous exercise protocol. For these patients, interval exercise represents an alternative because it offers the same benefit as high-intensity exercise. Besides, incremental exercise is better tolerated, as expressed by fewer breaks during the rehabilitation program and better adherence to exercise protocols (Puhan MA et al., 2006). Therapeutic intervention can be done in or out of water; the next section explains the therapeutic aquatic exercise intervention.

3.2 Therapeutic aquatic exercise intervention

This intervention is known for its power of prevention and treatment in different conditions, although not considered part of standard pulmonary rehabilitation. Therapeutic aquatic exercise intervention is a discipline that includes hydrotherapy, spa therapy, balneotherapy and physiotherapy, and is used for the prevention and treatment of diseases through water (Geytenbeek, 2008). Hydrotherapy is defined as a complementary therapy that uses the temperature and pressure of water as a therapeutic agent at a given temperature (Geytenbeek, 2002).

There is controversy in the scientific literature regarding the beneficial and harmful effects of water exercise for the respiratory system in people with respiratory problems. Different types of exercises can be carried out: walking, cycling, lifting weights in a swimming pool (figure 5), and so on. Previous studies show that hydrostatic pressure exerts on inspiratory muscle strength and limited chest expansion; this effect is enhanced as the temperature of the pool water decreases (Frontera, Herring, Micheli, & Silver, 2008). In addition, the diaphragm moves during diving due to compression by the abdomen, thus decreasing respiratory vital capacity (Greenleaf, 1984). Patients with chronic obstructive pulmonary disease benefit from the hydrostatic pressure exerted during immersion, which facilitates expiration and reduces the residual volume, decreasing the air trapped in this pathology (Asanuma, 1999; Dahlback, 1975; Schoenhofer, Koehler, & Polkey, 2004). Previous studies show that water exerts hydrostatic pressure on inspiratory muscle strength and limited chest expansion, this effect is enhanced with decreasing the temperature of the pool water (Agostoni, Gurtner, Torri, & Rahn, 1966). Therapeutic aquatic exercise intervention is known for its ability to prevent and treat different conditions. This intervention is a specialized field of physical training and therapy, used to achieve certain physical and functional goals using the properties of water (Geytenbeek, 2008).

The reviewed articles covered incremental therapeutic aquatic exercise with an intensity ranging from 50% to 90% of maximal oxygen consumption (VO_{2max}) with sessions of 30 to 50 minutes 2 to 5 days a week, for a total of 8 to 24 weeks at a temperature of 29 °C to 38 °C (Kurabayashi et al., 2000; Wadell, Sundelin, Henriksson-Larsen, Lundgren, 2004). COPD patients walked in water to the level of their shoulders, and they breathed out slowly through their mouth into water after sinking their nose 3-5 cm below the water level. The patients` eyes were not under the water. After exercise, patients dressed and rested on a chair in a comfortable room (25°C) for 30 minutes. Two studies showed clinical changes in the questionnaire of quality of life for respiratory patients. People who performed incremental exercise in the water showed functional changes in the distance walked in the walking test, in forced vital capacity and forced expiratory volume (Kurabayashi et al., 2000; Wadell, Sundelin, Henriksson-Larsen, & Lundgren, 2004). The aquatic intervention group that performed incremental exercise had improved health-related quality of life, compared to a control group without intervention (Wadell, Sundelin, Henriksson-Larsen, & Lundgren, 2004).

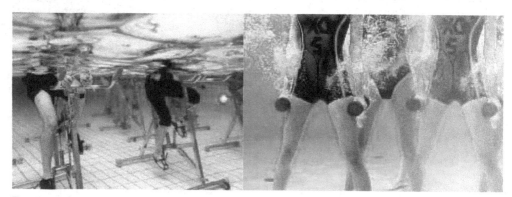

Fig. 5. Cycling and lifting weights

Physical therapy for COPD requires a certain duration and frequency in order to improve clinical parameters. Wadell et al. (2005a) indicated that training once a week (high intensity/low frequency) was not sufficient to sustain the improvements in physical capacity and quality of life achieved after a period of 3 months of high frequency aquatic exercise training with three sessions of 45 minutes each a week (high intensity/high frequency). However, high intensity physical training once a week for 6 months seemed to be enough to avoid deterioration compared to baseline. According to Kurabayashi's study, 6 consecutive days of exercise a week would be preferable to 3 alternative days of exercise a week, even if the cumulative exercise period was the same (Kurabayashi et al., 1998). The studies reviewed showed much heterogeneity with respect to the duration of treatment, ranging from 6 to 24 weeks. However, the typical duration of treatment was 8 to 12 weeks. Further studies should direct more attention to the specific duration, frequency and accuracy of aerobic intensity thresholds. Other authors found that exercise in water tends to provide even greater benefits than similar exercise training on land (Wadell, Sundelin, Henriksson-Larsen, & Lundgren, 2004).

Breathing exercises during immersion in water at 38 °C could be recommended as physical therapy after diagnosis of COPD. Elevation of the sub-peritoneal diaphragmatic pressure by the hydraulic pressure could help raise the diaphragm and assist in the evacuation of air during exhalation, resulting in a decrease in dead space. In addition, hydraulic pressure was reported to increase cardiac output, resulting in an improvement in blood gas exchange in lung capillaries. Besides these effects, inhalation of gas containing thermal hydrogen sulfate lowers the viscosity of sputum (Asanuma, Fujita, Ide, & Agishi, 1971). Only three studies (Kurabayashi et al., 2000; Kurabayashi et al., 1998; Perk, Perk, & Bodén, 1996) included breathing exercises during therapeutic aquatic exercise intervention.

3.3 Respiratory muscle training

In general, patients with COPD have weak inspiratory muscles (Polkey et al., 1996). This weakness may contribute to dyspnea and exercise limitation in patients with significant COPD. When evaluating the strength of respiratory muscles we should be aware that we are focusing primarily on the ability of these muscles to generate tension during a forced inspiratory or expiratory maneuver. The result of the maneuver can be measured with the mouth (Figure 6 Equipment to maneuver), and it is measured in centimeters H_2O. This primarily reflects a set of variables such as muscle mass (ability to generate force) and length-tension relationship.

The role of inspiratory muscle training (IMT) for individuals with stable COPD is unclear (Geddes, O'Brien, Reid, Brooks, & Crowe, 2008). The first systematic review on IMT found little evidence to support the use of IMT (Shoemaker, Donker, & Lapoe, 2009). The Amercian Thoracic Society/European Respiratory Society standards (Celli, MacNee et al., 2004) nor the Canadian Thoracic Society Recommendations for the Management of COPD (O'Donnell et al., 2008) recommend the incorporation of IMT into management plan. The Global Initiative for Chronic Obstructive Lung Disease (GOLD, 2010) states that "respiratory muscle training is beneficial, especially when combined with general exercise training" based on non-randomized trials and observational studies.

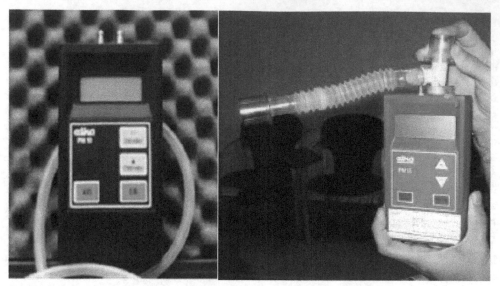

Fig. 6. Equipment to maneuver

In an attempt to reduce the severity of breathlessness and to improve exercise tolerance, IMT has been applied in many COPD patients (Weiner, Magadle, Beckerman, Weiner, & Berar-Yanay, 2003). Several different respiratory muscle training devices are available, ranging from sophisticated computerized systems to simple hand-held resistive devices. In addition, the relative benefits of strength versus endurance training, inspiratory versus expiratory training and effect in patients of differing severity are unknown (Garrod & Lasserson, 2007)

Types of intervention: Sham, low- and high-intensity IMT

There are studies comparing the effect of different types of intervention (Geddes, Reid, Crowe, O'Brien, & Brooks, 2005). In order to standardize studies that showed sham IMT and low intensity IMT at similar percentages of maximum inspiratory pression (PImax). Bégin et al., (Begin & Grassino, 1991) measured these loads using the tidal inspiratory pressure (PI) of individuals with COPD. Sham IMT was defined as that using the same type of device as the intervention group at an intensity less than or equal to the mean plus one standard deviation (SD). Since PI is directly proportional to the partial pressure of carbon dioxide in the arterial blood (PCO_2) of patients with COPD (Begin & Grassino, 1991), sham IMT for normocapneic individuals was defined as intensity p8.3 cm H_2O (mean PI +1 SD) and for individuals with moderate hypercapnia, as intensity p11.5 cm H_2O (Geddes et al., 2005).

Using IMT in combination with other interventions and using flow-dependent resistive training is important in the pulmonary rehabilitation program (Geddes et al., 2008). However, there are no established thresholds for what constitutes a clinically meaningful change in inspiratory muscle strength or endurance, other methods must be utilized to infer clinical benefit (Shoemaker et al., 2009). Geddes et al. (2005) recommended using IMT at least a total of 30 minutes daily but can be spread over more than one session a day. Training should occur at least 5 days a week. While gains may be measurable after as short as 5 weeks, IMT should become part of the individual´s exercise program. The minimal training intensity necessary could start as low as 22% PImax and be progressed to as high as 60% PImax using a targeted inspiratory resistive or threshold trainer (Geddes et al., 2005). Therefore, IMT significantly increased inspiratory muscle strength and inspiratory muscle endurance (Lotters, van Tol, Kwakkel, & Gosselink, 2002). In addition, research review found a clinically significant decrease in dyspnea sensation at rest and during exercise is observed after IMT (Lotters et al., 2002).

In conclusion, IMT improves inspiratory muscle strength and endurance, functional exercise capacity, dyspnea and quality of life. Inspiratory muscle endurance training was shown to be less effective than respiratory muscle strength training. In patients with inspiratory muscle weakness, the addition of IMT to a general exercise training program improved PImax and tended to improve exercise performance (Gosselink et al., 2011).

Furthermore, maximal inspiratory pressure is a volitional test and therefore open to criticism (Polkey & Moxham, 2004). Futher research is needed to explore the impact that different training protocols (frequency, intensity and duration of IMT, supervision) may have on outcomes and to determine the extent to which changes in outcomes associated with IMT translate into clinically important improvement for adults with COPD (Geddes et al., 2008).

4. Implications

In the research reviewed, there are strong arguments that pulmonary rehabilitation is beneficial for improving the quality of life related to health at the beginning of the program. Furthermore pulmonary rehabilitation reduces symptoms and increases participation in everyday activities. However, it is necessary to do more randomized controlled trials to clarify which components of the lung rehabilitation are essential. Future studies to discover the ideal length of treatment, the necessary degree of supervision, training intensity and how long the treatment effect persists.

Without no doubt, it is necessary to individualize programs for this population taking into account their different levels of severity. The prescription should begin at low intensity and short duration, for both parameters gradually increasing to the threshold of fatigue.

In summary, incremental aerobic resistance physical exercises are better than constant load physical exercises at an intensity range from 90% to 50 % of $VO_{2\,max}$, with a frequency of two or four days a week, the session is from 30 to 60 minutes during a period of treatment from eight to twelve weeks. Exercise training induces several symptomatic and functional adaptations resulting in an increased aerobic capacity, although clinical relevance is not collected in the study population. Maybe, for further studies we should take intrinsic patient factor (severity of COPD) into account over a longer period of time and how extrinsic factors of the exercises affect disease progression. Moreover, it is important to determine whether these physiological benefits of COPD patients who have performed an incremental aerobic resistance physical exercises program supervised justify the increased costs. Therefore, a cost/effectiveness analysis is necessary to determining whether the type of intervention program is supervised or not.

It is essential to investigate physical activity in daily life in patients with COPD in accordance to the GOLD stages. Pulmonary rehabilitation programs should incorporate the use of an accelerometer, the values of respiratory muscle strength and peripheral muscle strength (hand grip, knee- extension); also more sensitive tools for detecting changes in exercise tolerance should be included.

5. References

Agostoni, E., Gurtner, G., Torri, G., & Rahn, H. (1966). Respiratory mechanics during submersion and negative-pressure breathing. *Journal of Applied Physiology, 21*(1), 251-258.

American college of sports medicine position stand exercise and physical activity for older adults. (1998a). *Medicine and Science in Sports and Exercise, 30*(6), 992-1008.

American college of sports medicine position stand. The recommended quantity and quality of exercise for developing and maintaining cardiorespiratory and muscular fitness, and flexibility in healthy adults.(1998b). *Medicine and Science in Sports and Exercise, 30*(6), 975-991.

American Thoracic Society, & American College of Chest Physicians. (2003). ATS/ACCP statement on cardiopulmonary exercise testing. *American Journal of Respiratory and Critical Care Medicine, 167*(2), 211-277. doi:10.1164/rccm.167.2.211

Ancochea Bermúdez J, et al. (2009). *Estrategia en EPOC del sistema nacional de salud* Retrieved 2011, from
http://www.msc.es/organizacion/sns/planCalidadSNS/docs/EstrategiaEPOCS NS.pdf

Araujo, Z. T., & Holanda, G. (2010). Does the BODE index correlate with quality of life in patients with COPD? *Jornal Brasileiro De Pneumologia: Publicacao Oficial Da Sociedade Brasileira De Pneumologia e Tisilogia, 36*(4), 447-452.

Asanuma Y, Fujita S, Ide H, & Agishi Y. (1971). Improvement of respiratory resistane by hot water immersing exercise in adult asthmatic patient. *Clinical Rehabilitation, 1*, 211-217.

Asanuma Y. (1999). Influence of water immersion on lung volumes and pulmonary diffusing capacity. A comparison of healthy subjects and patients with chronic obstructive pulmonary disease. *Japanese Journal of Clinical Physiology, 29*(3), 187-192.

ATS Committee on Proficiency Standards for Clinical Pulmonary Function Laboratories. (2002). ATS statement: Guidelines for the six-minute walk test. *American Journal of Respiratory and Critical Care Medicine, 166*(1), 111-117.

Baraniak, A., & Sheffield, D. (2011). The efficacy of psychological based interventions to improve anxiety, depression and quality of life in COPD: A systematic review and meta-analysis. *Patient Education and Counseling, 83*(1), 29-36. doi:10.1016/ j.pec.2010.04.010

Barbera, J. A., Peces-Barba, G., Agustí, A. G., Izquierdo, J. L., Monsó, E., Montemayor, T., et al. (2001). Guía clínica para el diagnóstico y el tratamiento de la enfermedad pulmonar obstructiva crónica. *Archivos Bronconeumología, 37*(6), 297-316.

Bauldoff, G. S., Hoffman, L. A., Sciurba, F., & Zullo, T. G. (1996). Home-based, upper-arm exercise training for patients with chronic obstructive pulmonary disease. *Heart & Lung : The Journal of Critical Care, 25*(4), 288-294.

Bausewein, C., Farquhar, M., Booth, S., Gysels, M., & Higginson, I. J. (2007). Measurement of breathlessness in advanced disease: A systematic review. *Respiratory Medicine, 101*(3), 399-410. doi:10.1016/j.rmed.2006.07.003

Begin, P., & Grassino, A. (1991). Inspiratory muscle dysfunction and chronic hypercapnia in chronic obstructive pulmonary disease. *The American Review of Respiratory Disease*, 143(5 Pt 1), 905-912.

Berry, M. J., Rejeski, W. J., Adair, N. E., Ettinger, W. H.,Jr, Zaccaro, D. J., & Sevick, M. A. (2003). A randomized, controlled trial comparing long-term and short-term exercise in patients with chronic obstructive pulmonary disease. *Journal of Cardiopulmonary Rehabilitation*, 23(1), 60-68.

Borg, E., Borg, G., Larsson, K., Letzter, M., & Sundblad, B. M. (2010). An index for breathlessness and leg fatigue. *Scandinavian Journal of Medicine & Science in Sports*, 20(4), 644-650. doi:10.1111/j.1600-0838.2009.00985.x

Brooks, D., Solway, S., & Gibbons, W. J. (2003). ATS statement on six-minute walk test. *American Journal of Respiratory and Critical Care Medicine*, 167(9), 1287.

Burge, S., & Wedzicha, J. A. (2003). COPD exacerbations: Definitions and classifications. *The European Respiratory Journal.Supplement*, 41, 46s-53s.

Camargo, L. A., & Pereira, C. A. (2010). Dyspnea in COPD: Beyond the modified medical research council scale. *Jornal Brasileiro De Pneumologia: Publicacao Oficial Da Sociedade Brasileira De Pneumologia e Tisilogia*, 36(5), 571-578.

Casaburi, R., Porszasz, J., Burns, M. R., Carithers, E. R., Chang, R. S., & Cooper, C. B. (1997). Physiologic benefits of exercise training in rehabilitation of patients with severe chronic obstructive pulmonary disease. *American Journal of Respiratory and Critical Care Medicine*, 155(5), 1541-1551.

Casanova, C., Cote, C. G., Marin, J. M., de Torres, J. P., Aguirre-Jaime, A., Mendez, R., et al. (2007). The 6-min walking distance: Long-term follow up in patients with COPD. *The European Respiratory Journal: Official Journal of the European Society for Clinical Respiratory Physiology*, 29(3), 535-540. doi:10.1183/09031936.00071506

Celli, B. R., Cote, C. G., Marin, J. M., Casanova, C., Montes de Oca, M., Mendez, R. A., et al. (2004). the body-mass index, airflow obstruction, dyspnea, and exercise capacity index in chronic obstructive pulmonary disease. *The New England Journal of Medicine*, 350(10), 1005-1012. doi:10.1056/NEJMoa021322

Celli, B. R., MacNee, W., & ATS/ERS Task Force. (2004). Standards for the diagnosis and treatment of patients with COPD: A summary of the ATS/ERS position paper. *The European Respiratory Journal : Official Journal of the European Society for Clinical Respiratory Physiology*, 23(6), 932-946.

Clini, E., Foglio, K., Bianchi, L., Porta, R., Vitacca, M., & Ambrosino, N. (2001). In-hospital short-term training program for patients with chronic airway obstruction. *Chest*, 120(5), 1500-1505.

Conn, V. S., Hafdahl, A. R., Brown, S. A., & Brown, L. M. (2008). Meta-analysis of patient education interventions to increase physical activity among chronically ill adults. *Patient Education and Counseling*, 70(2), 157-172. doi:10.1016/j.pec.2007.10.004

Coppoolse, R., Schols, A. M., Baarends, E. M., Mostert, R., Akkermans, M. A., Janssen, P. P., et al. (1999). Interval versus continuous training in patients with severe COPD: A randomized clinical trial. *The European Respiratory Journal : Official Journal of the European Society for Clinical Respiratory Physiology*, 14(2), 258-263.

Cortopassi, F., Divo, M., Pinto-Plata, V., & Celli, B. (2011). Resting handgrip force and impaired cardiac function at rest and during exercise in COPD patients. *Respiratory Medicine, In Press, Corrected Proof* doi:DOI: 10.1016/j.rmed.2010.12.011

Couillard A, & Prefaut C. (2005). From muscle disuse to myopathy in COPD: Potencial contribution of oxidative stress. *European Respiratory journal*, 26(4), 703-719.

Dahlback, G. O. (1975). Influence of intrathoracic blood pooling on pulmonary air-trapping during immersion. *Undersea Biomedical Research*, 2(2), 133-140.

Eaton, T., Young, P., Nicol, K., & Kolbe, J. (2006). The endurance shuttle walking test: A responsive measure in pulmonary rehabilitation for COPD patients. *Chronic Respiratory Disease*, 3(1), 3-9.

Epstein, S. K., Celli, B. R., Martinez, F. J., Couser, J. I., Roa, J., Pollock, M., et al. (1997). Arm training reduces the VO2 and VE cost of unsupported arm exercise and elevation in chronic obstructive pulmonary disease. *Journal of Cardiopulmonary Rehabilitation*, 17(3), 171-177.

Esteban, C. (2009). Role of physical activity in chronic obstructive pulmonary disease. [Impacto de la actividad física en la EPOC] *Archivos de Bronconeumología*, 45 Suppl 5, 7-13. doi:10.1016/S0300-2896(09)72949-7

Esteban, C., Quintana, J. M., Aburto, M., Moraza, J., Egurrola, M., Perez-Izquierdo, J., et al. (2010). Impact of changes in physical activity on health-related quality of life among patients with COPD. *The European Respiratory Journal : Official Journal of the European Society for Clinical Respiratory Physiology*, 36(2), 292-300. doi:10.1183/09031936.00021409

Fishman, A. P. (2008). *Pulmonary diseases and disorders* (4th ed.). New York: McGraw-Hill.

Foy, C. G., Rejeski, W. J., Berry, M. J., Zaccaro, D., & Woodard, C. M. (2001). Gender moderates the effects of exercise therapy on health-related quality of life among COPD patients. *Chest*, 119(1), 70-76.

Frontera W.R., Herring S.A., Micheli L.J., & Silver J.K. (2008). *Medicina deportiva clínica: tratamiento médico y rehabilitación* Elsevier.

Garber, C. E., Blissmer, B., Deschenes, M. R., Franklin, B. A., Lamonte, M. J., Lee, I. M., et al. (2011). Quantity and quality of exercise for developing and maintaining cardiorespiratory, musculoskeletal, and neuromotor fitness in apparently healthy adults: Guidance for prescribing exercise. *Medicine and Science in Sports and Exercise*, 43(7), 1334-1359. doi:10.1249/MSS.0b013e318213fefb

Garrod, R., Marshall, J., Barley, E., & Jones, P. W. (2006). Predictors of success and failure in pulmonary rehabilitation. *The European Respiratory Journal : Official Journal of the European Society for Clinical Respiratory Physiology*, 27(4), 788-794. doi:10.1183/09031936.06.00130605

Garrod, R., & Lasserson, T. (2007). Role of physiotherapy in the management of chronic lung diseases: An overview of systematic reviews. *Respiratory Medicine*, 101(12), 2429-2436. doi:10.1016/j.rmed.2007.06.007

Geddes, E. L., Reid, W. D., Crowe, J., O'Brien, K., & Brooks, D. (2005). Inspiratory muscle training in adults with chronic obstructive pulmonary disease: A systematic review. *Respiratory Medicine*, 99(11), 1440-1458. doi:10.1016/j.rmed.2005.03.006

Geddes, E. L., O'Brien, K., Reid, W. D., Brooks, D., & Crowe, J. (2008). Inspiratory muscle training in adults with chronic obstructive pulmonary disease: An update of a systematic review. *Respiratory Medicine*, 102(12), 1715-1729. doi:10.1016/j.rmed.2008.07.005

Geytenbeek, J. (2002). Evidence for effective hydrotherapy. *Physiotherapy*, 88(9), 514-529. doi:DOI: 10.1016/S0031-9406(05)60134-4

Geytenbeek J. (2008). *Aquatic physiotherapy evidence-based practice guide*. Retrieved from http://www.npz-nrz.nl/downloads/files/Plenair%20Marijke%20HopmanRock2.pdf *Global iniciative for chronic obstructive lung disease (GOLD)*. (2010). Retrieved Marzo/23, 2011, from http://www.goldcopd.com

Gosselink, R., De Vos, J., van den Heuvel, S. P., Segers, J., Decramer, M., & Kwakkel, G. (2011). Impact of inspiratory muscle training in patients with COPD: What is the evidence? *The European Respiratory Journal : Official Journal of the European Society for Clinical Respiratory Physiology, 37*(2), 416-425. doi:10.1183/09031936.00031810

Green, R. H., Singh, S. J., Williams, J., & Morgan, M. D. (2001). A randomised controlled trial of four weeks versus seven weeks of pulmonary rehabilitation in chronic obstructive pulmonary disease. *Thorax, 56*(2), 143-145.

Greenleaf J E. (1984). Physiological responses to prolonged bed rest and fluid immersion in humans. *Journal of Applied Physiology, 57*(3), 619-633.

Gruffydd-Jones, K., & Loveridge, C. (2011). The 2010 NICE COPD guidelines: How do they compare with the GOLD guidelines? *Primary Care Respiratory Journal: Journal of the General Practice Airways Group, 20*(2), 199-204. doi:10.4104/pcrj.2011.00011

Guyatt, G. H., Berman, L. B., Townsend, M., Pugsley, S. O., & Chambers, L. W. (1987). A measure of quality of life for clinical trials in chronic lung disease. *Thorax, 42*(10), 773-778.

Hilberink, S. R., Jacobs, J. E., van Opstal, S., van der Weijden, T., Keegstra, J., Kempers, P. L., et al. (2011). Validation of smoking cessation self-reported by patients with chronic obstructive pulmonary disease. *International Journal of General Medicine, 4*, 85-90. doi:10.2147/IJGM.S15231

Jones, P. W., Quirk, F. H., Baveystock, C. M., & Littlejohns, P. (1992). A self-complete measure of health status for chronic airflow limitation. the st. george's respiratory questionnaire. *The American Review of Respiratory Disease, 145*(6), 1321-1327.

Jones, P. W. (2001). Health status measurement in chronic obstructive pulmonary disease. *Thorax, 56*(11), 880-887.

Jones PW. (2002). Interpreting thresholds for a clinically significant change in health status in asthma and COPD. *Eur Respir j., 19*, 398-404. doi:10.1183/09031936.02.00063702

Kurabayashi H, Machida I, Tamura K, Iwai F, Tamura J, & Kubota K. (2000). Breathing out into water during subtotal immersion: A therapy for chronic pulmonary emphysema. *American Journal of Physical Medicine & Rehabilitation, 79*, 150-153.

Kurabayashi, H., Machida, I., Hnda H., Akiba, T., Kubota, K., et al. (1998). Comparison of three protocols for breathing exercises during immersion in 38°C water for chronic obstructive pulmonary disease. *American Journal of Physical Medicine & Rehabilitation, 77*(2), 145-147.

Lacasse, Y., Goldstein, R., Lasserson, T. J., & Martin, S. (2006). Pulmonary rehabilitation for chronic obstructive pulmonary disease. *Cochrane Database of Systematic Reviews (Online), (4)*(4), CD003793. doi:10.1002/14651858.CD003793.pub2

Langer, D., Hendriks, E., Burtin, C., Probst, V., van der Schans, C., Paterson, W., et al. (2009). A clinical practice guideline for physiotherapists treating patients with chronic obstructive pulmonary disease based on a systematic review of available evidence. *Clinical Rehabilitation, 23*(5), 445-462. doi:10.1177/0269215509103507

Laszlo, G. (2006). Standardisation of lung function testing: Helpful guidance from the ATS/ERS task force. *Thorax, 61*(9), 744-746. doi:10.1136/thx.2006.061648

Lotters, F., van Tol, B., Kwakkel, G., & Gosselink, R. (2002). Effects of controlled inspiratory muscle training in patients with COPD: A meta-analysis. *The European Respiratory Journal: Official Journal of the European Society for Clinical Respiratory Physiology, 20*(3), 570-576.

Mahler, D. A., Mejia-Alfaro, R., Ward, J., & Baird, J. C. (2001). Continuous measurement of breathlessness during exercise: Validity, reliability, and responsiveness. *Journal of Applied Physiology (Bethesda, Md.: 1985), 90*(6), 2188-2196.

Mahler, D. A. (2006). Mechanisms and measurement of dyspnea in chronic obstructive pulmonary disease. *Proceedings of the American Thoracic Society, 3*(3), 234-238. doi:10.1513/pats.200509-103SF

Manual para la rehabilitación respiratoria para personas con EPOC. Retrieved from Manual_de_Rehabilitacion_Respiratoria_para_personas_con_EPOC.pdf

Maltais, F., LeBlanc, P., Jobin, J., Berube, C., Bruneau, J., Carrier, L., et al. (1997). Intensity of training and physiologic adaptation in patients with chronic obstructive pulmonary disease. *American Journal of Respiratory and Critical Care Medicine, 155*(2), 555-561.

Martín-Valero R, Cuesta-Vargas AI, & Labajos-Manzanares MT. (2010). Revisión de ensayos clínicos sobre rehabilitación respiratoria en enfermos pulmonares obstructivos crónicos. *Rehabilitación, 44*(2), 158-66.

May, D. B., & Munt, P. W. (1979). Physiologic effects of chest percussion and postural drainage in patients with stable chronic bronchitis. *Chest, 75*(1), 29-32.

National Clinical Guideline Centre. (2010) Chronic obstructive pulmonary disease: management of chronic obstructive pulmonary disease in adults in primary and secondary care. London: National Clinical Guideline Centre. Available from: http://guidance.nice.org.uk/CG101/Guidance/pdf/English

Miller, M. R., Hankinson, J., Brusasco, V., Burgos, F., Casaburi, R., Coates, A., et al. (2005). Standardisation of spirometry. *The European Respiratory Journal: Official Journal of the European Society for Clinical Respiratory Physiology, 26*(2), 319-338. doi:10.1183/09031936.05.00034805

Nelson, M. E., Rejeski, W. J., Blair, S. N., Duncan, P. W., Judge, J. O., King, A. C., et al. (2007). Physical activity and public health in older adults: Recommendation from the american college of sports medicine and the american heart association. *Circulation, 116*(9), 1094-1105. doi:10.1161/CIRCULATIONAHA.107.185650

Newton, D. A., & Bevans, H. G. (1978). Physiotherapy and intermittent positive-pressure ventilation of chronic bronchitis. *British Medical Journal, 2*(6151), 1525-1528.

Nici, L., Donner, C., Wouters, E., Zuwallack, R., Ambrosino, N., Bourbeau, J., et al. (2006). American thoracic Society/European respiratory society statement on pulmonary rehabilitation. *American Journal of Respiratory and Critical Care Medicine, 173*(12), 1390-1413. doi:10.1164/rccm.200508-1211ST

Normandin, E. A., McCusker, C., Connors, M., Vale, F., Gerardi, D., & ZuWallack, R. L. (2002). An evaluation of two approaches to exercise conditioning in pulmonary rehabilitation. *Chest, 121*(4), 1085-1091.

O'Donnell, D. E., Hernandez, P., Kaplan, A., Aaron, S., Bourbeau, J., Marciniuk, D., et al. (2008). Canadian thoracic society recommendations for management of chronic obstructive pulmonary disease - 2008 update - highlights for primary care. *Canadian Respiratory Journal : Journal of the Canadian Thoracic Society, 15 Suppl A*, 1A-8A.

Okubadejo, A. A., Jones, P. W., & Wedzicha, J. A. (1996). Quality of life in patients with chronic obstructive pulmonary disease and severe hypoxaemia. *Thorax, 51*(1), 44-47.

O'Shea, S. D., Taylor, N. F., & Paratz, J. (2004). Peripheral muscle strength training in COPD: A systematic review. *Chest, 126*(3), 903-914. doi:10.1378/chest.126.3.903

O'Shea, S. D., Taylor, N. F., & Paratz, J. (2009). Progressive resistance exercise improves muscle strength and may improve elements of performance of daily activities for people with COPD: A systematic review. *Chest*, 136, 1269-1283. Doi 10.1378/chest.09-0029

Pepin, V., Saey, D., Whittom, F., LeBlanc, P., & Maltais, F. (2005). Walking versus cycling: Sensitivity to bronchodilation in chronic obstructive pulmonary disease. *American Journal of Respiratory and Critical Care Medicine, 172*(12), 1517-1522. doi:10.1164/rccm.200507-1037OC

Pepin, V., Brodeur, J., Lacasse, Y., Milot, J., Leblanc, P., Whittom, F., et al. (2007). Six-minute walking versus shuttle walking: Responsiveness to bronchodilation in chronic obstructive pulmonary disease. *Thorax, 62*(4), 291-298. doi:10.1136/thx.2006.065540

Perk J, Perk L, & Bodén C. (1996). Cardiorespiratory adaptation of COPD patients to physical training on land and in water. *European Respiratory Journal, 9*(2), 248-252.

Polkey, M. I., Kyroussis, D., Hamnegard, C. H., Mills, G. H., Green, M., & Moxham, J. (1996). Diaphragm strength in chronic obstructive pulmonary disease. *American Journal of Respiratory and Critical Care Medicine, 154*(5), 1310-1317.

Polkey, M. I., & Moxham, J. (2004). Improvement in volitional tests of muscle function alone may not be adequate evidence that inspiratory muscle training is effective. *The European Respiratory Journal : Official Journal of the European Society for Clinical Respiratory Physiology, 23*(1), 5-6.

Puente-Maestu, L., Sanz, M. L., Sanz, P., Cubillo, J. M., Mayol, J., & Casaburi, R. (2000). Comparison of effects of supervised versus self-monitored training programmes in patients with chronic obstructive pulmonary disease. *The European Respiratory Journal: Official Journal of the European Society for Clinical Respiratory Physiology, 15*(3), 517-525.

Puente-Maestu, L., Sanz, M. L., Sanz, P., Ruiz de Ona, J. M., Rodriguez-Hermosa, J. L., & Whipp, B. J. (2000). Effects of two types of training on pulmonary and cardiac responses to moderate exercise in patients with COPD. *The European Respiratory Journal: Official Journal of the European Society for Clinical Respiratory Physiology, 15*(6), 1026-1032.

Puhan MA, Büsching G, Chünemann HJ, vanOort E, Zaugg C, & Frey M. (2006). Interval versus continuous high-intensity exercise in chronic obstructive pulmonary disease. A randomized trial. *Annals of Internal Medicine, 145*, 816-825.

Puhan, M., Scharplatz, M., Troosters, T., Walters, E. H., & Steurer, J. (2009). Pulmonary rehabilitation following exacerbations of chronic obstructive pulmonary disease. *Cochrane Database of Systematic Reviews (Online), (1)*(1), CD005305. doi:10.1002/14651858.CD005305.pub2

Rabe, K. F., Hurd, S., Anzueto, A., Barnes, P. J., Buist, S. A., Calverley, P., et al. (2007). Global strategy for the diagnosis, management, and prevention of chronic obstructive pulmonary disease: GOLD executive summary. *American Journal of Respiratory and Critical Care Medicine, 176*(6), 532-555. doi:10.1164/rccm.200703-456SO

Rabinovich, R. A., Ardite, E., Troosters, T., Carbo, N., Alonso, J., Gonzalez de Suso, J. M., et al. (2001). Reduced muscle redox capacity after endurance training in patients with chronic obstructive pulmonary disease. *American Journal of Respiratory and Critical Care Medicine, 164*(7), 1114-1118.

Rabinovich, R. A., & Vilaro, J. (2010). Structural and functional changes of peripheral muscles in chronic obstructive pulmonary disease patients. *Current Opinion in Pulmonary Medicine, 16*(2), 123-133. doi:10.1097/MCP.0b013e328336438d

Ramsey, S. D., & Sullivan, S. D. (2003). The burden of illness and economic evaluation for COPD. *The European Respiratory Journal.Supplement, 41*, 29s-35s.

Reda, A. A., Kotz, D., Kocks, J. W., Wesseling, G., & van Schayck, C. P. (2010). Reliability and validity of the clinical COPD questionniare and chronic respiratory questionnaire. *Respiratory Medicine, 104*(11), 1675-1682. doi:10.1016/j.rmed.2010.04.023

Ries, A. L., Bauldoff, G. S., Carlin, B. W., Casaburi, R., Emery, C. F., Mahler, D. A., et al. (2007). Pulmonary rehabilitation: Joint ACCP/AACVPR evidence-based clinical practice guidelines. *Chest, 131*(5 Suppl), 4S-42S. doi:10.1378/chest.06-2418

Ries, A. L. (2008). Pulmonary rehabilitation: Summary of an evidence-based guideline. *Respiratory Care, 53*(9), 1203-1207.

Rodrigues, F. (2010). Role of extra-pulmonary factors - depression, muscle weakness, health-related quality of life - in COPD evolution. *Revista Portuguesa De Pneumologia, 16*(5), 709-715.

Rose, C., Wallace, L., Dickson, R., Ayres, J., Lehman, R., Searle, Y., et al. (2002). The most effective psychologically-based treatments to reduce anxiety and panic in patients with chronic obstructive pulmonary disease (COPD): A systematic review. *Patient Education and Counseling, 47*(4), 311-318.

Schoenhofer, B., Koehler, D., & Polkey, M. I. (2004). Influence of immersion in water on muscle function and breathing pattern in patients with severe diaphragm weakness. *Chest, 125*(6), 2069-2074.

Schrier, A. C., Dekker, F. W., Kaptein, A. A., & Dijkman, J. H. (1990). Quality of life in elderly patients with chronic nonspecific lung disease seen in family practice. *Chest, 98*(4), 894-899.

Shoemaker, M. J., Donker, S., & Lapoe, A. (2009). Inspiratory muscle training in patients with chronic obstructive pulmonary disease: The state of the evidence. *Cardiopulmonary Physical Therapy Journal, 20*(3), 5-15.

Sinclair DJM, I. C. (1980). Controlled trial of supervised exercise training in chronic bronchitis. *BMJ, 1*, 519-521.

Sobradillo, V., Miravitlles, M., Jiménez, C. A., Gabriel, R., Viejo, J. L., Masa, J. F., et al. (1999). Estudio IBERPOC en españa: Prevalencia de sintomas respiratorios habituales y de limitación crónica al flujo aéreo. *Archivos Bronconeumologia, 35*(4), 159-166.

Storer, T. W. (2001). Exercise in chronic pulmonary disease: Resistance exercise prescription. *Medicine and Science in Sports and Exercise, 33*(7 Suppl), S680-92.

Sullivan, S. D., Ramsey, S. D., & Lee, T. A. (2000). The economic burden of COPD. *Chest, 117*(2 Suppl), 5S-9S.

Thompson, P. D., Buchner, D., Pina, I. L., Balady, G. J., Williams, M. A., Marcus, B. H., et al. (2003). Exercise and physical activity in the prevention and treatment of atherosclerotic cardiovascular disease: A statement from the council on clinical cardiology (subcommittee on exercise, rehabilitation, and prevention) and the council on nutrition, physical activity, and metabolism (subcommittee on physical activity). *Circulation, 107*(24), 3109-3116. doi:10.1161/01.CIR.0000075572.40158.77

Troosters, T., Gosselink, R., & Decramer, M. (2000). Short- and long-term effects of outpatient rehabilitation in patients with chronic obstructive pulmonary disease: A randomized trial. *The American Journal of Medicine, 109*(3), 207-212.

Troosters, T., Gosselink, R., Langer, D., & Decramer, M. (2007). Pulmonary rehabilitation in chronic obstructive pulmonary disease. *Respiratory Medicine: COPD Update, 3*(2), 57-64. doi:DOI: 10.1016/j.rmedu.2007.02.003

Troosters, T., Sciurba, F., Battaglia, S., Langer, D., Valluri, S. R., Martino, L., et al. (2010). Physical inactivity in patients with COPD, a controlled multi-center pilot-study. *Respiratory Medicine, 104*(7), 1005-1011. doi:DOI: 10.1016/j.rmed.2010.01.012

Vale F, Reardon JZ, ZuWallack RL. (1993). The long-term benefits of outpatient pulmonary rehabilitation on exercise tolerance and quality of life. *Chest, 103*, 42-45.

Verrill, D., Barton, C., Beasley, W., & Lippard, W. M. (2005). The effects of short-term and long-term pulmonary rehabilitation on functional capacity, perceived dyspnea, and quality of life. *Chest, 128*(2), 673-683. doi:10.1378/chest.128.2.673

Vilaró, J., Gimeno, E., Sánchez Férez, N., Hernando, C., Díaz, I., Ferrer, M., et al. (2007). Actividades de la vida diaria en pacientes con enfermedad pulmonar obstructiva crónica: Validación d. *Medicina Clínica, 129*(9), 326-332. Retrieved from http://external.doyma.es/pdf/2/2v129n09a13109543pdf001.pdf

Vu, K., & Mitsunobu, F. (2005a). Five year observation of the effects of spa therapy for patients with pulmonary emphysema, evaluated by %low attenuation area (%LAA) of the lungs on high-resolution CT, %Dlco and %residual volume (RV). *Alternative and Complementary Therapies, 11*(2), 89-93.

Vu, K., & Mitsunobu, F. (2005b). Spa therapy for chronic obstructive pulmonary disease. Studies at the Misasa medical center. *Alternative & Complementary Therapies,* (April), 89-93.

Wadell, K., Sundelin, G., Henriksson-Larsen, K., & Rune Lundgren. (2004). High intensity physical group training in water – an effective training modality for patients with COPD. *Respiratory Medicine, 98*, 428-438.

Wadell, K., Henriksson-Larsen, K., Lundgren, R., & Sundelin, G. (2005a). Group training in patients with COPD – long-   term effects after decreased training frequency. *Disability and Rehabilitation, 27*(10), 571-581. doi:10.1080/09638280400018627

Wadell, K., Sundelin, F., Lundgren, R., Henriksson-Larsén, K., & Lindström, B. (2005b). Muscle performance in patients with chronic obstructive pulmonary disease – effects of a physical training programme. *Advances in Physiotherapy, 7*, 51-59.

Weiner P, Magadle R, Beckerman M, Weiner M, & Berar-Yanay N. (2003). Specific expiratory muscle training in COPD. *Chest, 124*(2), 468-473.

White, A. J., Gompertz, S., & Stockley, R. A. (2003). Chronic obstructive pulmonary disease . 6: The aetiology of exacerbations of chronic obstructive pulmonary disease. *Thorax, 58*(1), 73-80.

Wijkstra, P. J., Ten Vergert, E. M., van Altena, R., Otten, V., Kraan, J., Postma, D. S., et al. (1995). Long term benefits of rehabilitation at home on quality of life and exercise tolerance in patients with chronic obstructive pulmonary disease. *Thorax, 50*(8), 824-828.

Yohannes, A. M., Baldwin, R. C., & Connolly, M. J. (2005). Predictors of 1-year mortality in patients discharged from hospital following acute exacerbation of chronic obstructive pulmonary disease. *Age and Ageing, 34*(5), 491-496. doi:10.1093/ageing/afi163

6

Hospital at Home for Elderly Patients with Acute Exacerbation of Chronic Obstructive Pulmonary Disease

Aimonino Ricauda Nicoletta[1], Tibaldi Vittoria[1],
Bertone Paola[1] and Isaia Giovanni Carlo[2]
[1]*Hospital at Home Service, San Giovanni
Battista Hospital of Torino*
[2]*University of Torino, Department of Medical
and Surgical Disciplines – Geriatric Section,
S. Giovanni Battista Hospital
Italy*

1. Introduction

Demographic, epidemiological, social, and cultural trends in European countries are changing the traditional patterns of care. The next decades will see increasing rates of care-dependent older people and non communicable diseases as the leading cause of chronic illness and disability. The break-up of the traditional large family group and urbanization will also lead to gaps in the care of older or disabled family members. These changes in needs and social structure require a different approach to health and social sector policy and services since a disease-oriented approach, alone, is no longer appropriate. An answer to these issues could be home care, a sustainable approach to prevent the need for unnecessary acute or long-term institutionalization and maintain individuals in their home and community as long as possible providing diagnostic, therapeutic and social support (Tarricone & Tsouros, 2008).

Home is a place of emotional and physical associations, memories and comfort. Although many people can be happy in assisted-living facilities, retirement communities or nursing homes – and for many people these are better options – leaving home can be disruptive and depressing for some people. Recent trends in health care favour alternatives to traditional hospital care for patients with acute or chronic diseases. Home care used appropriately decreases hospitalization and nursing home use without compromising medical outcomes. Moreover, patients generally prefer to remain in familiar surroundings. Physician support of home care services honors that preference (Levine et al., 2003).

Chronic Obstructive Pulmonary Disease (COPD) has been the focus of several hospital at home studies, however, most models studied have been early-discharge schemes that employed nursing care, without physician care in the home. There have been fewer studies of substitutive physician-led clinical unit model of hospital at home.

2. Ageing population: Demographics trends

Population ageing is progressing rapidly in many industrialized countries. For the world as a whole, the elderly will grow from 6.9% of the population in 2000 to a projected 19.3% in 2050 (Gavrilov & Heuveline, 2003).

Population ageing is a great challenge for the health care systems. As nations age, the prevalence of disability, frailty, and chronic diseases (Alzheimer's disease, cancer, cardiovascular and cerebrovascular diseases, COPD, etc.) is expected to increase dramatically.

Frailty is gaining attention in many fields because it increases the risk of hospitalization, falls, mortality and institutionalization. Geriatricians, gerontologists, and social scientists study frailty to better understand its impacts on health, individuals, and society. Frailty has been considered synonymous of disability or co-morbidity, but it is recognized that it is a biological syndrome identified by decreased reserves in multiple organ systems. The incidence of frailty increases with age, reaching more than 32% in those older than 90 years (Fried et al., 2001). Frailty can be a primary diagnosis, when the state is not associated directly with a specific disease, or a secondary diagnosis when the syndrome occur as a result of an acute event or the end stage of many chronic conditions, including severe congestive heart failure, stroke, chronic inflammatory diseases and dementia. The hospital, which is the "gold standard" for the delivery of acute medical care, is not an ideal environment for frail elderly patients. A new functional impairment and iatrogenic events such as nosocomial infections, pressure sores, falls and delirium are common during hospital stay.

Chronic obstructive pulmonary disease is a major cause of chronic morbidity and mortality. Patients with COPD usually have progressive airflow obstruction that is not fully reversible, which leads to a history of progressive, worsening breathlessness that can impact on daily activities and health-related quality of life. Winter outbreaks of COPD exacerbations, mostly occurring in elderly people with concurrent chronic co-morbidities, often generate dramatic increases in hospital emergency room admission. Such admissions have increased substantially over the past decade, comprising a significant proportion of all hospital admissions, and are associated with a high rate of readmission contributing to the high costs of care for COPD.

3. Chronic obstructive pulmonary disease: Epidemiological data

Chronic obstructive pulmonary disease is a leading cause of mortality and morbidity worldwide, affecting approximately 210 million people and leading to 3 million deaths annually (WHO, 2011).

The prevalence and morbidity data greatly understimate the total burden of COPD because the disease is usually not diagnosed until it is clinically apparent and moderately advanced. Furthermore, population-based estimates of COPD prevalence by region are problematic since the disease is progressive, measurement tools and definitions still vary among studies, and implementation of spirometry is often not feasible in developing regions (Lopez et al., 2006a).

A recent systematic review and meta-analysis on global burden of COPD reported a prevalence of physiologically defined COPD of 9-10% in adults (Halbert et al., 2006). These data agree with results from the BOLD study, a population-based prevalence study including participants from 12 sites worldwide (n=9425), reporting a prevalence of COPD stage II or higher of 10.1% overall, 11.8% for men and 8.5% for women (Buist et al., 2007).

In England the rate of COPD in the population is estimated at between 2% and 4%, representing between 982.000 and 1.96 million people. The diagnosed prevalence of COPD was 1.5% of the population in 2007/08 according to the Quality Outcome Framework (QOF) statistical bulletin. Approximately 835.000 people in England have been diagnosed with COPD in 2008/09. However, it is currently estimated that over 3 million people have the disease and that an estimated 2 million have undiagnosed COPD, among whom it is considered that 5.5% will have COPD at the mild end of the spectrum (NICE guidelines, update 2010).

Recent available data suggest that a pooled prevalence on spirometric basis is about 9% in European adults, with 4-6% of them suffering from a relevant clinical form of the disease. In Italy, prevalence of COPD is 4.5%, on average.

The reported total prevalence of chronic bronchitis in U.S. adults ranged from a high of 55 (2001) cases per 1.000 to a low of 34 (2007). The prevalence of chronic bronchitis appears to have peaked in 2001, followed by a subsequent decline from 2001 to 2007. In 2008, however, there was an increase in the prevalence (44 case per 1.000) compared to the previous year, and this prevalence was the same in 2009 (data from the U.S. National Health Interview Survey-NHIS, 1999-2009).

The epidemiology of COPD in five major Latin American cities (São Paulo, Santiago, Mexico city, Montevideo and Caracas) has been provided by the PLATINO project , launched in 2002: rates of COPD range from 7.8% in Mexico city to 19.7% in Montevideo, suggesting that COPD is a greater health problem in Latin America than previously realized (Menezes et al., 2005). COPD is emerging as public health problem also in the Middle Est and North Africa countries. In 2001, the prevalence of COPD in Africa was estimated 179/100.000 and 301/100.000 in eastern Mediterranean countries (Lopez et al., 2006b).

Currently, in the European Union COPD and asthma, together with pneumonia, are the third most common cause of death, while in North America COPD represents the fourth leading cause of death. Five year survival from diagnosis is 78% in men and 72% in women with clinically mild disease, but falls to 30% in men and 24% in women with severe disease. (NICE guidelines, update 2010). Due to an aging population, increase in COPD prevalence and mortality are expected in the coming decades. The World Health Organization (WHO) has estimated that COPD will be the third leading cause of death for both males and females worldwide by the year 2030, surpassed only by heart disease and stroke (WHO, 2011).

Burden of COPD can also be measured in disability-adjusted life years (DALYs). Worldwide, COPD is expected to move up from the 12th leading cause of DALYs in 1990 to the 5th leading cause in 2020 (Lopez et al., 2006 b).

In the United States COPD accounts for 15.4 million physician visits, 1.5 million emergency department visits and 636.000 hospitalizations each year (Dalal et al., 2011). In Italy, COPD is the fourth highest cause of hospital admission (130.000 admissions every year). In the UK COPD is the second largest cause of emergency admission and the most common cause for emergency admission to hospital due to respiratory disease. One fifth (21%) of bed days used for respiratory disease treatment are due to COPD, such that COPD accounts for more than one million "bed days" each year in hospitals in the UK (NICE guidelines, update 2010).

The impact of hospitalization for acute exacerbations is significant; mortality during admission is > 10% and mortality during the year after discharge following treatment for acute COPD exacerbation is 25-40% (Escarrabill, 2009).

An acute exacerbation of COPD is not an exceptional or unique event. The Risk Factors of COPD Exacerbation Study (EFRAM) found that 63% of patients were readmitted during the year following an exacerbation (Garcia-Aymerich et al., 2003). Patients with COPD experience exacerbations one to three times a year, with treatment often requiring emergency room care or hospitalization, which contributes substantially to the financial burden of the disease (Dalal et al., 2011).

Various observational studies have found that inpatient care accounts for 50-75% of the direct medical costs of COPD. This cost increases with disease severity: inpatient costs of patients with stage III (severe) disease are double those of patients with stage II (moderate) disease and 6.5 times greater than those of patients with stage I (mild) disease (Dalal et al., 2011).

The indirect cost of COPD are substantial with an impact on annual productivity amounting to an estimated 24 million lost working days per annum. There is little data available to quantify other indirect costs such as carer time and inability to carry out non-occupationally related activity (NICE guidelines, update 2010).

There continues to be high demand for acute care hospital beds for patients with an exacerbation of COPD. Recent reports highlight the fact that although the acute hospital is the standard venue for providing acute medical care, it may be hazardous for older persons, who commonly experience iatrogenic illness, functional decline, and other adverse events. One way to decrease or avoid admissions to hospital is to provide people with acute care treatment at home.

4. Current knowledge on home care for COPD exacerbations

COPD is often associated with exacerbations of symptoms. Exacerbations, particularly that result in admission to hospital, are significant events in the natural history of the disease. They are disruptive and distressing for patients, and account for a significant proportion of the total costs of caring for patients with COPD.

There is no generally agreed definition for an exacerbation of COPD. Definitions currently rely on clinical empiricism with little evidence-based scientific support (Caramori et al., 2009). Most common international guidelines and working groups provide very similar definition of a COPD exacerbation: "*an event in the natural course of the disease characterized by a change in the patient's baseline dyspnea, cough and/or sputum that is beyond normal day-to-day variations, is acute in onset, and may warrant a change in regular medication in a patient with underlying COPD*" (ATS/ERS guidelines, Celli et al., 2004; GOLD, 2009; BTS guidelines, 2007; CTS guidelines, O'Donnel et al., 2008; SEPAR/ALAT joint guidelines, Peces-Barba et al., 2008; Rodriguez-Roisin, 2000).

When an exacerbation of COPD has been diagnosed, to define its severity is essential. Quantification of severity is important in medical management as well as in determing the setting of care (Celli et al., 2004). At present, there is not a validated method for quantifying the severity of exacerbation. Generally, the intensity of the underlying COPD must be considered, as well as comorbidity and a history of previous exacerbations. In addition to these factors, the progression of the symptoms, response to therapy, and availability of adequate home care must be considered in order to decide whether hospitalization is necessary. However, grading of the severity of mild to moderate exacerbations remains contentious since they can be categorised either on clinical presentation (essentially symptoms) or healthcare use resources (Rodriguez-Roisin, 2006).

The most recent position paper of the American Thoracic Society and the European Respiratory Society (ATS/ERS task force) provide a three levels operational classification of severity of COPD exacerbations which allows to identify the best setting of care according to specific elements of clinical evaluation and diagnostic procedures. Level I: patient can be treated at home, Level II: requires hospitalization, Level III: leads to respiratory failure (Celli et al., 2004).

In the National Institute for Clinical Excellence (NICE) guidelines (update 2010), hospital-at-home and assisted-discharge schemes are recommended as a safe and effective alternative to conventional hospitalization (Grade A), particularly for patients with less severe exacerbations. The same authors admit that, currently, there are insufficient data to make firm recommendations about which patients with an exacerbation are most suitable for hospital-at-home or early discharge, and patient selection should depend on the resources available, absence of factors associated with worse prognosis and patient's preference (NICE guidelines, update 2010).

The joint guidelines of the Spanish Society of Pulmonology and Thoracic Surgery (SEPAR) and the Latin American Thoracic Society (ALAT) indicate home hospitalization only for patient without signs of severity such as diminished level of consciouness, abnormal chest radiograph, hypercapnia with acidosis, significant comorbidities, need of ventilatory support (Peces-Barba et al., 2008).

The Global Initiative for Chronic Obstructive Lung Disease (GOLD) guidelines (update 2009) state that "admission of patient with severe COPD exacerbations to intermediate or special respiratory care units may be appropriate if personnel, skills, and equipment exist to identify and manage acute respiratory failure successfully" (GOLD, 2009).

A first feasibility analysis of home-based services to prevent conventional hospitalization of COPD exacerbations was reported in 1999 by Gravil and collegues (Gravil et al., 1998). Subsequent controlled trials confirmed both safety and cost reduction when these types of services were applied to selected COPD patients (Cotton et al., 2000; Davies et al., 2000; Hernandez et al., 2003; Ojoo et al., 2002; Skwarska et al., 2000).

In a review and a meta-analysis including 7 robust RCTs (n=754 patients) Ram and collegues evaluated the overall efficacy of hospital at home schemes, showing that selected patients presenting to hospital emergency departments with acute exacerbation of COPD can be successfully treated at home when supported by visiting respiratory nurses at home. Authors suggested that approximately 25% of the patients with COPD who presented at the emergency department with acute exacerbations would be suitable for home treatment (Ram et al., 2003, 2004).

In conclusion, there is an international consensus on home care for COPD exacerbations, especially for less severe episodes, although data on specific characteristics of patients suitable for this form of care are currently insufficient. In addition, the confusion on definition of "home hospitalization" and "hospital at home" can make difficult to clear up this problem.

Intermediate care is a treatment model which bridges the interface between hospital and community care. A specific subtype of intermediate care is Hospital-at-Home. There is a consensus on defining "Hospital-at-Home" a model of care where "active treatment is provided by healthcare professionals in the patient's home for a condition that otherwise would require hospital care, always for a limited period" (Cochrane Database of Systematic Review, Shepperd et al., 2001). Many disparate models exist with the general nomenclature of "Hospital at Home", "Home hospitalization". These include usual community-based care, outpatient infusion centre, nurse-only outpatient care and the direct clinical unit model of care. These models have distinct features.

Established models for delivering hospital-level care in the home setting exist internationally, including United States, Canada, Israel, Australia, New Zeland, Spain, United Kingdom, Italy, France (Leff et al., 2005; Lemelin et al., 2007; Stessman et al., 1996; Caplan et al., 1999; Montalto, 2002; Richards et al., 2005; Cerrillo –Rodriguez et al., 2009; Pérez-Lopez et al., 2008; Kalra et al., 2008; Wilson et al., 1999; Myles et al., 1996; Aimonino Ricauda et al., 2008).

For patients with exacerbations of COPD, over the last few years there has been considerable interest especially in hospital-based rapid assessment units and early discharge or admission avoidance hospital at home schemes.

Rapid assessment units aim to identify those patients that can be safely be managed at home. These units generally involve a full assessment of the patient in the hospital by a multidisciplinary team and discharge to the community with appropriate support (e.g. nebuliser and compressor or oxygen concentrator, nursing and medical supervision from respiratory specialists, increased social support). Patients remains under the care of the hospital but General Pratictioners are made aware of the fact that their patients are receiving home care.

Early or assisted or supported discharge schemes aim to identify patients in hospital who could be discharge before they have fully recovered by providing increased support in their homes. These schemes involve getting people out of hospital as quickly as possible. In a recent review Shepperd and collegues have demonstrated that mortality and disability for patients recovering from stroke, COPD or surgical interventions are similar in hospital and in early/supported discharge services. Patients may also be more satisfied with their care at home, and at the same time their cares, in most cases, do not report additional burden. However, authors concluded that there is little evidence of cost savings to the health care system (Shepperd et al., 2009a).

The **admission avoidance schemes** provide active treatment by hospital health care professionals (doctors, nurses and other professional figures) in the patient's home, always for a limited time period. The key is that if the hospital at home service was not available, then the patient would need to be admitted to an acute hospital ward. In a systematic review of avoidance of admission through the provision of hospital care at home, 10 randomized trials involving elderly patients with medical condition were included (with a total of 1327 patients). For 5 of these trials individual patient data were obtained for meta-analysis, representing 87% of potentially eligible patients. Authors reported a significantly lower mortality at 6 months for patients who received hospital care at home, greater satisfaction and lower costs (if costs of informal care are excluded). (Shepperd et al., 2008; Shepperd et al., 2009b).

5. The Hospital at Home Service of Torino

In October 1984, with Resolution N. 1134/41/84, the Management Committee of the Local Health Unit 1/23 of Turin set up the 'Experimental Project of Home Hospitalisation'.

In October 1985 a team of doctors and nurses of the Turin Department of Geriatrics started an experiment that was unique in Italy at that time: medical treatment (including examinations and related medical and nursing services) at home rather than in hospital for patients with severe chronic or relapsing illnesses.

The Hospital at Home Service (HHS) is operating in Torino at S. Giovanni Battista Hospital, a large urban University teaching and tertiary-care hospital (Aimonino Ricauda et al., 2004, 2005, 2008; Tibaldi et al., 2004, 2009).

The HHS is a service that provides diagnostic and therapeutic treatments by health care professionals, in the patient's home, of a condition that otherwise would require acute hospital in-patient care. A quick admission to hospital is possible for examinations or interventions that cannot be carried out at home. Transport and acceptance are free for these patients, as part of the HHS service.

The HHS normally operates 12 hours a day (from 8 am to 8 pm), seven day a week. At night our Regional Emergency Unit ("118") can be contacted. For selected patients, medical staff is on-call 24 hours a day. Caregivers are instructed in the emergency plan and encouraged to telephone if problems arise.

The HHS team, equipped with 7 cars, is multidisciplinary and consists of 4 geriatricians, 13 nurses, 1 nurse coordinator, 2 physiotherapists, 1 social worker, 1 counsellor.

The main feature of HHS is that physicians and nurses work together as a team (Figure 1), with daily meeting to discuss the needs of each patient and to organize individualized medical care plans and day-to-day work. The three most important aspects of the nursing activity are:

- home visits to outpatients to give medical care as agreed with the doctors
- daily team meeting
- secretarial work, receiving applications for hospitalization, stocking pharmaceuticals and sanitary material, sending and collecting laboratory analysis, transporting patients for specialistic consultations or exams which can be done only in hospital

The team looks after 25 patients per day and 500 patients per year, on average. The most common diseases treated at home are cardiac, respiratory, cerebrovascular, metabolic and neoplastic diseases.

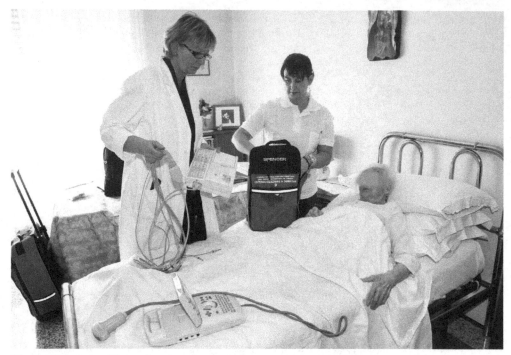

Fig. 1. Hospital at Home Service: doctor and nurse at patient's home

The HHS can be activated by a direct request of the general physician of the patient as an alternative to traditional hospital care, or by a request from hospital wards doctors to allow early and protected discharge from hospital.

Since 2001, a close collaboration has been started between the HHS and the Emergency Department (ED) of San Giovanni Battista Hospital, to propose, where possible, home care as an alternative to the traditional admission to hospital.

Now, approximately 60% of our patients are referred by the ED, 25% by hospital wards and 15% by specialist or general physicians in the community.

The relationship between the ED team and the "HHS mobile team" made up of 1 geriatrician and 1 nurse is very important. By using a multidimensional case sheet, the "HHS mobile team" carries out an assessment of the patient and his caregiver to evaluate the possibility of hospitalization at home and in order to give information on the service.

A "Module of interview with the family" was conceived and implemented to discover the willingness of the family to work together with HHS team, as a part of the patient's healthcare system.

When the availability is established, an "Informative Card" with information on the service has been given to the patient and his caregiver.

Then, the "HHS mobile team" together with the ED doctor writes a rough copy of patient's case sheet, which will be completed at home during the first HHS visit. In the ED all the necessary diagnostic tests (e.g., blood tests, radiography, ECG) are provided and then the patient moves home by ambulance, usually within a few hours.

Entry criteria for home hospitalization are: informed consent of patient and caregiver; stable, diagnosed medical conditions needing hospitalization but not expected to require emergency intervention; appropriate care supervision; telephone connection; living in the hospital catchment area (all the southern part of the city).

Exclusion criteria are: need of intensive monitoring or mechanical ventilation, a monitoring more frequent than every 2 hours of blood pressure or haemogasanalysis, patients with an heart attack or with very low levels of oxygen in the blood or with a serious acidosis or alkalosis or with a suspect of pulmonary embolism.

Many services or treatments can be provided at home, as shown in Table 1.

Assessment in Emergency Department and transport home via ambulance
Services and treatment provided: Physician and nursing visits   Standard blood tests   Pulse oximetry   Electrocardiogram   Spirometry   Echocardiogram   Internistic ecographies and Doppler ultrasonographies   Oral and intravenous medication administration, including antimicrobials and cytotoxic drugs   Oxygen therapy   Blood product transfusion   Central venous access (PICC, Midline)   Surgical treatment of pressure sores   X rays   Telemonitoring   Physical therapy   Occupational therapy   Counselling
Hospital-at-home patients are considered hospital patients, and all services are provided by the hospital, which retains legal and financial responsibility for care.

Table 1. Features of the Hospital at Home Service

A case history is made up for each patient and is always available at the patient's home, with an updated report available in the HHS office.

Medical consultation with other hospital specialists is possible in the hospital or at the home of the patient.

HHS has continued to increase its activity since its inception in 1985. Until now about 11000 admissions have been recorded. In 2010, 550 admissions were recorded, 9113 nursing visits and 4317 medical visits were conducted. The mean age of our patients was 80 years (range 30-101). Mean length of stay was 14 days.

In 2010 the Piedmont Region issued a decree to regulate this HHS model and acknowledged a refund of 165 Euros/day for DRG included in MDC number 1, 4, 5, 16, 17 (neurological, respiratory, cardiovascular, haematologic and neoplastic diseases), and 145 Euros for the other diseases.

6. The Hospital at Home approach to elderly patients with COPD exacerbation: Principles for patient selection and management

About 20% of patients admitted to the Emergency Department and referred to the HHS of Torino are affected by an exacerbation of COPD.

From an operational point of view, an acute exacerbation of COPD is defined on the basis of Anthonisen criteria as an increase in breathlessness, sputum volume, or purulence for at least 24 hours requiring acute hospitalization (Anthonisen et al., 1987).

Patients that can't be safely managed at home by HHS are those without a family or social support, with severe hypoxemia (PO_2 < 50 mmHg), severe acidosis or alkalosis (pH < 7.35 or > 7.55), suspected pulmonary embolism, suspected myocardial infarction.

In the ED all COPD patients undergo baseline standard clinical evaluation; blood tests (blood cell count, routine biochemical tests and arterial blood gas tensions); pulse oximetry; 12-lead electrocardiography; chest radiographs and hand-held spirometry. Further investigations (including pneumologist's assessment) are performed when required, according to the clinical judgement of the ED physician. Patients eligible for HHS are immediately transferred home by ambulance.

HHS patients receive hospital-level treatments and services at home as dictated by their condition. Treatment of COPD exacerbations is based on the optimized use of bronchodilators as well as the administration of systemic corticosteroids and antibiotics, when requested, administered intravenously in about 90% of patients, and oxygen therapy by nasal cannula or Venturi mask. Non-invasive mechanical ventilation is administered at home in collaboration with pneumologists. Acute administration of nutritional support is possible at home, if requested.

The home care program emphasize patient and caregiver education on the knowledge of the disease giving advices about smoking cessation, nutrition, management of activities of daily living and energy conservation, understanding and use of drugs, health maintenance and early recognition of triggers of exacerbation that required medical intervention. Protocols for prevention of nosocomial infections, bed sores, immobilization, dysphagia are routinely adopted for frail patients. Moreover, a counselling service is offered to the most frail patients and caregivers . Aim of the counselling process is to offer to users the opportunity of exploring, discovering and clarify thought and action patterns, thus enabling them to make a better use of their resources in that specific situation of need. Within a situation of crisis and complexity, the counsellor aims at obtaining a safe, confident and cooperative environment capable of transmitting information, implementing support, modifying attitudes, promoting health education to the patient and the family and finally enabling them to better cope with the situation. The counsellor do not provide standardized information to increase the caregiver's skill in caregiving; rather, counselors focused on helping caregivers understand and resolve their reactions to caregiving process.

In the first days after admission in HHS each patient is visited at home on a daily basis by physicians and nurses. In the following days the patients is seen every day by a nurse and at intervals of 2-3 days or less by the doctor, as required by the patient's clinical condition. Hospital at home staff is available at all times for urgent home visits, which occur within 20-30 minutes by the telephone call. Home visit include: physical examination, measurement of vital signs (pulse, blood pressure, respiratory rate, temperature, oxygen saturation), administration and revision of therapy, if necessary. Essential skills for members of the HHS team are the ability to take a comprehensive clinical history and assess clinical condition, familiarity with pharmacological and non-pharmacological approaches, good communication skills, understanding of airway clearance techniques.

Upon admission, for each patients are recorded: blood pressure, spirometric parameters (FEV_1, FVC, $FEV_1/FVC\%$), hematocrit, blood glucose, serum creatinine concentration, serum hepatic enzymes, serum nutritional parameters (e.g, total proteins, albumin, transferrin, lymphocytes) and electrolytes, arterial blood gas levels (pH, partial pressure of oxygen, partial pressure of carbon dioxide, bicarbonate, pulse oximetry), sputum culture if possible. During the HHS admission clinical assessment and routine observations are useful in assessing the rate of recovery from an exacerbation. Blood tests, including arterial blood gases measurement and spirometry are repeated according to the clinical condition of the patient. A chest X ray at home is possible, if necessary.

At home, a multidimensional geriatric assessment is conducted using validated instruments. The multidimensional geriatric assessment include the evaluation of comorbidity using the Cumulative Illness Rating Scale (Conwell et al., 1993), severity of illness using the Acute Physiology And Chronic Health Evaluation (Knaus et al., 1985), depression status using the Geriatric Depression Scale (Yesavage et al., 1982), functional status using Katz Activities of Daily Living and Lawton Instrumental Activities of Daily Living (Katz et al., 1963; Lawton & Brody, 1969), cognitive status using the Mini-Mental State Examination (Folstein et al., 1975), quality of life using the Nottingham Health Profile (Hunt et al., 1985), nutritional status using the Mini Nutritional Assessment (Guigoz et al., 1997), characteristics of caregiver with special attention to the level of stress using the Relatives' Stress Scale (Greene et al., 1982), and satisfaction using an "ad hoc" questionnaire for customer satisfaction (Figure 2).

The HHS patients undergo acute rehabilitative care at home, including pulmonary rehabilitation when needed, and their caregivers are encouraged to actively participate in the rehabilitation process. Education and psychological support are important for the overall success of rehabilitation. Education improves knowledge, coping and self-management, actively engaging patients to maintain strategies that reduce dyspnoea, maintain good lifestyle habits and participate in decision-making when acute exacerbation occur.

When patients recover from an acute exacerbation of COPD the dimission is planned, making arrangements with General Pratictioner. District Health Services are activated if required.

Recently, two papers on hospital- at-home treatment of elderly patients with an acute exacerbation of COPD have been published by HHS of San Giovanni Battista Hospital of Torino (Aimonino Ricauda et al., 2007, 2008). Between April 2004 and April 2005 a prospective randomized controlled single-blind trial was conducted to evaluate hospital readmission rates and mortality at 6 month follow up in selected elderly patients with acute exacerbation of COPD. One hundred and four elderly patients admitted to hospital for acute exacerbation of COPD were randomly assigned to General Medical Ward (GMW, n=52) or to Hospital at Home Service (HHS, n=52). Baseline sociodemographic information, clinical data, functional, cognitive, nutritional status, depression and quality of life were obtained (Table 2). All patients were elderly, multimorbid, and functionally and cognitively impaired.

Characteristic	Geriatric Home Hospitalization Service (n=52)	General Medical Ward (n=52)	P-Value
Age, mean ± SD	80.1± 3.2	79.2± 3.1	.20
Male, n (%)	29 (56)	39 (75)	.06
Married, n (%)	27 (52)	29 (56)	.84
Family support at home, n (%)	52 (100)	52 (100)	.89
Smoking history, n (%)			
Current smoker, n (%)	7 (13)	6 (11)	.97
Ex-smoker, n (%)	34 (65)	35 (67)	.95
Nonsmoker, n (%)	11 (21)	11 (21)	.81
Number of cigarettes/d ± SD	20 ± 11	21 ± 15	.83
FEV1, mean ± SD	0.92 ± 0.4	1.04 ± 0.5	.18
Percentage of predicted FEV1	38	47	
Respiratory rate, mean ± SD	24 ± 5	25 ± 7	.32
Home oxygen use before admission, n (%)	18 (35)	12 (23)	.45
Arterial blood gas, mean ± SD			
pH	7.40 ± 0.04	7.41 ± 0.03	.19
Partial pressure of oxygen	69 ± 19	65 ± 14	.23
Partial pressure of carbon dioxide	44 ± 12	46 ± 12	.47
Activities of Daily Living score, mean ± SD*	2.3 ± 2.2	1.9 ± 2.2	.36
Instrumental Activities of Daily Living score, mean ± SD†	7.1 ± 4.9	8.1 ± 4.2	.27
Geriatric Depression Scale score, mean ± SD‡	16.1 ± 6.1	17.2 ± 6.8	.45
Mini Nutritional Assessment, mean ± SD§	17.1 ± 6.5	18.3 ± 6.2	.37
Mini-Mental State Examination score, mean ± SD‖	21.8 ± 6.9	21.8 ± 6.3	.89
Cumulative Illness Rating Scale score, mean ± SD			
Comorbidity index#	2.6 ± 1.5	3.0 ± 1.8	.24
Severity index**	2.5 ± 0.5	2.6 ± 0.5	.19
Acute Physiology and Chronic Health Examination II score, mean ± SD††	9.5 ± 4.0	10.3 ± 4.0	.29
Nottingham Health Profile score, mean ± SD‡‡	20.6± 9.6	19.3± 8.2	.46

Normal range * 0-6, † 0-14, ‡ 0-30, § 0-30, ‖ 0-30, # 0-14, **1-5, †† 0-100, ‡‡ 0-38.
SD = standard deviation; FEV1 = forced expiratory volume in 1 second.

Table 2. Baseline Characteristics of the Study Populations

QUESTIONNAIRE ON CUSTOMER'S SATISFACTION

Please, answer to the following questions.
Your answers will enable us to improve the quality of our care.
The questionnaire is anonimous and will be processed in a sealed envelope.
You may be helped by a family member or a friend.
Thank you for your comments on the back side of this sheet.

What I think about:

	Excellent	Very good	Poor	Unsatisfactory
1. Medical care				
2. Nursing care				
3. Medical explanations on diagnosis				
4. Medical explanations on disease course and treatment				
5. Nursing advice				
6. Medical and nurses attitudes				
7. Feeling of safety and protection about home hospital/inpatient treatment				
8. Satisfaction about your home hospital/inpatient treatment				

Detailed comments

Positive aspects

....
....

Issues to be improved

....
....

Date,......../......../........

Fig. 2. Questionnaire on customer's satisfaction

Patients in both groups received COPD-related treatment at similar rates. The incidence of selected medical complications did not differ between the two setting of care, with the exception of urinary tract infections, which were observed in about 6% of GMW patients and only in 1% of HHS patients (p=.049). There was a lower incidence of hospital readmission for HHS patients compared with GMW patients at 6-month follow-up (42% versus 87%, p<0.001). Cumulative mortality at six months was 20.2% in the total sample, without significant differences between the two study groups. Patients managed in HHS had a longer mean length of stay than those cared for in GMW (15.5 $\pm$ 9.5 v 11.0 $\pm$ 7.9 days, p = 0.010). It is important to highlight that all patients discharged from HHS had completed the care program at home, whereas 11.5% of GMW patients continued their care in long-term facility after hospital discharge, with an average daily cost of $ 174.7 for a mean period of 25 + 8.7 days. Only HHS patients experienced improvements in depression and quality of life scores. Satisfaction at discharge was very good or excellent for 94% of HHS patients and 88% of acute hospital patients (p=0.83). On a cost per patient per day basis, HHS costs were lower than costs in GMW ($ 101.4 ± 61.3 versus $ 151.7 ± 96.4, p=0.002). Analysis of costs for hospital-at-home patients revealed that 79% of costs were due to drugs, durable medical equipment, diagnostic procedures, medications, and other nonstaff costs.

7. New key aspects of COPD management at home: Telemonitoring and teleradiology

The challenges that are posed to the health care sector in terms of using innovative tools and methods are relevant. Issues like the growing of ageing population and of citizens in chronic conditions are the focus of the last medical progress, which offer new and better treatments.

Telecare and telemedicine are promising if considered as solutions for different particular conditions, such as rural regions and all the situations where the healthcare services could cope with a shortage of specialists or equipments.

Telemedicine, moreover, connecting hospital and homes could - in some cases - contribute to avoiding the traditional hospital admission, resulting less stressful for patients, and money saving as well. Technology can also improve the quality of life by supporting informal carers, making it more likely that people receiving care and their informal carers can continue to stay active at home and in the community instead of being institutionalized. With developments in medical and other technologies, people with very complex conditions may increasingly be treated at home rather than in hospital or institutional care. In San Diego, California, physicians arrive at patients' homes with a new version of the black bag that includes a mobile x-ray machine and a device that can perform more than 20 laboratory tests at the point of care. Landers recent opinion is that "the venue of care for the future is the patient's home, where clinicians can combine old-fashioned sensibilities and caring with the application of new technologies to respond to major demographic, epidemiologic, and health care trends. Five major forces are driving health care into the home: the aging population, epidemics of chronic diseases, technological advances, health care consumerism, and rapidly escalating health care costs" (Landers, 2010).

Telemonitoring devices have been tested on an elderly HHS population in Torino. In November 2008 Telecom Italia (TI), "San Giovanni Battista" Hospital and "Mario Boella" Institute (ISMB) of Torino started a project called *MyDoctor@Home*, for telemonitoring patients affected by an acute exacerbation of COPD or acute heart failure, managed at home by the HHS of "San Giovanni Battista" Hospital.

MyDoctor@Home (Figure 3) is an e-health service that enables the patient to measure at home, with portable and Bluetooth connected medical devices, his own physiological parameters and to transmit them in real time, through a mobile phone, to a platform operating in a TI data center, accessed by the sanitary structure. The patients use the mobile phone in order to transmit the measures, and they may also receive messages reminding them to take measurements and/or to follow their medication schedule.

Through the web platform "MyDoctor@Home", physicians or nurses can monitor in real time or from remote the received measures and can interact with the patient in different modalities (telephone, video-calling, visit at home) (Figure 4).

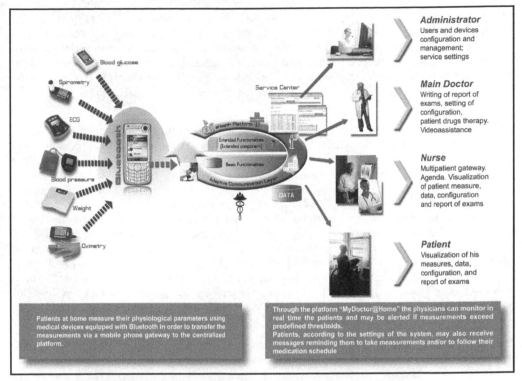

Fig. 3. The MyDoctor@Home Platform

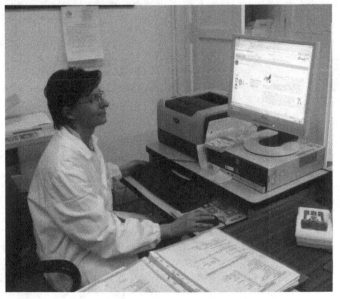

Fig. 4. MyDoctor@Home: Computer work station at HHS office

The system enables the physician to the definition of value thresholds that can be personalized on the basis of single clinical situations. The platform informs the physician on recent measures by sending an SMS so that he can activate quickly the appropriate actions. There is a reduction of reaction times also when the nurse, during the visit at home, sends to the doctor measures performed with professional devices, like for example the ECG or the spyrometer, receiving, quickly, the feedback of the exams and instructions such as for example the variation of the therapy.

Eighteen patients have been involved in the study between June 2009 and June 2010 (27% with a COPD exacerbation), with a mean age of 86 years. All patients were functionally and cognitively impaired, with a poor quality of life. Instruments for telemonitoring resulted easy to use. The use of the equipment of telemonitoring had the benefit to avoid 24 visits by nurses and doctors on the sample in exam. Of them, 15 were substitued by phone contacts on therapy adjustments due to clinical parameter alterations registered by telemonitoring and 9 were substitued by phone counselling. Our preliminary data suggest that the use of our devises could have a reassuring role on the caregivers. Moreover, it has been demonstrated a significantly progressive reduction in the stress levels of caregivers from the baseline to the discharge (Aimonino Ricauda et al., 2011). Nevertheless, the sample size was small and the findings may not be generalizable, given that the study was conducted at only one centre and by an operationally mature hospital-at-home unit. There is the need for better quality studies in the future that can establish a clear role for telemonitoring as an adjunct to intermediate care.

Transporting radiology to the patient's home is challenging. Preliminary experiences indicate that the coupling of simple, light-weight X-ray equipment with an advanced CR-detector system proves effective for externalization of radiographic service. The image and examination quality has been proved to be the same or insignificantly lower than those performed with a stationary equipment and analysis on safety of radio-protection systems show a very low risk exposure for health staff as well as for the general population.

The study of Laerum and collegues showed that mobile, digital radiography service prove better for the nursing home patients at a compatible examination and imagine quality, and a substantially reduced cost for society (Laerum et al., 2005). The study of Sawyer concluded that domiciliary radiography services could be suitable for selected groups of patients (Sawyer et al., 1995).

A pilot study on domiciliary teleradiology service has been conducted at the HHS of Torino between June 2008 and June 2009. Acutely ill HHS patients in need of a radiological examination were randomly assigned to perform imaging at home (Intervention group, n=34) or in hospital (Control group, n=35). Inclusion criteria were: immobilization or chairbound, need for chest, pelvis/hips, joints, upper and lower limbs, hands and feet, abdomen X-rays, absence of definite delirium at enrollment according to the Confusion Assessment Method (CAM) (Inouye et al., 1990) and presence of intermediate or high risk of delirium according to the criteria of Inouye (Inouye et al., 1993), . The radiological examinations were performed at home by two qualified Radiology Technicians (RT) using a portable high frequency X-ray tube, improved cassettes (with imaging plate inside) and a mobile radiological station (Computed Radiography POC 260, Carestream) with visualization and real-time processing of acquired images (Figure 5, Figure 6). Using the Picture Archive and Communication System (PACS) of our hospital acquired images were

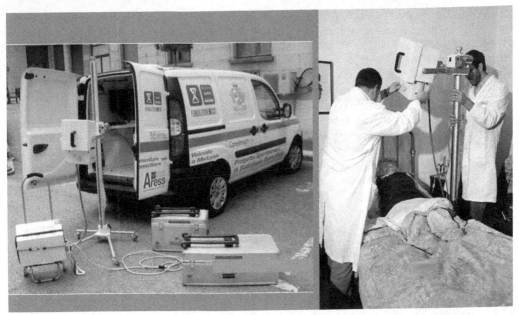

Fig. 5. Mobile tele-radiology station: equipment and Radiology Technicians at patient's home

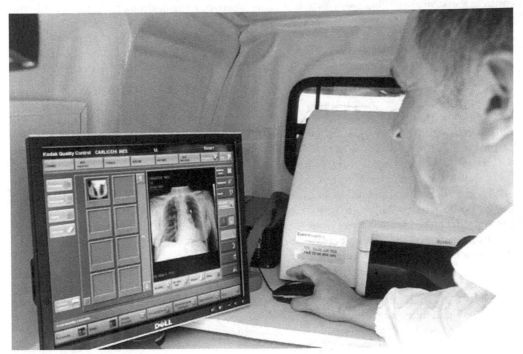

Fig. 6. Mobile tele-radiology station: computed radiography system

transmitted directly via wireless broadband Internet to the radiologists in the hospital who were able to read a radiograph in real time. A firewall hardware has been used in order to protect the confidentiality of patient data. Only one radiography was performed at home in all patients, mainly a chest X-ray. All patients were very old (mean age 78 years in the entire sample), mostly multimorbid, functionally and cognitively impaired, at high risk of developing delirium in 62%. After radiological examinations an acute confusional status, according to the CAM criteria, requiring pharmacological treatment (antipsychotic drugs) appeared in 17% of patients in the Control group, whereas no one in the Intervention group developed delirium. Customer satisfaction for domiciliary X-rays was very good/excellent for 94%. This study demonstrates that a mobile, digital radiography service could be a good option for frail, vulnerable elderly and immobile patients at a compatible examination and image quality, and, due to our analysis, at a substantially reduced cost for the health care system (data in press in Arch Int J, August 2011).

8. Conclusion

Acute exacerbations of COPD are the most common cause of admission to hospital for respiratory illnesses. This causes an increased demand on hospital beds especially during the winter months. Increased provision of services in the community is one proposed method for reducing the pression on acute hospitals.

Intermediate care is a treatment model which bridges the interface between hospital and community care. It often involves cooperation between hospital doctors, general praticitioners, nurses, physioterapists and other healthcare professionals. A specific subtype of intermediate care is Hospital-at-home, were active treatment is provided by healthcare professionals in the patient's home for a condition that otherwise would require hospital care, always for a limited period. Providing acute hospital-level care in a patient's home can be a safe end efficacious alternative to hospital care, especially for frail elderly patients.

The physician-led substitutive "clinical unit" hospital-at home model of Torino provides care that substitutes entirely for an inpatient acute hospital admission; an intensity of care, including medical and nursing care, similar to that provided in the hospital, commensurate with the severity of illness treated; and care that usual community-based home care services cannot provide. Some prior studies of hospital at home for COPD have been of early discharge hospital at home models that treat patients at home with nursing care after they have been admitted to and stabilized in the acute hospital. Davies and collegues in their study of substitutive hospital at home care for COPD employed a nurse-based model that provided only twice daily nursing visits for a period of 3 days and although responsibility for patients rested with hospital physicians, patient's clinical condition did not necessarily require hospital physician's visits at home (Davies et al., 2000). Our intervention targeted very elderly patients with multiple comorbid illnesses, functional impairments and a fairly elevated degree of clinical severity, as shown by the APACHE mean score. These patients need frequent home visits by doctors, nurses and physiotherapists who work together as a team. In our experience HHS care was associated with a reduction in hospital readmission for COPD patients. In addition, HHS care was associated with improvements in quality of life and depression symptoms and a reduction in costs of care. HHS is appropriate for this target population that is especially susceptible to iatrogenic consequences of hospital care and to disruption in their common routines.

The importance of targeting appropriate interventions to appropriate patients has been seen in studies of home care services in which more intensive interventions that included multidimensional assessment were associated with positive outcomes.

Despite the evidence supporting hospital-at-home care, it has had relatively limited dissemination worldwide. Hospital-at-home care is a complex clinical model and, as such, faces substantial dissemination barriers (Leff, 2009).

Our experience suggests that a mature, physician-led, substitutive clinical unit model of hospital-at-home for elderly patients with acute exacerbation of COPD is feasible and is associated with reduction in hospital readmissions and better quality of life.

To date, the evidence base is focused nearly exclusively on patient-related outcomes, rather than on outcomes of interest to potential adopter organizations. There is a need for further studies that include a larger number of patients and an economic evaluation of direct and indirect costs. Moreover, the costs of implementation and the adoption process required within an health organization are to be well delineated.

Hospital at Home of Torino is a part of a comprehensive *continuum of services* at one end of which lies the hospital system and at the other end of which lie community services. Our model is well delineated from an organizational and administrative point of view, and may be considered an example for dissemination.

9. References

Aimonino Ricauda N., Bo M., Molaschi M., Massaia M., Salerno D., Amati D., Tibaldi V. & Fabris F. (2004). Home hospitalization service for acute uncomplicated first ischemic stroke in elderly patients: a randomized trial. *J Am Geriatr Soc* , 52, 278-283.

Aimonino Ricauda N., Isaia G., Rocco M., Tibaldi V., Bergonzini M., Fiorano T., Marinello R., Bertone P. & Isaia G.C. (2011). Il telemonitoraggio in pazienti affetti da BPCO e scompenso cardiaco acuto ospedalizzato a domicilio. *G Gerontol*, 59, 163-166. (Italian)

Aimonino Ricauda N., Isaia G., Tibaldi V., Bestente G., Frisiello A., Sciarappa A., Cavallo S., Ghezzi M. & Larini G. (2010). Telecare and Telemedicine in home care practice: field trial results, In: *Distributed Diagnosis and Home Healthcare*, Rajendra Acharya U, American Scientific Publishers.

Aimonino Ricauda N., Tibaldi V., Barale S., Bardelli B., Pilon S., Marchetto C., Zanocchi M. & Molaschi M. (2007). Depressive symptoms and quality of life in elderly patients with exacerbation of chronic obstructive pulmonary disease or cardiac heart failure: preliminunary data of a randomized controlled trial. *Arch Gerontol Geriatr*, Suppl. 1, 7-12.

Aimonino Ricauda N., Tibaldi V., Leff B, Scarafiotti C., Marinello R., Zanocchi M & Molaschi M. (2008). Substitutive "Hospital at Home" versus inpatient care for elderly patients with exacerbations of chronic obstructive pulmonary disease: a prospective randomized, controlled trial. *J Am Geriatr Soc*, 56, 493-500.

Aimonino Ricauda N., Tibaldi V., Marinello R., Bo M., Isaia G., Scarafiotti C. & Molaschi M. (2005). Acute ischemic stroke in elderly patients treated in hospital at home: a cost minimization analysis. *J Am Geriatr Soc*, 53, 1442-1443.

Anthonisen N.R., Manfreda J., Warren C.P.W., Hershfield E.S., Harding G.K.M. & Nelson N.A. (1987). Antibiotic therapy in exacerbations of chronic obstructive pulmonary disease. *Ann Intern Med*, 106, 196-204.

British Thoracic Society Guideline Development Group. (2007). Intermediate care –Hospital-at-Home in chronic obstructive pulmonary disease: British Thoracic Society guideline. *Thorax*, 62, 200-210.

Buist A.S., McBurnie M.A., Vollmer W.M., Gillespie S., Burney P., Mannino D.M., Menezes A.M.B., Sullivan S.D., Lee T.A., Weiss K.B., Jensen R.L., Marks G.B., Gulsvik A. & Nizankowska-Mogilnicka E., on behalf of the BOLD Collaborative Research Group. (2007). International variation in the prevalence of COPD (the BOLD Study): a population-based prevalence study. *Lancet*, 370, 741-750.

Burge S. & Wedzicha J.A. (2003). COPD exacerbations: definitions and classifications. *Eur Respir J*, 21, suppl. 41, 46s-53s.

Caplan G.A., Ward J.A., Brennan N.J., Coconis J., Board N. & Brown A. (1999). Hospital in the home: a randomised controlled trial. *Med J Aust*, 170, 156-160.

Caramori G. Adcock I.M. & Papi A. (2009). Clinical definition of COPD exacerbations and classification of their severity. *South Med J*, 102, 3, 277-282.

Celli B.R., , MacNee W. & committee members ATS/ERS Task Force. (2004). Standards for the diagnosis and treatment of patients with COPD: a summary of the ATS/ERS position paper. *Eur Respir J*, 23, 932-946.

Cerrillo-Rodríguez M., Alvarez-Arcaya A., Fernández-Díaz E,.& Fernández-Cruz A. (2009). A prospective study of the management of non-massive pulmonary embolism in the home. *Eur J Intern Med*, 20, 598-600.

Conwell Y., Forbes N.T., Cox C. & Caine E.D. (1993). Validation of a measure of physical illness burden at autopsy: the Cumulative Illness Rating Scale. *J Am Geriatr Soc*, 41, 38-41.

Cotton M.M., Bucknall C.E., Dagg K.D., Johnson M.K., MacGregor G., Stewart C. & Stevenson R.D. (2000). Early discharge for patients with exacerbations of chronic obstructive pulmonary disease: a randomised controlled trial. *Thorax*, 55, 902-906.

Dalal A.A., Shah M., D'Souza A.O. & Rane P. (2011). Costs of COPD exacerbations in the emergency department and inpatient setting. *Respir Med*, 105, 454-460.

Davies L., Wilkinson M., Bonner S., Calverley P.M.A. & Angus R.M . (2000). "Hospital at home" versus hospital care in patients with exacerbations of chronic obstructive pulmonary disease: a prospective randomised controlled trial. *BMJ* 321, 1265-1268.

Escarrabill J. (2009). Discharge planning and home care for end-stage COPD patients. *Eur Respir J*, 34, 507-512.

Folstein M.F., Folstein S.E. & McHugh P.R. (1975). "Mini Mental State". A practical method for grading the cognitive state of patients for the clinician. *J Psychiatr Res*, 12, 189-198.

Fried L.P., Tangen C.M., Walston J., Newman A.B., Hirsch C., Gottdiener J., Seeman T., Tracy R., Kop W.J., Burke G. & McBurnie M.A.; Cardiovascular Health Study Collaborative Research. (2001). Frailty in older adults: evidence for a phenotype. *J Gerontol A Biol Sci Med Sci*, 56, M146-M156.

Garcia-Aymerich J., Farrero E., Félez M.A., Izquierdo J., Marrades R.M. & Antò J.M., on behalf of the EFRAM investigators. (2003). Risk factors of readmission to hospital for a COPD exacerbation: a prospective study. *Thorax*, 58, 100-105.

Gavrilov L.A., Heuveline P. (2003). Aging of population, In: *The encyclopedia of population*, Paul Demeny and Geoffrey McNicoll (Eds), Macmillian Reference USA, New York.

Global strategy for the diagnosis, management, and prevention of COPD. Global Initiative for Chronic Obstructive Lung Disease (GOLD), 2009. Available at: www.goldcopd.org.

Gravil J.H., Al-Rawas O.A., Cotton M.M., Flanigan U., Irwin A. & Stevenson R.D. (1998). Home treatment of exacerbations of chronic obstructive pulmonary disease by an acute respiratory assessment service. *Lancet, 351*, 1853-1855.

Greene J.G., Smith R., Gardiner M. & Timbury G.C. (1982). Measuring behavioral disturbance of elderly demented patients in the community and its effects on relatives: a factor analytic study. *Age Ageing*, 11, 121-126.

Guigoz Y., Vellas B. & Garry P.J. (1997). Mini Nutritional Assessment: a practical assessment tool for grading the nutritional state of elderly patients. *Facts, Researche and Intervention in Geriatrics*, Suppl, 15-32.

Halbert R.J., Natoli J.L., Gano A., Badamgarav E., Buist A.S. & Mannino D.M. (2006). Global burden of COPD: systematic review and meta-analysis. *Eur Respir J*, 28, 523-532.

Hernandez C., Casas A., Escarrabill J., Alonso J., Puig-Junoy J., Farrero E., Vilagut G., Collvinent B., Rodriguez-Roisin R., Roca J. & partners of the CHRONIC project. (2003). Home hospitalisation of exacerbated chronic obstructive pulmonary disease patients. *Eur Respir J*, 21, 58-67.

Hunt S.M., McEwen J. & McKenna S.P. (1985). Measuring health status: a new tool for clinicians and epidemilogists. *J Royal Coll Gen Pract*, 35, 185-188.

Inouye S.K., van Dyck C.H,. Alessi C.A., Balkin S., Siegal A.P. & Horwitz R.I. (1990). Clarifying confusion: the confusion assessment method: a new method for detecting delirium. *Ann Intern Med*, 113, 941-948.

Inouye S.K., Viscoli C.M., Horwitz R.I., Hurst L.D. & Tinetti M.E. (1993). A predictive model for delirium in hospitalized elderly medical patients based on admission characteristics. *Ann Intern Med*, 119, 474-481.

Kalra L., Evans A., Perez I., Knapp M., Donaldson N., Swift C.G. (2000). Alternative strategies for stroke care: a prospective randomised controlled trial. *Lancet, 356*, 894-899.

Katz S., Ford A.B., Moskowitz R.W., Jackson B.A. & Jaffe M.W. (1963). Studies of illness in the aged. The index of ADL: a standardized measure of biological and psychosocial function. *JAMA*, 185, 914-919.

Knaus W.A., Draper E.A., Wagner D.P. & Zimmerman J.E. (1985). APACHE II: a severity disease classification system. *Crit Care Med*, 13, 818-829.

Laerum F., Amdal T., Kirkevold M. Kirkevold M., Engedal K., Hellund J.C., Oswold S., Borthne K., Sager E.M. & Randers J. (2005). Moving equipment, not patients: mobile, net-based digital radiography to nursing home patients. *Int Congr, 1281,* 922-925.

Landers S.H. (2010). Why health care is going home. *N Engl J Med* 363, 18, 1690-1691.

Lawton M.P. & Brody E.M. (1969). Assessment of older people: self-maintaining and instrumental activities of daily living. *Gerontologist*, 9, 179-186.

Leff B. (2009). Defining and disseminating the hospital-at-home model. *CMAJ*, 180, 2, 156-157.

Leff B., Burton L., Mader S.L., Naughton B., Burl J., Inouye S.K., Greenough W.B., Guido S., Langston C., Frick K.D., Steinwachs D. & Burton J.R. (2005). Hospital at home: feasibility and outcomes of a program to provide hospital-level care at home for acutely ill older patients. *Ann Intern Med*, 143, 798-808.

Lemelin J., Hogg W.E., Dahrouge S., Armstrong C.D., Martin C.M., Zhang W., Dusseault J.A., Parsons-Nicota J., Saginur R. & Viner G. (2007). Patient, informal caregiver and care-provider acceptance of a hospital in the home program in Ontario, Canada. *BMC Health Services Research*, 7, 130.

Levine S.A., Boal J. & Boling P.A. (2003). Home care. *JAMA*, 290, 9, 1203-1207.

Lopez A.D., Mathers C.D., Ezzati M., Jamison D.T. & Murray C.G. Global and regional burden of disease and risk factors, 2001: systematic analysis of population health data. (2006b). *Lancet*, 367, 9524, 1747-1757.

Lopez A.D., Shibuya K., Rao C., Mathers C.D., Hansell A.L., Held L.S., Schmid V. & Buist S. (2006a). Chronic Obstructive Pulmonary Disease: current burden and future projection. *Eur Respir J*, 27, 397-412.

Menezes A.M.B., Perez-Padilla R., Jardim J.R., Muino A., Lopez M.V., Valdivia G., Montes de Oca M., Talamo C., Hallal P.C. & Victora C.G., for the PLATINO Team. (2005). Chronic obstructive pulmonary disease in five Latin American cities (the PLATINO study): a prevalence study. *Lancet*, 366, 1875-1881.

Montalto M. (2002). *Hospital in the Home: Principles and Practice*. ArtWords Publishing, Melbourne.

Myles J.W., Pryor G.A., Parker M. & Anand JK. (1996). Hospital at home. Scheme in Peterborough is expanding. *BMJ*, 313, 232-233.

National Clinical Guideline Centre. (2010). Chronic obstructive pulmonary disease: management of chronic obstructive pulmonary disease in adults in primari and secondary care. London: National Clinical Guideline Centre. Available at: http://guidance.nice.org.uk/CG101/Guidance/pdf/English.

O'Donnel D.E., Hernandez P., Kaplan A., Aaron S., Bourbeau J., Marciniuk D., Balter M., Ford G., Gervais A., Lacasse Y., Maltais F., Road J., Rocker G., Sin D., Sinuff T. & Voduc N. (2008). Canadian Thoracic Society recommendations for management of chronic obstructive pulmonary disease – 2008 update – highlights for primary care. *Can Respir J*, 15 (SupplA), 1A-8A.

Ojoo J.C., Moon T., McGlone S., Martin K., Gardiner E.D., Greenstone M.A. & Morice A.H. (2002). Patients' and cares' preferences in two models of care for acute exacerbations of COPD: results of a randomised controlled trial. *Thorax*, 57, 167-169.

Peces-Barba G., Barbera J.A., Agustì À., Casanova C., Casas A., Izquierdo J.L., Jardim J., Varela V.L., Monsò E., Montemayor T. & Viejo J.L. (2008). Joint guidelines of the Spanish Society of Pulmonology and Thoracic Surgery (SEPAR) and the Latin American Thoracic Society (ALAT) on the diagnosis and management of chronic obstructive pulmonary disease. *Arch Bronconeumol*, 44, 5, 271-281.

Pérez-López J., San Josè Laporte A., Pardos-Gea J., Tapia Melenchón E., Lozano Ortín E., Barrio Guirado A. & Vilardell Tarrés M. (2008). Safety and efficacy of home intravenous antimicrobial infusion therapy in older patients: a comparative study with younger patients. *Int J Clin Pract*, 62, 1188-1192.

Ram F.S.F., Wedzicha J.A., Wright J. & Greenstone M. (2004). Hospital at home for patients with acute exacerbations of chronic obstructive pulmonary disease: systematic review of evidence. *BMJ,* 329, 315-319.

Ram F.S.F., Wedzicha J.A., Wright J.J. & Greenstone M. (2003). Hospital at home for acute exacerbations of chronic obstructive pulmonary disease. *Cochrane Database of Systematic Reviews,* Issue 4, Art. No.: CD003573. DOI: 10.1002/14651858.CD003573.

Richards D.A., Toop L.J., Epton M.J., McGeoch R.B., Town G.I., Wynn-Thomas S.M., Dawson R.D., Hlavac M.C., Werno A.M. & Abernethy P.D. (2005). Home management of mild to moderately severe community-acquired pneumonia: a randomised controlled trial. *Med J Aust,* 183, 235-238.

Rodriguez-Roisin R. (2000). Toward a consensus definition for COPD exacerbations. *Chest ,* 117, 398s-401s.

Rodriguez-Roisin R. (2006). Review Series. COPD exacerbations. 5: Management. *Thorax,* 61, 535-544.

Sawyer R.H., Patel U. & Horrocks W. (1995). Domiciliary radiography: an important service? *Clin Radiol,* 50, 51-55.

Shepperd S., Doll H., Angus M.R. Clarke M.J., Iliffe S., Kalra L., Aimonino Ricauda N., Tibaldi V. & Wilson A.D. (2009b). Avoiding hospital admission through provision of hospital care at home: a systematic review and meta-analysis of individual patient data. *CMAJ,* 180, 175-82.

Shepperd S., Doll H., Angus R.M., Clarke M.J., Iliffe S., Ricauda N. & Wilson A.D. (2008). Hospital at home admission avoidance. *Cochrane Database of Systematic Reviews,* Issue 4, Art. No.: CD007491. DOI: 10.1002/14651858.CD007491.

Shepperd S., Doll H., Broad J., Gladman J., Iliffe S., Langhorne P., Richards S., Martin F. & Harris R. (2009a). Early discharge hospital at home. *Cochrane Database of Systematic Reviews,* Issue 1, Art. No.: CD000356. DOI: 10.1002/14651858.CD000356.pub3.

Shepperd S., Iliffe S. (2001). Hospital at home versus in-patient hospital care. *The Cochrane Database of Systematic Reviews.* Issue 2. Art. No.: CD000356. DOI: 10.1002/14651858.CD000356.

Skwarska E., Cohen G., Skwarski K.M., Lamb C., Bushnell D., Parker S. & MacNee W. (2000). Randomised controlled trial of supported discharge in patients with exacerbations of chronic obstructive pulmonary disease. *Thorax,* 55, 907-912.

Smith S.M., Brame A., Kulinskaya E. & Elkin S.L. (2011). Telemonitoring and Intermediate care. *Chest,* 139, 731-732.

Stessman J., Ginsberg G., Hammerman-Rozenberg R., Friedman R., Ronen D., Israeli A. & Cohen A. (1996). Decreased hospital utilization by older adults attributable to a home hospitalisation program. *J Am Geriatr Soc,* 44, 591-598.

Tarricone R. & Tsouros A.D. (2008). *Home care in Europe. The solid facts.* Bocconi University. ISBN 978 92 890 4281 9. Milano, Italy.

Tibaldi V., Aimonino N., Ponzetto M., Stasi M.F., Amati D., Raspo S,. Roglia D., Molaschi M. & Fabris F. (2004). A randomized controlled trial of a home hospital interventions for frail elderly demented patients: behavioral disturbances and caregiver's stress. *Arch Gerontol Geriatr,* (9), 431-436.

Tibaldi V., Aimonino Ricauda N., Costamagna C., Obialero R., Ruatta C., Stasi M.F. & Molaschi M. (2007). Clinical outcomes in elderly demented patients and caregiver's stress: a 2-year follow-up study. *Arch Gerontol Geriatr,* 44 (Suppl.1), 401-406.

Tibaldi V., Isaia G., Scarafiotti C., Gariglio F., Zanocchi M., Bo M., Bergerone S. & Aimonino
    Ricauda N. (2009). Hospital at home for elderly patients with acute
    decompensation of chronic heart failure. A prospective randomized controlled
    trial. *Arch Intern Med*, 169, 17, 1569-1575.
Wilson A., Parker H., Wynn A., Jagger C., Spiers N., Jones J. & Parker G. (1999). Randomised
    controlled trial of effectiveness of Leicester hospital at home scheme compared
    with hospital care. *BMJ*, 319, 1542-1546.
World Health Organization (WHO). (2011). Chronic obstructive pulmonary disease (COPD).
    Fact sheet no. 315. Available at:
    www.who.int/mediacentre/factsheets/fs315/en/index.html
Yesavage J.A., Brink T.L., Rose T.L., Lum O., Huang V., Adey M. & Leirer V.O. (1982).
    Development and validation of a geriatric depression screening scale: a preliminary
    report. *J Psychiatr Res*, 17, 37-49.

7

Antipneumococcal Vaccination in COPD Patients

Angel Vila-Corcoles and Olga Ochoa-Gondar
Research Unit of the Primary Care Service of Tarragona-Valls,
Institut Català de la Salut, Tarragona, Catalonia
Spain

1. Introduction

Streptococcus Pneumoniae, the most common cause of community-acquired pneumonia (CAP), remains a major cause of morbidity and mortality worldwide. Despite appropriate antibiotic therapy and intensive care treatment, mortality rates due to pneumococcal infections remain considerable, especially in elderly and high-risk individuals such as patients with chronic heart or pulmonary disease (Kyaw 2005).

The main reservoir of pneumococci is the nasopharynx, and the possible outcomes after colonisation are clearance by the organism, asymptomatic persistence of infection (carrier state), or progression to disease. Disease presentation depends on whether the bacteria spreads to adjacent mucosal tissues causing mucosal infections (otitis, sinusitis, bronchitis and nonbacteraemic pneumonias) or whether it invades the bloodstream, or other sterile sites, resulting in invasive pneumococcal disease (IPD), principally bacteraemic pneumonia, meningitis and sepsis. The outcome is a complex process that depends on interactions between factors related to the host, therapy and microorganism (Feikin 2000, Baddour 2004). Figure 1 illustrates the overlap between overall community-acquired pneumonia, pneumococcal pneumonia and IPD.

The reported incidences of IPD have widely varied in different studies. These differences probably reflect different rates of obtaining blood cultures from patients with pneumonia. The incidence of bacteremic pneumococcal pneumonia ranged from 9 to 18 cases per 100.000 adults-year in a multicentre study carried out in five countries (Kalin 2000). The true incidence of nonbacteremic pneumococcal pneumonia is unknown, but it is probably 3-4 fold higher considering that it has been estimated that 80% of all pneumococcal pneumonias happen without bacteremia (Orqvist 2005).

Chronic obstructive pulmonary disease (COPD) is a major risk factor for community-acquired pneumonia, and smoking (the most common cause of COPD) has been reported as an important risk factor for IPD (Torres 1996, Nuorti 2000).

Nowadays, COPD is a leading cause of morbidity and mortality worldwide. The prevalence of COPD increases with increasing age (approximately 1-3% in middle aged adults *vs* 6-10% in elderly people) and it is approximately three-fold higher in men than in women (Murtagh 2005). Likely, the prevalence of COPD is underestimated given the absence of systematic

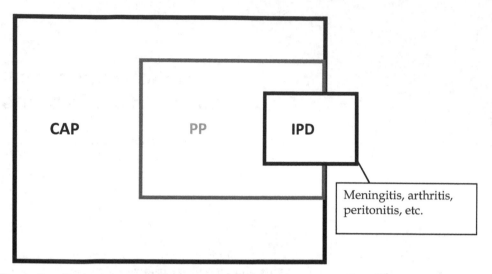

Fig. 1. Overlap between overall community-acquired pneumonia (CAP), pneumococcal pneumonia (PP) and Invasive Pneumococcal Disease (IPD).

investigations in clinical practice for those patients with apparently non-severe or trivial symptoms. It has been estimated that approximately 15-25% people over 45 years-old have a moderate obstructive ventilatory disorder (GOLD 2008). If we consider mortality, a according to World Health Organization estimates, COPD is the fourth leading cause of death worldwide, with more than 2.7 million deaths in 2000 (NHLBI 2001).

Incidence data of pneumococcal infections focused on COPD patients is scarce but, given these persons are considered to be at risk of pneumococcal infections, incidence is believed to be very large. Among patients with pneumonia, COPD is the most commonly reported comorbidity. Among COPD patients with pneumonia, hospital admission increases with the intensity of airflow obstruction. The incidence of all-cause pneumonia among people with COPD is around 40-50 cases per 1000 patients-year (approximately 3-4 fold greater than in the general population). In the United States, the reported annual incidence of hospitalisation for CAP was 11 cases per 1000 among the general population over 65 years-old and 41 cases per 1000 among those patients with chronic lung diseases (Jackson 2003). In Europe, incidences of 14 and 46 episodes per 1000 person-year have been reported among the general population and COPD patients, respectively (Vila-Corcoles 2006, Ochoa-Gondar 2008). Pneumococcus remains the most common microorganism identified among patients with chronic respiratory diseases with CAP (Liebermen 2002, Mandell 2007) although Gram-negative bacilli are increasing in patients with severe obstruction (Restrepo 2008, Ko 2008). Incidences of laboratory-confirmed pneumococcal CAP ranged from 0.5 to 2.1 per 1000 in the general population and 0.7 to 5.9 per 1000 among patients with chronic pulmonary disease (Jackson 2003, Vila-Corcoles 2006, Alfegeme 2006, Ochoa-Gondar 2008) of which approximately 25% were bacteremic and 75% non-bacteremic cases. These figures are likely to be an underestimation of the true incidence of pneumococcal bacteremia because they do not take into account persons from whom blood cultures were never obtained or those where the culture was performed after the start of antibiotic therapy. In addition, those patients with COPD who develop pneumonia have more severe pneumonia and therefore are admitted to the intensive care unit more frequently and have significantly higher 30-day mortality than non-COPD patients (Restrepo 2008, Molinos 2009).

Acute exacerbations (although they represent a less serious illness than CAP) are also an important cause of morbidity and mortality in COPD patients (NICE 2004, Papi 2006, GOLD 2008). Approximately 50% of acute exacerbations in chronic bronchitis are triggered by bacterial infection (Sethi 2000) being pneumococcus responsible for almost a third of bacterial acute exacerbations (Saint 2001). There is an increased risk of exacerbations in COPD patients with persisting bacterial colonisation in the respiratory tract, especially in COPD patients with pneumococcal colonisation. It has been reported that pneumococcus was recovered from sputum in 33% of patients with COPD exacerbation (Bogaert 2004).

Immunizations with influenza and pneumococcal vaccines (together with smoking cessation, inhaled long-acting bronchodilators or inhaled corticosteroids) are a variety of strategies that may be effective in order to reduce incidence of pneumonia and acute exacerbations in COPD patients (CDC 1997, Black 2004, Poole 2009, Varkey 2009).

2. Types of antipneumococal vaccines

The pneumococcus is surrounded by a polysaccharide capsule, and differences in this capsule permit serological differentiation into distinct serotypes (Hausdorff 2005). However, the existence of more than 90 distinct serotypes (differing in their chemical composition, potential immunogenicity and epidemiological impact on different population groups) has greatly complicated the development and evaluation of anti-pneumococcal vaccines.

At the moment, there are 3 established approaches to anti-pneumococcal vaccination: capsular polysaccharide pneumococcal vaccines (PPV), protein-polysaccharide conjugate pneumococcal vaccines (PCV) and protein-based pneumococcal vaccines (PBPV) (Fedson 2003, Abraham Van-Parijs 2004, Tai 2006). At present, only the "old" PPV-23 for use in adults and two "new" PCVs (PCV-10 and PCV-13), both licensed in 2010 for use in children, are available in clinical practice.

2.1 Pneumococcal polysaccharide vaccine

The currently available PPV-23 was licensed in 1983 and is usually recommended for all elderly people and some at-risk groups including those with chronic respiratory diseases. The vaccine contains capsular polysaccharide antigens from the 23 most dominant serotypes among clinical isolates of S. pneumoniae, accounting for approximately 80-90% of overall invasive infections in the adult population. These antigens induce type-specific antibodies (by a T cell-independent mechanism) that enhance opsonization, phagocytosis and killing of pneumococci by phagocytic cells (Fedson 2003).

Antibody response is generally satisfactory after vaccination, but children aged <2 years and immunodeficient persons do not consistently develop immunity, and certain high-risk individuals (including some people with medical co-morbidities and elderly individuals) may respond poorly (Sankilampi 1996, CDC 1997, Fedson 2003). Following vaccination there is a slow but steady decline in serotype-specific antibody titres, and pre-vaccination levels are generally reached within 5-10 years. An anamnestic response does not occur at revaccination, although there is a significant increase in antibody levels (sometimes slightly lower than after the primary dose) (Sankilampi 1996, Artz 2003). Revaccination is only recommended for those persons who received PPV-23 before 65 years of age (CDC 1997) but its clinical effectiveness has not been clearly proved (Artz 2003).

Despite many studies of PPV efficacy in different populations, few randomized-controlled trials (RCTs) to date were focused on COPD patient (Leech 1987, Davis 1987, Alfageme 2006, Steentoft 2006, Ya Tseimakh 2006, Teramoto 2007, Furumoto 2008) and they have reported unconclusive results. Outcome measures in the different trials were very heterogeneous and included pneumonia, acute exacerbations, change in lung function, hospital admissions or visits to the emergency department and mortality (includes mortality from respiratory disease, causes other than respiratory disease and all-cause mortality). The heterogenity of outcomes reported in the distinct trials, together with the low accuracy of the criteria diagnosis for COPD (not verified by spirometric data in some trials), largely limits the comparison of the different results and their interpretation.

In two earlier RCTs published in 1987 evaluating a 14-valent PPV, Davis et al and Leech et al did not observe any efficacy of pneumococcal vaccination, but these negative results were attributed to the small number of patients included in the series and the low rate of pneumococcal bacteremia. Importantly, before vaccination, antibody titers were higher among the COPD patients than among the healthy control subjects in both trial, which suggests previous pneumococcus exposure and largely limits possible conclusions on vaccine efficacy in this population (Leech 1987, Davis 1987).

In the largest RCT on PPV efficacy in COPD patients published to date, Alfageme et al analysed the efficacy of PPV in a RCT including 596 Spanish patients with spirometric diagnosis of COPD (298 receiving PPV-23 and 298 receiving placebo), concluding that the efficacy of vaccination depends on the age and the severity of airflow obstruction. Considering overall study population, in Alfageme's trial, no differences in the risk of all-cause pneumonia was observed in vaccinated as compared with control subjects (OR: 1.03; 95% CI: 0.64-1.67). In subgroup analyses including only cases due to pneumococcus (5 cases) or unknown etiology (53 cases) pneumococcal vaccination appeared effective among subjects under 65 years (OR:0.24; 95% CI: 0.07-0.80), but it did not appear efficacious among COPD patients 65 years or older (OR: 1.14; 95% CI: 0.62-2.07). Among those patients with severe functional obstruction (forced expiratory volume in 1 second <40%) vaccination appeared to be more efficacious (OR: 0.52; 95% CI: 0.20-1.07), with greatest efficacy in younger patients with severe airflow obstruction (OR: 0.09; 95% CI: 0.01-0.65) (Alfageme 2006).

In a short trial including 49 COPD patients, Steentoft et al observed that a rise in antibody levels after PPV-23 occurred among patients with COPD despite the use of systemic steroid treatment, but a statistically significant clinical effect of vaccination was not demonstrated. In fact, no differences between vaccinated and control subjects were observed for the risk of pneumonia (OR: 0.59; 95% CI: 0.15-2.32), acute exacerbations (OR: 1.44; 95% CI: 0.29-7.14) or hospital admission (OR: 0.95; 95% CI: 0.26-3.48) (Steentoft 2006).

In 2006, Granger et al published the first Cochrane systematic review and meta-analysis on PPV efficacy focused on COPD patients, concluding that PPV was not effective in this population to reduce all-cause pneumonia (OR: 0.89; 95% CI: 0.58-1.37) or all-cause mortality (OR: 0.94; 95% CI: 0.67-1.33) (Granger 2006).

In 2010, Walters et al uptated the Cochrane review including a total of 7 RCTs in their meta-analysis specifically focused on COPD patients. According this meta-analysis, in six studies involving 1372 people, the reduction in the risk of developing pneumonia among vaccinated compared to control did not achieve statistical significance (OR: 0.72; 95% CI: 0.51-1.01). The reduction in likelihood of acute exacerbations of COPD from two studies involving 216 people neither reached statistical significance (OR: 0.58; 95% CI: 0.30-1.13). Of the secondary outcomes for which data were available there was no statistically significant effect for reduction in hospital admissions (two studies) or emergency department visits (one study). Considering mortality, according to three studies involving 888 people followed during periods up to 48 months post-vaccination, there was no significant reductions in the risk of all-cause death (OR: 0.94; 95% CI: 0.67-1.33), or death from cardiorespiratory causes (OR: 1.07; 95% CI: 0.69-1.66). The authors concluded that, while it is posible that PPV may provide some protection against morbidity in persons with COPD, no significant effect on any of the outcomes was shown in the meta-analysis, recomending that further large RCTs in this population would be needed to confirm the effectiveness of the vaccine suggested by results from some individual studies (Walters 2010).

In the present authors opinion, all RCTs on PPV efficacy focused in COPD patients has been largely underpowered considering that the most large RCT (Alfageme 2006) included less than six hundred patients (with only five definitive pneumococcal pneumonias observed during 3-year follow-up). Furthermore, given the effectiveness of the vaccine in protecting individuals against IPD, commencing new RCTs in populations at risk where vaccine effectiveness and disease burden is known would create ethical difficulties. Thus, although nonRCTs have inherent limitations (especially the possibility of selection bias), they can provide interesting data on the effectiveness and impact of the vaccination. In this way, several observational studies have reported benefits using the PPV-23 in patients with chronic respiratory diseases (Nichol 1999, Ochoa-Gondar 2008, Watanuki 2008, Sumitani 2008).

On other hand, given COPD is not a cause of immunodepression (apart from the impairment of local defences) and the reported antibody response is compatible with a vaccine efficacy despite its relatively rapid decline, data on efficacy in the general population can also be used to establish vaccine recommendations for these persons. Figure 2 shows point estimates of PPV efficacy against IPD, pneumonia and death according to the two last published meta-analyses (Moberley 2008, Huss 2009).

The last Cochrane review on PPV efficacy/effectiveness among the general population recommends the use of PPV to prevent IPD in adults (particularly otherwise healthy adults), but it also concluded that the meta-analysis did not provide compelling evidence to support the routine use of PPV to prevent pneumonia or death. This meta-analysis demonstrates strong evidence of protection against IPD, with an efficacy of 74% (95% CI 56% to 85%) in RCTs and an effectiveness of 52% (95% CI 37% to 61%) in observational studies (case-controlled and cohort studies). Vaccine efficacy appears poor amongst the subgroup of adults with chronic diseases, where vaccination efficacy did not reach statistical significance. In relation to all-cause pneumonia (the most reported outcome in the Cochrane review, the meta-analysis showed that the PPV provides an apparent protective efficacy of 29%, although substantial statistical heterogeneity was observed (OR: 0.71; 95% CI: 0.52-0.97) (Moberley 2008).

We note the limited amount of data regarding persons with chronic pulmonary diseases. Considering RCT's data, vaccination of younger patients with COPD appears best supported, while the evidence of a benefit to older patients is weaker. However, given

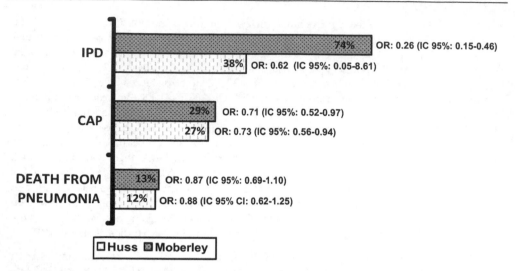

Fig. 2. Estimation of PPV efficacy against IPD, pneumonia and death according to the two last published meta-analyses (Moberley 2008, Huss 2009).

observational studies, PPV also appears effective in older patients with COPD. Because the risks of immunization are believed to be very small, public policy at this time continues to support immunization of all patients with chronic lung diseases regardless of age (CDC 1997, CDC 2010). New CDC's recommendations for using the PPV in adults have been publihsed in 2010. The CDC's new recommendations include some changes from 1997 recommendations.the indications for which PPV-23 vaccination is recommended now include smoking and asthma(CDC 2010).

2.2 Pneumococcal conjugate vaccines

Given the poor immunogenicity of PPV in children, extensive efforts have been made to develop a new generation of pneumococcal vaccines with good immunogenicity in infants. The result was a protein-polysaccharide combination, known as pneumococcal conjugate vaccine (PCV), which contains selected polysaccharides bound to a protein carrier. This renders the vaccine T-cell-dependent, and thus capable of stimulating antibody responses and priming for a memory response on rechallenge. The firstly available PCV contained specific antigen for the 7 most common pneumococcal serotypes in children, and was licensed for paediatric use in 2000 (Black 2000).

In contrast to the PPV-23, which only had a limited impact on the overall disease burden, the introduction of the PCV-7 as routine vaccination for infants has provided very encouraging results, even reducing incidences of pneumococcal disease in unvaccinated people (by herd immunity reducing the transmission of PCV-7 strains in the population) (Whitney 2003, Hicks 2007). In addition, an important reduction in drug-resistant Streptococcus pneumoniae isolates has been observed in all-age groups after the introduction of PCV-7 for children (Kyaw 2005).

Among people over 50 years in the United States, IPD declined by 28% (from 40.8 to 29.4 per 100,000 person-year between 1998-2003) (CDC 2005) with further reductions in recent years

(Pilishvili 2010). Nevertheless, it must be noted that for some groups of older adults the reduction was somewhat lower. There was only a very modest reduction in the number of cases in subjects with comorbid conditions, such as chronic renal disease, heart disease and chronic pulmonary disease (Lexau 2005, Lockhart 2006).

Considering the good immune response and efficacy shown in children, it has been proposed that the use of the conjugate vaccine could improve antibody responses and clinical efficacy in high-risk adults with poor response to PPV (Fry 2002, Lockhart 2006, Jackson 2008). An important immunological consequence of conjugation of polysaccharide antigen with a carrier protein is that the CD4+ helper T-cell fraction contributes to the immunological response. Thus a T-cell-dependent response is generated, with predominant IgG1 and IgG3 antibodies, instead of the T-cell-independent antibody response that occurs with simple polysaccharide antigens (Wuorimaa 2001). This is an important advantage for the conjugated vaccine, given that the response to polysaccharide antigens is much more varying and age-dependent, and antibody levels therefore more uncertain than with conjugated antigens. Thus, as in young children, adult population groups could obtain benefit from using a conjugate vaccine in the future.

Until now, the low serotype coverage has been a very important shortcoming for the "old" PCV-7, bbut he new PCVs including more serotypes (especially the PCV-13, which has broad serotype coverage for both children and adults) could be a good future alternative for all age groups (Scott 2008).

However, at the moment, there are important factors to consider before PCV could ever be used in adult populations. There are only limited immunogenicity data and no data on clinical efficacy in adults. Furthermore, it is not known how many doses of conjugate vaccine adults would require, what age groups should receive the vaccine, and what would be the optimal timing for pneumococcal conjugate vaccination (Abraham Van-Parijs).

2.3 Protein-based pneumococcal vaccines

Although the virulence of Streptococcus pneumoniae is largely dependent on its polysaccharide capsule, it has been demonstrated that numerous protein virulence factors are involved in the pathogenesis of pneumococcal disease (Orihuela 2004), and currently extensive efforts are being made to develop a new generation of pneumococcal vaccines. These vaccines, known as protein-based pneumococcal vaccines (PBPV), are composed of pneumococcal proteins or virulence factors, together with antibodies to them to neutralize their function and reduce the virulence of the infecting bacteria (Tai 2006).

Several formulations of experimental PBPV candidates containing different pneumococcal proteins (eg, PspA, PspC, Ply, or PsaA) have shown protective effects against invasive infections and nasopharyngeal carriage in animal models, and some studies assessing the development of natural antibodies after carriage and invasive disease in humans have reported development of an immune response against some of them (Tai 2006). It has been reported that the combination of various proteins with different protective functions may provide a broader protection (Ogunniyi 2007). Furthermore, other pneumococcal proteins identified very recently by exploiting molecular immunological techniques suggest interesting new vaccine directions (Giefing 2008).

Theoretical major advantages for a future PbPV could be the serotype-independent protection, the possibility of oral or intranasal administration, and probably a less complex production process and a lower cost than conjugate vaccines. However, at the moment, information on humans is scarce, and many studies and several years will be needed to elucidate the true potential of PbPV in human prevention. If finally these proteins can not provide sufficient protection as a sole component of the vaccine, it is posssible that they could be used either as a carrier protein for a conjugate vaccine or as a supplement component for the current vaccines to provide additional protection against pneumococcal infections (Wright 2008).

3. Conclusions

S. pneumoniae remains a major cause of morbidity and mortality worldwide. There are different preventive options but, at the moment, none is optimal. Among patients with chronic respiratory diseases, pending other more effective antipneumococcal vaccines, the PPV-23 (together with influenza vaccine) is currently the only preventive approach that has demonstrated an effect, even if it does not match up to expectations (Gaillat 2009).

COPD patients are commonly described as an at-risk population for pneumococcal infections, but RCTs on PPV efficacy in such patients are very limited and largely underpowered to obtain a reliable conclusion about the efficacy of the vaccine. Among the general population, most meta-analyses have concluded that the PPV is effective against IPD among immunocompetent persons. Recommendations for vaccinating COPD patients are based on this data, although the evidence for vaccine efficacy is less clear among persons with comorbidities.

Among COPD patients, the effectivenes of vaccination in preventing pneumonia and/or acute infective exacerbations is unclear. Two meta-analyses focused on COPD patients concluded that, although it is possible that PPV may provide some protection in persons with COPD, no significant protective effects were demonstrated in the meta-analysis. Considering nonRCTs, the clinical effectivenes of vaccination is also uncertain, but several studies have reported distinct benefits from pneumococcal vaccination in preventing distinct respiratory infections (using the PPV-23 alone and/or together with influenza vaccine).

Several studies have shown that the PPV-23 is cost-effective for preventing IPD among the general population over 65 years in developed counttries, but there is no data about cost-effectiveness of vaccination among COPD patients given the lack of efficacy data in these persons. Current CDC's recommendations for using PPV-23, besides COPD, include smoking and asthma. Revaccination (5-10 years after prime dose) is recommended for those persons who received PPV-23 before 65 years of age. It must not be forgoten, however, that the PPV-23 provides incomplete protection, it does not elicit long-lasting immunity, and no anamnestic effect occurs at revaccination. So, more effective vaccination strategies are needed.

In the next few years, the results of ongoing trials evaluating the efficacy of the PCVs in adults will be critical in determining the position of the conjugate vaccine in the prevention of pneumococcal diseases in patients with chronic respiratory diseases. In coming years, new PCVs including progressively more serotypes (most likely emerging types due to epidemiological changes) will probably be needed. However, the serotype replacement phenomenon can not be fully overcome by increasing the number of serotypes, so new technologies, such as protein-based or genomic vaccines, will be greatly needed. Experimental protein-based pneumococcal vaccine candidates offer the potential advantage of serotype-independent protection and several are in various stages of development in animal models, but none can be expected to be available in clinical practice for several years at least.

Until better options are available, the PPV-23 should continue to be used in high-risk individuals, including younger and older adults with COPD. Although only moderately effective, the burden of pneumococcal disease is greatest in these persons and they can obtain benefit from vaccination.

4. References

Abraham-Van Parijs B. Review of pneumococcal conjugate vaccine in adults: implications on clinical evelopment. Vaccine 2004; 22: 1362-71.

Alfageme I, Vazquez R, Reyes N et al. Clinical efficacy of anti-pneumococcal vaccination in patients with COPD. Thorax 2006; 61: 189-195.

Artz AS, Ershler WB, Longo DL. Pneumococcal vaccination and revaccination of older adults. Clin Microbiol Rev 2003 ; 16: 308-18.

Baddour LM, Yu VL, Klugman KP, Feldman C, Ortqvist A, Rello J, Morris AJ, Luna CM, Snydman DR, Ko WC, Chedid MB, Hui DS, Andremont A, Chiou CC; International Pneumococcal Study Group. Combination antibiotic therapy lowers mortality among severely ill patients with pneumococcal bacteremia. Am J Respir Crit Care Med 2004; 170:440-4.

Black S, Shinefield H, Fireman B et al. The Northern California Kaiser Permanent Vaccine Study Center Group. Efficacy, safety and immunogenicity of heptavalent pneumococcal conjugate vaccine in children. Pediatr Infect Dis J 2000; 19: 187-95.

Black PN, McDonald CF. Interventions to reduce the frequency of exacerbations of chronic obstructivepulmonary disease.Postgrad Med J 2009; 85(1001):141-7.

Centers for Disease Control and Prevention. Prevention of pneumococcal disease: recommendations of the Advisory Committee on Immunization Practice (ACIP). MMWR Morb Mortal Wkly Rep 1997; 46(RR-8): 1-24.

Centers for Disease Control and Prevention. Direct and indirect effects of routine vaccination of children with 7-valent pneumococcal conjugate vaccine on incidence of invasive pneumococcal disease--United States, 1998-2003. MMWR Morb Mortal Wkly Rep 2005; 54: 893-7.

Centers for Disease Control and Prevention. Advisory Committee on Immunization Practices (ACIP). Prevention of pneumococcal disease among infants and children-use of 13valent pneumococcal conjugate vaccine and 23-valent pneumococcal polysaccharide vaccine. MMWR Recommendations 2010; Reports 59(RR11), 1–18.

Davis A, Aranda CP, Schiffman G, Christianson LC. Pneumococcal infection and immunologic response to pneumococcal vaccine in chronic obstructive pulmonary disease. Chest 1987; 92(22): 204-212.

Fedson DS, Musher DM. Pneumococcal polysaccharide vaccine. In: Plotkin SA, Orenstein WA, eds. Vaccines. 4th ed. Philadelphia: Saunders, 2003: 529-88.

Feikin DR, Schuchat A, Kolczak M, Barrett NL, Harrison LH, Lefkowitz L, McGeer A, Farley MM, Vugia DJ, Lexau C, Stefonek KR, Patterson JE, Jorgensen JH. Mortality from invasive pneumococcal pneumonia in the era of antibiotic resistance, 1995-1997. Am J Public Health 2000; 90: 223-9.

Fry AM, Zell ER, Schuchat A, Butler JC, Whitney CG. Comparing potential benefits of new pneumococcal vaccines with the current polysaccharide vaccine in the elderly. Vaccine 2002; 21: 303-11.

Furumoto, Ohkusa Y, Chen M et al.Additive effect of pneumococcal vaccine and influenza vaccine on acute exacerbation in patients with chronic lung disease.Vaccine 2008; 26: 4284-4289.

Gaillat J. Should patients with chronic obstructive pulmonary disease be vaccinated against pneumococcal diseases?. Expert Rev Respir Med 2009; 3(6):585-96.

Giefing C, Meinke AL, Hanner M et al. Discovery of a novel class of highly conserved vaccine antigens using genomic scale antigenic fingerprinting of pneumococcus with human antibodies. J Exp Med 2008; 205: 117-31.

GOLD Executive Committee. Global strategy for diagnosis, management, and prevention of COPD [updated 2008]. Available from: http://www.goldcopd.com/ 2008.

Granger R, Walters J, Poole PJ, Lasserson TJ, Mangtani P, Cates CJ, Wood-Baker R. Injectable vaccines for preventing pneumococcal infection in patients with chronic obstructive pulmonary disease. Cochrane Database Syst Rev. 2006 Oct 18;(4):CD001390. Review. Update in: Cochrane Database Syst Rev. 2010;11:CD001390.

Hausdorff WP, Feikin DR, Klugman KP. Epidemiological differences among pneumococcal serotypes. Lancet Infect Dis 2005; 5: 83-93.

Hicks L, Harrison L, Flannery B, et al. Incidence of pneumococcal disease due to non-pneumococcal conjugate vaccine (PCV7) serotypes in United States during the era of widespread PCV7 vaccination, 1998-2004. J Infect Dis 2007; 196:1346-54.

Huss A, Scott P, Stuck AE, Trotter C, Egger M. Efficacy of pneumococcal vaccination in adults: a meta-analysis. CMAJ 2009; 180: 48-58.

Jackson L, Neuzil K, Yu O, Benson P, Barlow W, Adams A, et al.Effectiveness of pneumococcal polysaccharide vaccine in older adults. New England Journal of Medicine 2003;348(18):1747-55.

Jackson LA, Janoff EN. Pneumococcal vaccination of elderly adults: new paradigms for protection. Clin Infect Dis 2008; 47: 1328-38.

Kalin M, Örtqvist A, Almela M et al. Prospective study of prognostic factors in community-acquired bacteremic pneumococcal disease in 5 countries. J Infect Dis 2000; 182: 840-7.

Ko FW, Ip M, Chan PK, Ng SS, Chau SS, Hui DS. A one year-prospective study of infectious etiology in patients hospitalized with acute exacerbations of COPD and concomitant pneumonia. Resp Med 2008; 102: 1109-1116.

Kyaw MH, Rose CE Jr, Fry AM, Singleton JA, Moore Z, Zell ER, Whitney CG. The influence of chronic illnesses on the incidence of invasive pneumococcal disease in adults. J Infect Dis 2005; 192: 377-86.

Lee TA, Weaver FM, Weiss KB. Impact of pneumococcal vaccination on pneumonia rates in patients with COPD and asthma. J Gen Intern Med 2007; 22(1):62-7.

Leech JA, Gervais A, Ruben FL. Efficacy of pneumococcal vaccine in severe chronic obstructive pulmonary disease. CMAJ 1987; 136, 361-365.

Lexau CA, Lynfield R, Danila R, et al. Changing epidemiology of invasive pneumococcal disease among older adults in the era of pediatric pneumococcal conjugate vaccine. JAMA 2005; 294 (16): 2043-51.

Lieberman D, Gelfer Y, Varshavsky R, Dvoskin B, Leinonen M, Friedman MG. Pneumonic vs nonpneumonic acute exacerbations of COPD. Chest 2002; 122(4): 1264-70.

Lockhart SP, Hackell JG, Fritzell B. Pneumococcal conjugate vaccines: emerging clinical information and its implications. Expert Rev Vaccines 2006; 5: 553-64.

Mandell LA, Wunderink RG, Anzueto A, Bartlett JG, Campbell GD, Dean NC, et al.Infectious Diseases Society of America/American Thoracic Society consensus guidelines on the management of community-acquired pneumonia in adults.Clinical Infectious Diseases 2007;44(Suppl 2): S27-72.

MMWR Morb Mortal Wkly Rep. 2010 Sep 3; 59(34):1102-6. Updated recommendations for prevention of invasive pneumococcal disease among adults using the 23-valent pneumococcal polysaccharide vaccine (PPSV23). Centers for Disease Control and Prevention; Advisory Committee on Immunization Practices.

Moberley SA, Holden J, Tatham DP, Andrews RM. Vaccines for preventing pneumococcal infection in adults. Cochrane Database Syst Rev 2008; (1): CD000422.

Molinos L, Clemente MG, Miranda B, Alvarez C, del Busto B, Cocina BR, Alvarez F, Gorostidi J, Orejas C; ASTURPAR Group. Community-acquired pneumonia in patients with and without chronic obstructive pulmonary disease. J Infect. 2009; 58(6):417-24.

Murtagh E, Heaney L, Gingle J, Sheperd R et al. Prevalence of obstructive lung disease in a general population sample: the NICECOPD study. Eur. J. Epidemiol. 20,443-453 (2005).

National Heart Lung and Blood Institute. Global strategy for the diagnosis, management, and prevention of chronic obstructive pulmonary disease. Bethesda: National Heart, Lung and Blood Institute; 2001. NIH Publication No 2701: 1-100.

National Institute of Clinical Excellence. COPD: National clinical guideline on management of chronic obstructive pulmonary disease in adults in primary and secondary care. Thorax 2004;59(Suppl 1): 181-272.

Nichol KL, Baken L, Wuorenma J, et al. The health and economic benefits associated with pneumococcal vaccination of elderly persons with chronic lung disease. Arch Intern Med 1999; 159: 2437-42.

Nuorti P, Butler J, Farley M, et al. The active bacterial core surveillance team. Cigarette smoking and invasive pneumococcal disease. N Engl J Med. 2000; 342:681-9.

Ochoa-Gondar O, Vila-Corcoles A, Ansa X. Effectiveness of pneumococcal vaccination in older adults with chronic respiratory diseases: results of the EVAN-65 study. Vaccine 2008; 26: 1955-1962.

Ogunniyi AD, Grabowicz M, Briles DE, Cook J, Paton JC. Development of a vaccine against invasive pneumococcal disease based on combinations of virulence proteins of Streptococcus pneumoniae. Infect Immun 2007; 75: 350-7.

Orihuela CJ, Gao G, Francis KP, Yu J, Tuomanen EI. Tissue-specific contributions of pneumococcal virulence factors to pathogenesis. J Infect Dis 2004; 190: 1661-9.

Ortqvist A, Hedlund J, Kalin M. Streptococcus pneumoniae: epidemiology, risk factors, and clinical features. Semin Respir Crit Care Med 2005; 26: 563-74.

Papi A, Bellettato CM, Braccioni F, Romagnoli M, Casolari P, Caramori G, et al.Infections and airway inflammation in chronic obstructive pulmonary disease severe exacerbations. American Journal of Respiratory & Critical Care Medicine 2006; 173(10): 1114-21.

Pilishvili T, Lexau C, Farley MM et al; Active Bacterial Core Surveillance/Emerging Infections Program Network. Sustained reductions in invasive pneumococcal disease in the era of conjugate vaccine. J Infect Dis 2010; 201(1): 32-41.

Poole PJ, Chacko E, Wood-Baker RW, Cates CJ. Influenza vaccine for patients with chronic obstructive pulmonary disease (Cochrane review). Cochrane Database of Systematic Reviews 2009, Issue 4. [DOI: 10.1002/14651858.CD002733.pub2].

Restrepo MI, Mortensen EM, Pugh JA, Anzueto A. COPD is associated with increased mortality in patients with community-acquired pneumonia. Eur Resp J 2008; 28: 346-351.

Saint S, Flaherty KR, Abrahamse P et al. Acute exacerbation of chronic bronchitis: disease-specific issues that influence the cost-effectiveness of antimicrobial therapy. Clin. Ther. 23, 499-512 (2001).

Sankilampi U, Honkanen PO, Bloigu A, Herva E, Leinonen M. Antibody response to pneumococcal capsular polysaccharide vaccine in the elderly. J Infect Dis 1996; 173: 387-393.

Scott D, Ruckle J, Dar M, Baker S, Kondoh H, Lockhart S. Phase 1 trial of 13-valent pneumococcal conjugate vaccine in Japanese adults. Pediatr Int. 2008; 50(3): 295-9.

Sethi S. Infectious etiology of acute exacerbations of chronic bronchitis. Chest 2000; 117(Suppl. 2): 380S-385S.

Steentoft J, Konradsen HB, Hilskov J, Gislason G, Andersen JR. Response to pneumococcal vaccine in chronic obstructive lung disease: the effect of ongoing, systemic steroid treatment. Vaccine 2006; 24: 1408-1412.

Sumitani M, Tochino Y, Kamimori T, Fujiwara H, Fujikawa T. Additive inoculation of influenza vaccine and 23-valent pneumococcal polysaccharide vaccine to prevent lower respiratory tract infections in chronic respiratory disease patients. Int Med 2008; 47: 1189-1197.

Tai SS. Streptococcus pneumoniae protein vaccine candidates: properties, activities and animal studies. Crit Rev Microbiol 2006; 32: 139-53.

Teramoto S, Yamamoto H, Yamaguchi Y, Hanaoka Y, Ishil M, Ouchi Y, et al.Clinical efficacy of anti-pneumococcal vaccination in elderly patients with COPD [Abstract]. American Thoracic Society International Conference, May 18-23, 2007, San Francisco, California, USA. 2007; Vol. 175: A137.

Torres A, Dorca J, Zalacain R, et al. Community- acquired pneumonia in chronic obstructive pulmonary disease. A Spanish multicenter study. Am J Respir Crit Care Med 1996; 154: 1456-61.

Varkey JB, Varkey AB, Varkey B. Prophylactic vaccinations in chronic obstructive pulmonary disease: currentstatus. Curr Opin Pulm Med 2009;15(2):90-928.

Vila-Corcoles A, Ochoa-Gondar O, Hospital I et al. Protective effects of the 23-valent pneumococcal polysaccharide vaccine in the elderly population: the EVAN-65 study. Clin Infect Dis 2006; 43: 860-868.

Walters JA, Smith S, Poole P, Granger RH, Wood-Baker R. Injectable vaccines for preventing pneumococcal infection in patients with chronic obstructive pulmonary disease. Cochrane Database Syst Rev. 2010 Nov 10; 11: CD001390.

Watanuki Y, Miyazawa N, Kudo M, Inoue S, Goto H, Takahashi H, Kaneko T and Ishigatsubo Y. Effects of pneumococcal vaccine in patients with chronic respiratory disease. Eur Respir Rev 2008; 17: 107, 43-45.

Whitney CG, Farley MM, Hadler J, et al. Decline in invasive pneumococcal disease after the introduction of protein- polysaccharide conjugate vaccine. N Engl J Med 2003; 348: 1737-46.

Wright AK, Briles DE, Metzger DW, Gordon SB. Prospects for use of interleukin-12 as a mucosal adjuvant for vaccination of humans to protect against respiratory pneumococcal infection. Vaccine 2008; 26: 4893-903.

Wuorimaa T, Dagan R, Väkeväinen M et al. Avidity and subclasses of IgG after immunization of infants with an 11-valent pneumococcal conjugate vaccine with or without aluminum adjuvant. J Infect Dis 2001; 184: 1211-5.

Ya Tseimakh I, Martynenko I, Paraeva S. Prophylactic efficacy of pneumococcal vaccination for chronic obstructive pulmonary disease (COPD) [Abstract]. European Respiratory Journal 2006; 28 (Suppl 50): 178s [P1091].

8

Chest Mobilization Techniques for Improving Ventilation and Gas Exchange in Chronic Lung Disease

Donrawee Leelarungrayub
Department of Physical Therapy,
Faculty of Associated Medical Sciences, Chiang Mai University
Thailand

1. Introduction

The clinical treatment and rehabilitation of chronic lung disease such as Chronic Obstructive Pulmonary Disease (COPD) is very challenging, as the chronic and irreversible condition of the lung, and poor quality of life, causes great difficulty to the protocol for intervention or rehabilitation. Most of the problems are, for example, air trapping and destroyed parenchymal lung, which cause chest wall abnormalities and respiratory muscle dysfunction that relate to dyspnea and decreased exercise tolerance (ATS/ERS 2006). Many intergrated problems such as increased airflow resistance, impaired central drive, hypoxemia, or hyperinflation result in respiratory muscle dysfunction, for instance, lack of strength, low endurance level, and early fatigue. Lung hyperinflation in COPD increases the volume of air remaining in the lung and reduces elastic recoil, thus giving rise to air trapping, which results in alveolar hypoventilation (Ferguson 2006). Thus, poor biomechanic chest movement and weak respiratory muscles affect respiratory ventilation (Jones & Moffatt, 2002). Furthermore, in COPD, the combination of V/Q mismatch, diffusion limitation, shunt and hypoventilation or hyperventilation is presented commonly, which leads to gas exchange impairment (West 2003). To solve inefficient ventilation from thoracic pump dysfunction, thoracic mobility exercise or mobilization techniques can be performed (Rodrigues & Watchie, 2010). Chest mobilization is one of many techniques and very important in conventional chest physical therapy for increasing chest wall mobility and improving ventilation (Jennifer & Prasad, 2008). Either passive or active chest mobilizations help to increase chest wall mobility, flexibility, and thoracic compliance. The mechanism of this technique increases the length of the intercostal muscles and therefore helps in performing effective muscle contraction. The techniques of chest mobilization are composed of rib torsion, lateral stretching, back extension, lateral bending, trunk rotation, etc. This improves the biomechanics of chest movement by enhancing direction of anterior-upward of upper costal and later outward of lower costal movement, including downward of diaphragm directions. Maximal relaxed recoiling of the chest wall helps in achieving effective contraction of each intercostal muscle. Thus, chest mobilization using breathing, respiratory muscle exercise or function training allows clinical benefit in chronic lung disease, especially COPD with lung hyperinflation or barrel-shaped chest (Jones & Moffat,

2002). Therefore, the technique of chest mobilization helps in chest wall flexibility, respiratory muscle function and ventilatory pumping, and results from this relieve both dyspnea symptoms and accessory muscle use. This technique is still controversial because it lacks clinical evidence, but it does show clinical benefit , especially in COPD by improving pulmonary function, breathing pattern and weaning from a ventilator.

2. Biomechanics of chest movement and thoracic spine

Movement of the thorax is like the pump-handle pattern (Hammon, 1978). Movement of the chest wall is a complex function within the rib cage, sternum, thoracic verterbra, and muscles. Basic observation reveals chest configuration for abnormality of the spine or chest shape, for example, scoliosis, kyphoscoliosis, barrel, or pectus excavatum (Bates, 1987). Normally, in all joint movement at the end of expiration, the intercostal muscles are at a suitable length before contraction during inspiration.

In assessment, chest stiffness may be caused by muscle structure being applied directly in the supine, side lying or sitting position. Stretching the rib cage, rotating the trunk or lateral flexion of the trunk can be evaluated. Furthermore, suitable lengthening of soft tissue around the chest wall and respiratory muscles is related to the efficency of contraction force and chest movement. In the case of emphysematus lung or air trapping in COPD, abnormal chest configurature and reduced chest movement with shortened muscle length and weakness are experienced (Malasanos et al., 1990).

Finally, increasing chest movement with stronger contraction of respiratory muscles can help in gaining lung volume, breathing control and coughing efficiency, and reducing symptoms by improving aerobic capacity, endurance, functional ability, and quality of life.

2.1 Functional movement

The thoracic cage is composed of three parts: thoracic spine, ribs, and sternum, which connect to costovertebral and condrosternal joints, and so movement occurs in three dimensions; transverse, antero-posterior and vertical directions (Landel et al., 2005). True ribs (2nd to 8th rib) move more flexibly because of no clavicle obstruction, whereas the 11th and 12th ribs connect to the cartilage, therefore causing less freedom to move.

1.   Flexion and extension

The basic structure of the costovertebral joint comprises both the angle and neck articulation of the rib with the spine, and is attached to costotransverse and radiate ligaments. In the direction of thorax flexion (Grant, 2001), there is anterior sagittal rotation, when the costovertebral joint moves as anterior gliding that slightly rotates, whereas downward rotation and gliding occur during extension. The lower thoracic spine moves more freely than the upper one. The sternum is composed of the manubrium, body, and xiphoid process, and is anterior with upward expansion when breathing deeply. In fact, when it comes to movement, the manubrium is somewhat fixed to the first rib, whereas the body is more flexible around the 2nd to 7th rib. Thus, movement of the sternum looks like a hinge joint during deep inspiratory and relaxed expiratory phases. For extension, the extensor muscle group is the most active, with a motion range of approximately 20-25 degrees. Thorax extension presents the opposite movement to flexion, with backward sagittal rotation by posterior translation and slight distraction of the spine (Neumann, 2002).

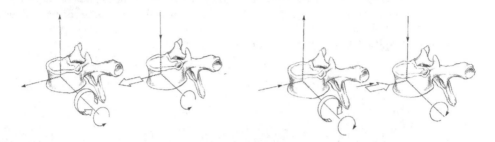

Fig. 1. Anterior rotation of the spine during flexion, and posterior rotation during extension. (Grant, 2001; Lee, 2002)

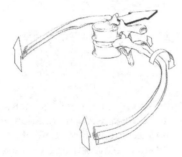

Fig. 2. Extension of the thorax; showing the movement in superior upward and posterior gliding of the costotransverse joint. (Grant, 2001; Lee, 2002)

2. Lateral flexion

In flexion direction, the thoracic body rotates slightly on the flexion side, while the posterior rotates in the opposite direction so that the costovertebral joint is opened and inferior

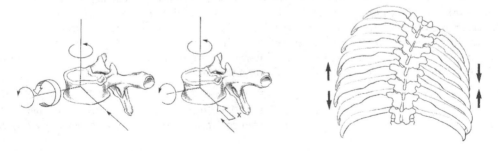

Fig. 3. Biomechanics of lateral flexion to the right; showing the movement of thoracic body and costovetebral joint on both sides. (Grant, 2001; Lee, 2002)

gliding occurs to increase rib space. Mobility of the thorax on flexion, either to the right or left, is found more in lower than upper thoracic parts. Thus, stretching of the lower thorax is rather more successful than that of the upper part. A normal range of motion is approximately 45 degrees: 25 degrees at the thorax and 20 degrees at the lumbar spines. During flexion to the left, the inferior facet of T6 on the left side moves above the superior facet of the T7 spine. In thorax movement, lateral flexion directly affects the rib space in both approximation and stretch away (Figure 3), which results in the transverse process, when the head of the rib glides in the opposite direction (Figure 4).

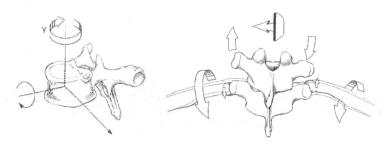

Fig. 4. Rotation of the trunk and thorax, with rib cage and costovertebral joint movement. (Grant, 2001; Lee, 2002)

3. Trunk rotation

Trunk rotation is a complex movement that involves many joints. For example, during rotation to the three left events are shown as; 1) rib rotation with costotransverse posterior gliding on the rotating side, whereas anterior rotation of the rib and gliding are on the opposite side, 2) thoracic body that is elevated and depressed in each segment, and 3) vertical asymmetrical torsion. Upper thoracic spine can move like pure axial rotation as well as thoracolumbar and cervicothoracic rotation. However, sometimes movement of the upper and lower thoracic spines also co-move with lateral flexion or rotation. Thus, articular facet between high and low spines is a sliding movement (Grant, 2001; Lee, 2002).

In conclusion, the chest wall, which is composed of spine, sternum, and ribs, moves in synchronization, no matter whether it is lateral flexion, flexion, extension, or rotation. However, the quality of movement affects individual direction because the costovertebral joint makes contact with the vertebral body, so that lateral expansion is affected more than anterior movement. Whereas, the 2nd to 8th ribs connect to the sternum anteriorly, thus expanding the chest in an anterior direction with pumping handle or anterior and superior motion, as well as bucket handle with lateral and superior motion (Norkin & Levangie, 1992) that occur in regular breathing (Greenman, 1996).

The chest mobilization technique is preferred in cases of COPD or chronic lung disease, with the basic theory of mainly improving ventilation. In addition, aging, prolonged use of a ventilator and chronic illness with neuromuscular dysfunction also concern chest wall mobility.

Rib torsion, passive stretching, trunk rotation, back extension, lateral flexion and thoracic mobilization are practiced to improve chest flexibility.

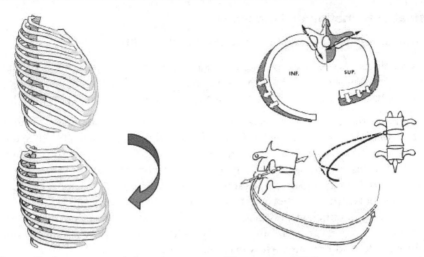

Fig. 5. Pump-Bucket pattern of chest movement. (Greenman, 1996)

3.1 Soft tissue flexibility

The theory of Laplace's law suggests that the length of muscle relates to the maximal force of either diaphragm or intercostal muscles, which affect ventilation in the lung (Kisner et al., 1996; Grossman et al., 1982). Previous evidence showed that stretching the anterior deltoid and pectoralis major muscles, including the sternocleidomastoid, scalenes, upper and middle fibers of trapezius, levaytor scapulae, etc., can increase vital capacity (Putt & Paratz, 1996). In the case of a patient with COPD, the lower diaphragm is depressed horizontally in a contracted length, thus, the resting length is insufficient for contraction. Tachypnea and dyspnea is then a common sign (Cane, 1992). This phenomenon still presents in patients who use a mechanical ventilator for a long period of time (Guerin, 1993). Muscle around the chest wall can be divided into two dimensions; anteriorly with pectoralis major and internal or external intercostal muscles; and posteriorly with erector spinae, latissumus dorsi, serratus posterior superior or serratus posterior inferior muscles, which are important for lung ventilation (Kacmarek et al., 2005). Thus, retraction or spasm of these soft tissues, or muscles, limits chest expansion.

Impairment or disease relates to ineffective chest wall movement

1. Scoliosis or kyphosis (Leong et al., 1999)
2. Osteoporosis or ankylosing spondylitis (Neill et al., 2005)
3. Nerve injury as spinal cord injury (Baydur et al., 2001)
4. Skin disease such as scleroderma, multiple sclerosis etc. (Woo et al., 2007)
5. Myofacial pain or chest pain (Wise et al., 1992)
6. Post thoracic surgery for lung or heart operation (Macciarini et al., 1999)
7. Prolonged use of a mechanical ventilator (Gillespine et al., 1985)
8. Chronic lung disease or pneumonia (Hoare & Lim, 2006)
9. Proloned bed rest (Suesada et al., 2007) or aging (Chaunchaiyakul et al., 2004)
10. Other factors; pain, posture, diaphragm dysfunction (Vibekk, 1991).

4. Physical examination and outcomes

Observation of respiratory symptoms and chest wall mobility

General screening of respiratory problems can be assessed from the signs or symptoms of respiratory depression such as tachypnea, use of accessory muscles, abnormal breathing pattern, cyanosis, nasal flaring etc. which refer to hard work in breathing (Irwin & Tecklin, 1995).

Normal shape of the chest can be observed by the diameter of anterior and lateral views, where the ratio of diameter between anterior and lateral measurement should be more than 1.0. However, in the case of COPD, this ratio may be less than 1.0 and the shape is called barrel chest (Jardins & Tietsort, 1997). In COPD, the barrel chest is shown simply from intrapulmonary air trapping or emphysema, which depresses the diaphragm downward and intercostal outward in a shortened position. The shortening of muscle length before inspiration causes insufficient contractile force. Shortness of breath and decreased chest expansion can be observed clinically. Finally, aggressive dyspnea and low ventilation induce physical deconditioning via low exercise performance (Celli, 2000).

Dyspnea intensity is quantified most easily by using the modified Brog (0-10) category ratio scale (Borg, 1982). This tool evaluates also within other protocols such as the Medical Research Council (MRC) scale, New York Heart Association (NYHA) scale, London Chest Activity of Daily Living scale and Pulmonary Functional Status and Dyspnea Questionnaire (Meek, 2004). Many reports and studies used a Brog scale for identification the dyspnea symptoms and interprets the effectiveness of program.

Palpation on chest expansion

Evaluation of chest expansion is very comfortable for the clinician. Various protocols such as the three levels of upper, middle, and lower lobes (Cherniack, 1983) can be performed manually. Circumferential change from full expiration to maximal inspiration at supine position can be applied with a tape at the axilla (upper lung) and xiphoid (lower lung) levels, as suggested by previous reports (Carlson, 1973), and this protocol has shown good reliability (Lapier et al., 2000). For example, 3 ¼ inches ± ¼ inch could be increased at the axillary level of 20-to 30-year old women (Carlson, 1973). Another level that can be measured to present chest expansion by tape is the 4th intercostal rib space (Fisher et al., 1990). Furthermore, the chest caliper is a new tool that can be used to evaluate chest expansion. Previous evidence has shown that application of the chest caliper enables measurement of thoracic diameters at rest and during activity, but it could not refer to the normal data for chest expansion (Davis & Troup, 1966).

Original palpable examination is of chest expansion in the respiratory system, and less expansion may reflect intrapulmonary lesion such as secretion obstruction or atelectasis. Sometimes, incomplete recoiling from expiration results in many issues such as mass, emphysema, or air trapping. Although, no scientific data have shown normal length of complete recoiling in chest expiration, clinical experience can adjust muscle tightness or shortening around the chest wall. Palpation of the chest wall for flexibility can be evaluated in sitting, side lying, supine, or prone position. Conventional chest movement can be performed with manual evaluation.

Upper costal chest expansion (Figure 6)

Position: Sitting.

Handling: All finger tips are placed at the upper trappezius with whole plamar on the upper chest above the 4th rib at the mid clavicle line, and the tips of both thumbs close to the midline at the mid-sternum line.

Command: Gentle compression and order the subject to breathe in deeply and release following chest expansion.

Results: Approximate calculation of different distances between the tips of thumbs in centimeters (cm) before an after full inspiration.

Direction: Upper costal expansion should be upward with anterior expansion.

Middle costal chest expansion (Figure 6)

Position: Sitting or lying supine.

Handling: All finger tips placed at the posterior axillary line with tips of both thumbs close to the horizontal mid line. The whole plamar should be placed on the middle chest area (4th to 6th rib anteriorly at the mid-clavicle line).

Command: Gentle compression and order the subject to breathe in deeply and release following chest expansion.

Results: Approximate calculation of different distances between the tips of thumbs in centimeters (cm) before an after full inspiration.

Direction: Middle chest expansion should be outward and slightly up ward.

Lower costal chest expansion (Figure 6)

Position: Sitting.

Handling: All finger tips placed at the anterior axillary line with tips of both thumbs close to the horizontal mid line. The whole plamar placed on the lower chest area (below the scapular line and not lower than the 10th rib posteriorly).

Command: Gentle compression and order the subject to breathe in deeply and release following chest expansion.

Results: Approximate calculation of different distance between the tips of thumbs in centimeters (cm) before an after full inspiration.

Direction: Lower costal expansion should be outward.

Sternocostal Movement Evaluation (Figure 6)

Position: Sitting

Handling: Palm placed to cover all sternum (head and body).

Command: Gentle compression and order the subject to breathe deeply.

Result: Anterior expansion during sternum expansion, then upward expansion during sternum (head part) movement.

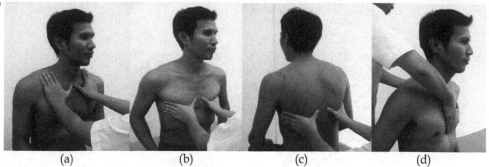

(a)   (b)   (c)   (d)

Fig. 6. Three levels of manual evaluation for upper (above the 4th rib anteriorly) (a), middle (between the 4th and 6th ribs anteriorly) (b), lower lung expansion (below the scapulae and above the 12th thoracic vertebrae, posteriorly) (c), and sternum flexibility (d).

Tape and Caliper Evaluation (Fisher et al., 1990; Carlson, 1973)(Figure 7)

Both of these methods can be applied in a sitting position, which is better than lying supine. From the author's experience, the three levels: upper, middle and lower, can be measured at the axillary, nipple line, and xiphoid process. The latest report on measuring the thoracic excursion or expansion was carried out by Bockenhauer and coworker (2007) (Bockenhauer et al., 2007). It suggests anatomic landmarks on the chest wall as follows;

Upper thoracic expansion is seen as the third intercostal space at the midclavicular line and the fifth thoracic spineous process.

Lower thoracic expansion is seen at the tip of the xiphoid process and the 10th thoracic spineous process.

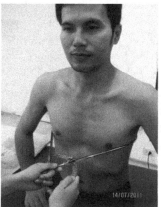
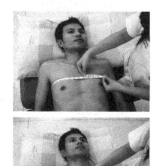

Fig. 7. Application of cloth tape for measuring the upper (right above), lower (right below) thoracic expansion and hand position, and use of the caliper to measure chest expansion (left).

The cloth tape method has been modified by placing the circumference on the specific landmarks transversly and measuring the different changes between full expiration and full inspiration. Although results were studied in 9 healthy subjects, the mean of upper and lower expansion ranged from 1.0 to 7.0 cm, and 1.5 to 7.98 cm, respectively. For the chest caliper, there was no report or data for the range of normal chest expansion.

Thoracic Flexibility Evaluation (Figure 8)

The thoracic or chest wall flexibility is not determined or evaluated exactly for standard value or comparison between healthy and chronically ill subjects. Thus, many practitioners make decisions individually from clinical experience. Thoracic or chest wall flexibility can be evaluated by many procedures in different positions.

In supine or side lying positions, the examiner can evaluate in various directions, but the result is concerned with the lateral intercostal part.

A. Position: Supine with head supported with or without a pillow at the mid-thorax (Figure 8)

Handling: Two hands on the lateral lower chest (6th to 8th rib at the mid -axillary line).

Direction: 1. Hemi-cross counterpressure.
2. Hemi-caudal stretching force.
3. Bilater-caudal stretching force.

B. Position: Side lying position with or without a pillow in the mid-thorax, combined with hand elevation (Figure 8)

Handling: Two hands on the lateral lower chest (6th to 8th rib at the mid axillary line). One hand holding the subject's hand and the other on the lateral lower chest.

Direction: Hemi-caudal stretching force with two hands, and opposite and cephalic stretching.

C. Position: Sitting position without support (Figure 9)
Sternum movement and upper chest expansion
Trunk rotation test
Lateral bending test or anterioposterial flexion test
Trunk flexion and extension test.

Chest X-ray film: Evaluation of lung volume from a chest X-ray (CXR) film is measured possibly from previous evidence of using manual illustration for free hand tracing (May et al., 2009) or calculating total lung capacity from the thoracic roentgen image (Dieterich et al., 1990). In fact, improvement of air entry or volume can be observed from clinically increasing the dark field on the film. In COPD, silhouette sign and secretion retention are identified commonly, including atelectasis from a secretion block (Reid & Chung, 2004), which is the main problem in decreasing lung volume or resorptive atelectasis (Harden, 2009). Thus, the effectiveness of chest mobilization to improve lung ventilation can be reassessed by increasing the aeroted areas or resolving the lung collapse on the chest film.

Dynamic lung ventilation: In the case of lung volume evaluation, functional residual capacity (FRC), tidal volume (Vt) and forced vital capacity (FVC) from the pulmonary function test are challenging outcomes (Dexter, 2010). FRC decreases when there is an

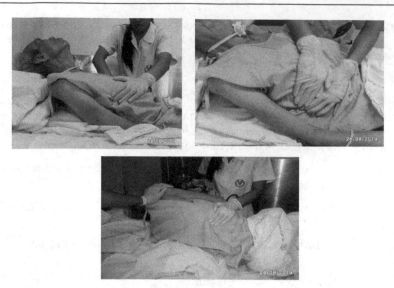

Fig. 8. Rib torsion (right above) and trunk extension (left above) and lateral stretching technique (below). (Leelarungrayub et al., 2009)

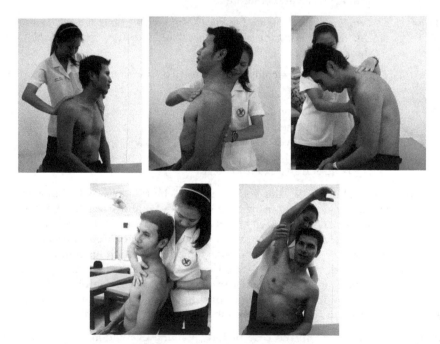

Fig. 9. Functional trunk test as flexion (right above), extension (middle above), rotation(left above), lateral flexion(right below), combined extension, and rotation tests (left below).

imbalance between the lungs and chest wall. Both atelectasis and kyphoscoliosis from abnormal posture affect the elastic recoil of the chest. A barrel chest affects the muscle length of the chest wall or diaphragm by either increasing or decreasing it , and a reduction in force results, which reduces vital capacity (VC) (Henderson & Clotworthy, 2009). In the case of patient who used a ventilator, improvement in lung volume or ventilation can be evaluated from tidal volume (Vt), expiratory tidal volume (ETV), or minute ventilation (VE). In the early exacerbation stage, evaluation of lung volume is difficult because of dynamic hyperinflation, but if the patient is on a ventilator with SMIV or CPAP modes, minute ventilation (VE) and FRC is very easy to measure (Vines, 2010). Finally, the weaning time from a ventilator is the final outcome that presents the improvement clinically.

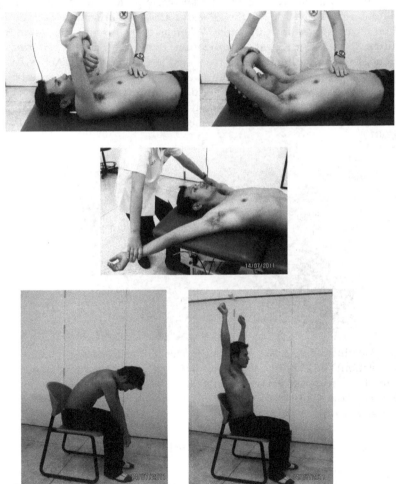

Fig. 10. Passive stretching of the pectoralis major (above and middle) and active stretching of the pectoralis muscles with inspiration with exhalation during flexion and breathing in during extension (below).

From the overall outcomes, chest expansion, dyspnea, chest radiography, and dynamic lung ventilation are most important in representing the effectiveness of a technique. Other parameters can be evaluated such as breathing pattern, respiratory rate, oxygen saturation, etc., and respiratory muscle strength if protocol training is included.

5. Chest mobilization techniques

Chest mobilization techniques are the original protocol used in chronic lung disease, which has the tendency to cause poor posture, rigidity, or lack of thoracic spine and rib cage movement (Vibekk, 1991). These techniques are divided into passive and active chest mobilization, which depends on the patient's condition. In the case of an unconscious patient, as seen in an intensive care unit (ICU) where prolonged treatment is carried out with or without ventilator support, the" **Passive Chest Mobilization Technique**" can be performed on the chest wall by a therapist. Whereas, in the case of a patient in recovery or good condition, the "**Active Chest Mobilization Technique**" can be performed. In some general practices, patients who have just recovered can have modified Active-Passive Chest Mobilization to improve flexibility of the chest wall. The aim of these techniques is to improve thoracic mobility at the upper, middle or lower parts of the chest. Furthermore, these techniques need to be selected carefully to minimize dyspnea, and they should be applied in sitting, sitting leaning forward or high side lying positions (Lee, 2002; Rodrigues & Watchie, 2010).

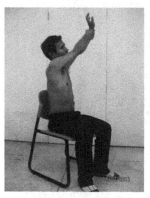 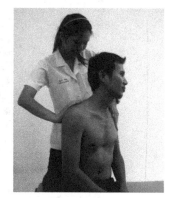

Fig. 11. Chest Mobilization Techniques for improving thoracic mobility at the postero-lateral parts (trunk rotation) (Vibekk, 1991) by active and passive trunk rotation on both sides. Exhalation in a forward position is carried out at the beginning of flexion, and rotation of the left side is performed laterally with inspiration. However, an exhalation phase is carried out during passive trunk rotation.

5.1 Antero-posterior upper costal chest wall mobilization

The original technique is similar to the previously mentioned protocol (Frownfelter, 1987). This pattern is suitable for giving benefit in cases of shortening pectoralis muscles. Some evidence has shown that winging and trunk rotation can improve vital capacity (Pryor et al., 2000). The benefits of this pattern improve both ventilation in upper lobes of boths and also stretches the pectoralis muscle that may tight.

5.2 Postero-lateral chest wall mobilization

This technique has many procedures such as trunk torsion, rotation, and lateral bending (Frownfelter, 1987). It not only affects the ribs and tissue, but also moves the costovertebral and facet joints. This pattern is very useful in ordet to improve the ventilation around in the lower lobe of both lungs.

5.3 Lateral chest wall mobilization (Figure 12)

This technique can be applied in cases of unconsciousness and good consciousness. This part can be mobilized either by therapist likes lateral flexion on the bed, or rib torsion. Other procedures can be performed by passive stretching in sitting position. The last choice that is very strong and give the best result in order to stretching by side lying on the pillow and passive stretching. This pattern helps to improve the chest wall flexibility around the lower thoracic and improves the ventilation in both lower lungs. Sometime, lateral chesl wall stretching effects to the thoracic joints either sterocostal or costovertebral joints.

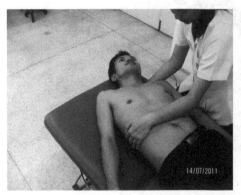
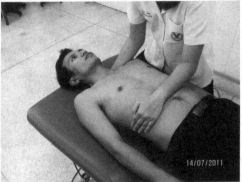
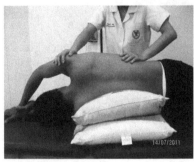
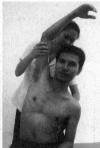
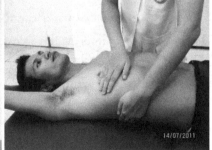

Fig. 12. Chest Mobilization Techniques for improving lateral thoracic mobility; Passive lateral flexion (above), passive rib torsion (right below) (Wetzel et al., 1995), and trunk flexion (middle below), including passive lateral flexion in side lying position on the pillows (left below)

5.4 Thoracic joint mobilization (Figure 13)

From the biomechanics of chest movement, vertebral joints connect to the ribs and sternum with a complex unit that promotes chest expansion. Although this movement is very hard to observe, it also is very effective for ventilation. Therefore, this joint movement is promoted for improving ventilation (Vibekk, 1991).

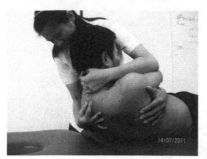 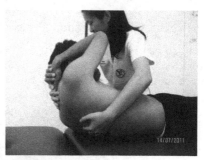

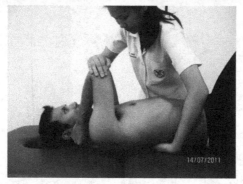

Fig. 13. Mobilization of the facet joint by flexion and extension (Vibekk, 1991), direct rib stretching at the supine lying (left above), facet joint (right above), and costovertebral joint (below).

6. Indication and contra-indication of chest mobilization techniques

There has been no information on the indication for chest mobilization before, which gives a tendency for limitation of chest movement; either structurally or physiologically. However, this technique can be used for various conditions such as COPD, prolonged bed rest, abnormal spine, deconditioning and aging.

The contra-indications for using this method are listed (Viekk, 1991) below:

- Severe and unstable rib fracture
- Metastasis bone cancer
- Tuberculosis spondylitis
- Severe osteoporesis
- Herination
- Severe pain
- Unstable vital signs

7. Clinical analysis on the effectiveness of programs

The clinical procedure for representing the efficiency of this treatment is very difficult because of the low number of cases. Representation of improvement using statistical analysis is limited by either parametric or non-parametric evaluation. In clinical rehabilitation, matching age and disease condition to set up a control or treated group is very difficult. Furthermore, presentation of a positive outcome in clinical improvement is very important.

Many reports of case studies from rehabilitation have shown results with explanations such as postural restoration from physical therapy (Spence, 2008). However, an interesting procedure for evaluating a single system was designed by Bloom and Fischer (1982). This system was designed basically to involve an individual or a single system by repeatedly taking recordings of dependent variables (Ottenbacher, 1986). The components of this design are composed of only sequential application and withdrawal or variation of intervention, with the use of frequent and repeated measures. Thus, this design is not a fixed procedure and can be applied in various study proposals.

The design of a case study has many models; A-B, A-B-A, A-B-A-B, and B-A-B, where A is the baseline period and B the treatment period. There is also an A-B-C model for use in different treatments. Various repeated data recordings are performed in each period, and more than 4 are enough for clinical analysis when a Bloom Table is used. Clinical explanation can be presented by visual inspection and raw data analysis. A simple line graph is an easy procedure for presenting the changes and tendency in each period. Improvement or deterious results in pre-treatment, during treatment or post-treatment can be explained from a changing or trend line. In addition, comparison of mean levels in each period is also a very important evaluation. Statistical analysis of this system can be performed using the Bloom Table (Bloom, 1975), which observes the proportion during baseline and number of treatments above or below the celeration line. Important analysis of data in each period involves changes in all parameters that must evaluate autocorrelation, which helps to separate changes between condition and treatment. Other procedures that present the statistical difference between baseline and treatment use the two standard deviation band method and C-statistic (Ottenbacher, 1986). Some researches have used this design such as the study of Cleland and Palmer (2004), who showed the effectiveness of manual physical therapy, therapeutic exercise, and patient education on bilateral disc displacement in a single-case A1 (control period) –B (intervention period) -A2 (withdrawal of the intervention) design, and also presented the results by visual analog scale and the two standard deviation band method (Cleland & Palmer, 2004). Overall, representation of effective rehabilitation or treatment in rare or few cases can be performed with a single case design.

8. Clinical implementation

Case 1: Chest mobilization treatment in the sub-acute stage

Illness history and medical treatment: A sixty years old man, diagnosed with aspirated pneumonia and underlying cysticercosis from obstructive hydrocephalus, was admitted to hospital with respiratory failure. A physician treated him with tracheostomy and on a ventilator (tidal volume = 450 mL, I:E = 2.1, and respiratory rate = 16 bpm). A hematology test showed low haemoglobin (8.9 g/dL) and haematocrite (27.7%), and the chemistry lab test showed hyponatermia and hypoglycemia.

Chest X-ray: Interstitial infiltration of the left and right upper lobe (Figure 14).

Physical examination: A thin man, with general muscle atrophy, moderate dyspnea, use of accessory muscles during inspiration, decreased chest expansion on the left more than right side, dullness at the left lung, decrease of air entry with bronchovesicular breath sound and coarse crepitation in both lungs (Figure 14 right)

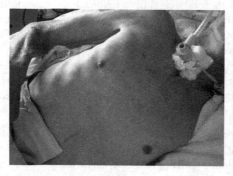 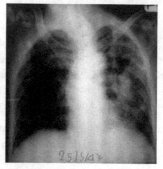

Fig. 14. Chest radiograph before treatment showing infiltration in the left lung and upper area of the right upper lobe (right), and general configurature of the chest wall showing very tight or stiff movement (left).

Treatment: Passive rib torsion at the left lung was added to the general chest physical therapy program; postural drainage, percussion, and breathing exercise (Figure 15) twice daily for 7 days.

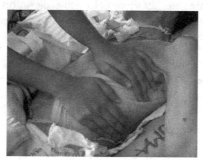

Fig. 15. Passive rib torsion at the left chest wall 10 times per session during ventilation.

Progession: After treatment, repeated chest radiography showed improvement of aerotion and less infiltration in the left lung (Figure 16). Medical treatment could stop using a ventilator to supplement oxygen at 10 Lpm, with a T-piece for 1 hr alternately in a 4 hr period, because hypoglycemia, hyponatermia and malnutrition, dyspnea and use of some accessory muscles were present.

Remaining problems: General weakness, ineffective breathing, shortness of breath, minimized chest expansion and stiffness, and air entry reduction without crepitation.

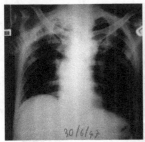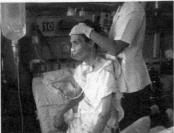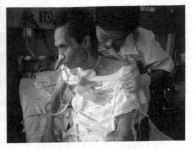

Fig. 16. Chest radiograph after 7 days of treatment (left) and Chest mobilization in sitting position with sternum compression, trunk extension and rotation (middle and right).

Progressive treatment: Passive chest mobilization in a sitting position by stimulating chest expansion in an anterio-posterior direction with sternum compression, back extension and trunk rotation.

Final outcomes: In this case, chest mobilization in anterio-posterior direction or stimulated sternum movement increased chest expansion by evaluating the expiratory tidal volume (TVE), tidal volume, and SpO_2. Patients who have stopped using a ventilator and are only on an O_2 with T-piece can be discharged from hospital after 2 weeks treatment with chest mobilization. However, there is more intensive treatment such as sitting, standing and walking training, and weight training to increase the upper and lower limbs' strength.

Case 2: Chest mobilization treatment in the acute stage

History of illness and medical treatment: A sixty-three years old man was diagnosed with chronic lung disease, pneumonia and sepsis. A physician treated him with an orotracheal tube on a ventilator (Pressure support= 12 cmH_2O, O_2 = 35%, VTE = 150 mL). Blood gas results showed respiratory acidosis and moderate hypoxia with metabolic compensation. Medical problems after treatment were prolonged use of a ventilator (for one month), with recurrent infection and pneumothorax at the right lung, which was resolved by intercostal drainage (ICD). Then, the medical program for weaning off the ventilator was unsuccessful.

Chest X-ray: Left lung atectasis and pneumothorax at the right lung with ICD (Figure 17 left)

Physical examination: A thin man was using a ventilator and presenting general weakness, muscle atrophy and malnutrition. He produced very little chest expansion on either side. Dullness presented at the left lung and hyperresonance at the right one.

Treatment: Initially, an upright position was combined with a chest mobilization technique on the left chest wall, and percussion to remove secretion was performed 3 times daily.

Progession: After 3 days of treatment, chest radiography was evaluated repeatedly (Figure 17), showing improvement of aerotion in the left lung, but atelectasis at the lower lung. The physician could not reduce pressure support while the patient was on the ventilator, but the expiratory tidal volume improved from 155 to 366 mL and an ICD was removed successfully. Unfortunately, remaining problems presented because of respiratory muscle weakness, and malnutrition, and the final goal of stopping the ventilator still had to be reached.

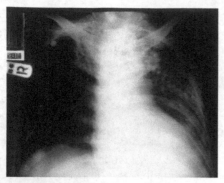
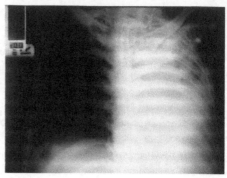

Fig. 17. Chest radiograph showing atelectasis of the left lung, and pneumothorax at the right lung with ICD before treatment (right) and after 3 days of treatment showing improvement of aerotion in the left lung with atelectasis of the left lower lobe (left).

Progressive treatment: An extensive program was carried out from previous treatment with passive chest mobilization in supine position because of weakness. Passive pectoralis muscle and breathing exercise were performed combined with diaphragmatic and intercostal muscle contraction by relearning.

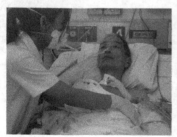
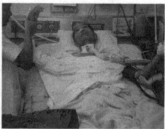
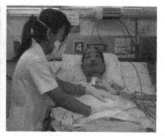

Fig. 18. Passive chest mobilization being combined with breathing exercise of the intercostal and diaphragmatic muscles.

Final outcomes: For this case in the ICU stage, benefits of chest mobilization presented improvement of ventilation at the left lung, and more advantageous treatment was shown when combining other techniques such as breathing exercise with intercostal muscle and diaphragm relearning. However, treatment was unsuccessful in other factors such as pneumothorax, malnutrition and the patient's overall condition.

Case 3: Chest mobilization treatment in the chronic stage

Illness history and medical treatment: A sixty years old man was diagnosed with stable COPD and acute exacerbation because of prolonged use of a ventilator, no rehabilitation for 3 months, and unsuccessful weaning from the ventilator with recurrent infection and much secretion. Ventilator mode was maintained with pressure control (pressure support = 25 cmH_2O, rate = 15 bpm, I:E = 1:2, FiO_2 = 0.45, and PEEP =10 cmH_2O. Blood gas showed moderate hypoxemia (PaO_2 = 85 mmHg) with hypercapnea ($PaCO_2$ = 55 mmHg) and completed compensation. Berodual forth for preventing bronchospasm and Fluimucil A600 for diluting the secretion were administered routinely.

Chest X-ray: CXR shows specific atelectasis at the right lower lobe and hyperaerotion in the left lung before treatment (Figure 19 left).

Physical examination: A thin man using a ventilator presented with muscle weakness, atrophy and malnutrition. BMI was 13.5 kg/m². Chest expansion was very small on both sides. Dullness presented in the left lung and hyperresonance at the right lung.

Treatment: For general chest physical therapy with postural drainage, percussion and breathing exercises were carried out in the ward, such as upright position combined with a chest mobilization technique and compression on sternum, and trunk rotation was used to improve chest wall flexibility. An additional program of passive rib torsion, trunk extension and lateral stretching on a pillow was carried out as well. All programs were performed 3 times daily (Figure 19 middle and right).

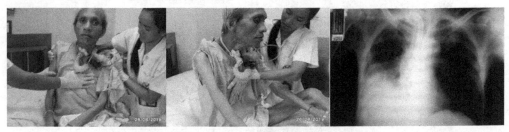

Fig. 19. Chest radiograph showing atectasis of the right lower lobe and hyperaerotion in the left lung before treatment (right), Chest mobilization being performed with compression on sternum, trunk rotation of both sides, sterum and trunk rotation of both sides (middle and left) (Leelarungrayub et al., 2009).

Clinical evaluation: Efficiency of treatment was monitored using various parameters such as expiratory tidal volume, chest expansion at the mid axillary line with a tape and dyspnea, and followed up by CXR after treatment. This effective treatment used the single-case research design with the A (Pre-CPT), B (CPT treatment), and A (Post-CPT) model for 7 day periods.

Results (Figure 20): A 7 day control period (Pre-CPT) showed low expiratory tidal volume (ETV) (mean = 195± 30 mL) and chest expansion (mean = 2.1± 0.54 cm), and during the 7 days of treatment (CPT) benefits were shown by increased mean of ETV (260±49 mL) and chest expansion (3.6±0.22 cm). The dyspnea score was reduced from 6.4±1.14 to 4.4± 0.54. Statistical comparison using the Bloom Table showed significant changes in ETV, with 5 points, 4 points, and all points above the trend line from a Pre-CPT period. However, the Post-CPT and ETV showed deterious effects when treatment was stopped and all points went below the trend line, except for the dyspnea score and chest expansion, which maintained the same level. In both the Pre-CPT and CPT period, all data showed non-significant results of autocorrelation, which meant that the changes in each period did not come from disease progression, especially during treatment (CPT).

Clinical implementation: The chest mobilization technique is very important for improving ventilation and gas exchange in cases that are measured by lung volume and chest expansion, including dyspnea. In figure 20 shows the significant changes of this technique by increasing in a mean of all paprameter when compared to the before treatment of

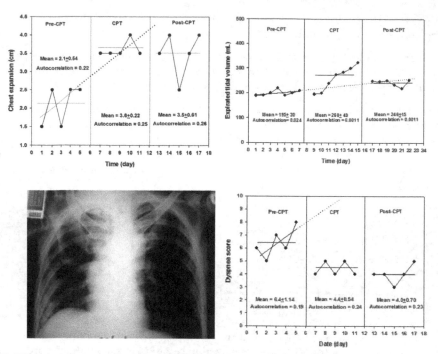

Fig. 20. Visual analog graphs of expired tidal volume (ETV) (right above), chest expansion (left above), dyspnea score (right below) with their autocorrelation with trend lines, and CXR showed an improvement of aeration in the right lower lobe on the 7th day of treatment (left below). (Leelaraungrayub et al., 2009)

baseline. Expirated tidal volume and chest expansion were significant difference, and dyspnea score reduced. Moreover, chest radiography of post-treatment showed increasing in the lung volume and less infiltration.

9. Conclusion

Chest mobilization techqniues are very useful in clinical practice for improving lung ventilation and gas exchange. They also can be applied in various cases, for example, chronic obstructive pulmonary disease (COPD), pneumonia, chronic illness from stroke, spinal injury, prolonged use of a ventilator, etc. These techniques can be applied with others such as breathing exercise, cough training, or exercise in regular pulmonary rehabilitation. Before and after intervention, assessments of observations, palpation or chest expansion measurement,, including X-ray recheck and lung function test, are very important for confirmation of clinical improvement with a single case research design. Improvement of ventilation and gas exchange is very important in gaining health status or quality of life in ICU, or sub-acute or chronic stages. Efficiency of aerobic capacity directs the function and physical performance in daily life. However, this chapter is an example of interesting theory that needs more study to confirm its results. It is hoped that there will be more reports or wider application of chest mobilization in hospitals and communities for improving health status and pulmonary rehabilitation.

10. References

American Thoracic Society/European Respiratory Society Statement on Pulmonary Rehabilitation. (2006). *American journal of respiratory and critical care medicine*, Vol.170, pp. 1390-1413, ISSN 1535-4970.

Bates, B. (1987). *A guide to physical examination and history taking*. 4th edition, Lippincott. ISBN 0397546238, Philadelphia.

Baydur, A.; Adkins, R.H. & Milic-Emili, J. (2001). Lung mechanics in individuals with spinal cord injury: effects of injury level and posture. *Journal of Applied Physiology*, Vol.90, No.2, pp. 405-411, ISSN 8750-7587.

Bloom, M, & Fischer, J. (1982). *Social service: Evaluation research (Social action programs); evaluation*, Prentice-Hall, ISBN 0132923181, New Jersy.

Bloom, M. (1975). *The parasox of helping: Introduction to the philosophy of scientific practice*, John Wiley & Sons, Inc, ISBN-10: 0023108908, New Jersy.

Bockenhauer, S.E.; Chen, H.; Julliard, K.N. & Weedon, J. (2007). Measuring thoracic excursion: Reliability of the cloth tape measure technique, *Journal of the American osteopathic assocation*, Vol.107, No.5, pp.191-196. ISSN 0098-6151.

Brog, G.A.V. (1982). Psychophysical basis of perceived exertion, *Medicine and science in sports and exercise*, Vol.14, pp.377-381, ISSN 0195-9131.

Cane, L.D. (1992). Functional anatomy and physiology of ventilation In: *Pulmonary management in physical therapy*. Zadai CC, (Ed), Churchill livingstone, pp.13-18, ISBN 0443087415, Tokyo.

Carlson, B. (1973). Normal chest excursion. *Physical Therapy*, Vol.53, No.1, pp. 10- 14, ISSN ISSN 0031-9023.

Celli, B.R. (2000). Exercise in the rehabilitation of patients with respiratory disease, In: *Pulmonary rehabilitation*. Guideline to success, Hodgkin, J.E., Celli, B.R., Connors, G.L (Eds). Lippincott, Williams&Wilkins, pp.156-157. ISBN 9780781719896, Philadelphia.

Chaunchaiyakul, R.; Groeller, H.; Clarke, J.R. & Taylor, N.A.S. (2004). The impact of aging and habitual physical activity on static respiratory work at rest and during exercise. *Americal Journal of Physiology Lung Cellular and Molecular Physiology*, Vol.287, pp.L1098-L1106, ISSN 1040-0605.

Cherniack, R.M. & Cherniack, L. (1983). *Respiration in health and disease*, 3th edition, WB. Saunders, pp. 311-316, ISBN 0721625274, Philadelphia.

Cleland, J. & Palmer, J. (2004). Effectiveness of manual phyiscal therapy, therapeutic exercise, and patient education on bilateral dise displacement without reduction-of the temporomandibular joint: a single-case design, *Journal of Orthopeadic Sports Physical Therapy*, Vol.34, pp.535-548, ISSN 0190-0611.

Davis, P.R. & Troup, J.D.G. (1966). Human thoracic diameters at rest and during activity. *Journal of Anatomy*, Vol.100, pp.387-410, ISSN 0021-8782.

Dexter, J.R. (2010). Pulmonary function test. In: *Clinical assessment in respiratory care*, Wilkins, R.L., Dexter, J.R., Heuer, A.J, (Eds). 6th edition. pp. 166-175, St. Louis, ISBN 978-1-4160-5923-3, Missouri.

Dieterich, W.R. & Schneider, W.D. (1990). Determination of total lung capacity from the thoracic roentgen image, *Zeitschrift fur erkrankungen der atmungsorgane*, Vol.174, pp.67-72, ISSN 0303-657x.

Ferguson, G.T. (2006). Why dose the lung hyperinflate?. *Proceedings of the American Thoracic Society*, Vol.3, pp.176-179, ISSN 1546-3222.

Fisher, L.R.; Cawley, M.I.D. & Holgate, S.T. (1990). Relation between chest expansion, pulmonary function, and exercise tolerance in patients with ankylosing spondylitis, *Annals of the Rhumatic disease*, Vol.49, pp.921-925, ISSN 00034967.

Frownfelter, D.(1987). *Chest Physical therapy and pulmonary rehabilitation*, 2nd edition, pp. 170-177, Year book medical publishers, ISBN 0-8151-3340-5, Chicago.

Gillespie, D.J.; Hyatt, R.E. & Schroeder, M.A. (1985). Effect of ventilation by high-frequency oscillation on lung and chest wall mechamics in the dog, *Lung*, Vol.163, pp.317-325. ISSN 0341-2040.

Grant, R. (2001). *Physical therapy o the cervical and thoracic spine*, 3rd edition, Churchill Livingstone, pp. 45-60, ISBN 0-443-07155-1, New York.

Greenman, P. (1996). *Principles of manual medicine*, 2nd edition, Williams& Wilkins, ISBN 0683035584, Baltimore.

Grossman, M.; Sahrmann, S. & Rose, S. (1982). Review of length-associated changes in muscle, *Physical Therapy*, Vol.62, pp.1799-1808, ISSN 0031-9023.

Guerin, C.; Coussa, M.L.; Eissa, N.T.; Corbeil, C.; Chasse, M.; Braidy, J.; Matar, N.& Milic-Emili, L. (1993). Lung and chest wall mechanic in mechanically ventilated COPD patients. *Journal of Applied Physiology*, Vol.74, pp.1570-1580, ISSN 8750-7587.

Hammon, L. (1978). Review of respiratory anatomy, In: *Chest physical therapy and pulmonary rehabilitation*. Frownfelter, D.L (Ed), Year Book Medical Publishers, Inc. pp.3-18, ISBN 0815132964, London.

Harden, S. (2009). Chest X-ray interpretation, In: *Respiratory Physiotherapy*, 2nd edition, Harden, B., Cross, J., Broad, M.A,, Quint, M,, Ritson, P., Thomas, S, (Eds). pp.51-59, Churchill Liveingstone, ISBN 978-0-7020-3003-1, Toronto.

Henderson, B. & Clotworthy, N. (2009). The management of volume loss, In: *Respiratory Physiotherapy*, 2nd edition, Harden, B., Cross, J., Broad, M.A., Quint, M., Ritson, P., Thomas, S., (Eds), Churchill Liveingstone, pp.83-91, ISBN 9780080449852, Toronto.

Hoare, Z. & Lim, S. (2006). Pneumonia: update on diagnosis and management. *British Medine Journal*, Vol.332, pp.1077-1079, ISSN 0959-8138.

Irwin, S. & Tecklin, J.S. (1995). *Cardiopulmonary physical therapy*, 3rd edition, Mosby, ISBN 080162908x, Toronto.

Jardins, T.D. & Tietsort, J.A. (1997). Assessment skills core to practitioner success, In: *Respiratory care*, 4th edition, Burton, G.E., Hodgkin, J.E., Ward, J.J., (Eds), Lippincott Raven, p.168-200, ISBN 1-56238-545-3, Philadelphia.

Jennifer, A. & Prasad, S.A. (2008). Physiotherapy techniques, In: *Physiotherapy for respiratory and cardiac problems*, 4th ed, Pryor, JA., Prasad, S.A (Eds), pp. 188-190, Churchill Livingstone, ISBN 9780080449852, Toronto.

Jones, M. & Moffatt, F. (2002). *Cardiopulmonary physiotherapy*. BIOS Scientific publishers limited, ISBN 1-85996-297-1, Guidford.

Kacmarek, R.M.; Dimas, S. & Mack, C.W. (2005). *The essentials of respiratory care*, 4th edition, Elsevier Mosby, pp.92-94, ISBN 0323027008, Missouri.

Kisner, C. & Colby, L.A. (1996). *Therapeutic exercise: foundations and technique*, 3rd edition, FA Davis Company, pp.143-182, ISBN 0-683-04576-8, Philadelphia.

Landel, R.; Hall, C.; Moffat, M. & Smith, S.R.(2005). The thoracic spine, In: *Therapeutic exercise*. 2nd edition, Hall, C.M.,& Brody, L.T (Eds), Lippincott, Williams&Wilkins, pp. 610-615, ISBN 0-397-55260-2, Philadelphia.

LaPier, T,K.; Cook, A.; Droege, K.; Oliverson, R.; Rulon, R.; Stuhr, E.; Yates, D. & Devine, N.(2000). Intertester and Intratester Reliability of chest excursion measurements in subjects without impairment. *Cardiopulmonary Physical Therapy Journal*, Vol.11, No.3, pp.94-98, ISSN 1541-7891.

Lee, D. (2002). Biomechanics of the thorax, In: *Physical therapy of the cervical and thoracic spine*. 3rd edition, Grant R (Ed), Churchill Livingstone, pp. 45-60, ISBN 0443065640, Philadelphia.

Leelarungrayub, D.; Pothongsunan, P.; Yankai, A. & Pratanaphon, S (2009). Acute clinical benefits of chest wall-stretching exercise on expired tidal volume, dyspnea and chest expansion in a patient with chronic obstructive pulmonary disease, Journal of Bodywork and Movement Therapies, Vol.13, pp.338-343, ISSN 1360-8592.

Leong, J.C., Lu, W.W., Luk, K.D., Karlberg, E.M. (1999). Kinematics of the chest cage an spine during breathing in healthy individuals and in patients with adolescent idiopathic scoliosis, *Spine*, Vol. 24, pp.1310-1315, ISSN 0887-9869.

Lin, K.C.; Dizner-Golab, A.; Thurer, R.L. & Loring, S.H. (2004). Mediastinal and chest wall limitations to asymmetry of lung inflation, *Journal of Applied Physiology*, Vol.96, No.3, pp. 999-1004, ISSN 8750-7587.

Macciarini, P.; Ladurie, F.L.R.; Cerrina, J.; Fadel, E.; Chpelier, A. & Philippe, D. (1999). Clamshell or sternotomy for double lung or heart-lung transplantation?, *European Journal of Cariothoracic Surgery*, Vol.15, pp.333-339, ISSN 1010-7940.

Malasanos, L.; Barkauskas, V. & Stoltenberg-Allen, K. (1990). *Health assessment*, 4th edition, St.Louis:Mosby, ISBN 0801604788,Toronto.

May, C.; Prendergast, M.; Salman, S.; Rafferty, G.F. & Greenough, A. (2009). Chest radiograph thoracic areas and lung volumes in infants developing bronchopulmonary dysplasia, *Pediatric pulmonology*, Vol.4, pp80-85, ISSN 1099-0496.

Meek, P.M. (2004). Measurement of dyspnea in chronic obstructive pulmonary disease, *Chronic respiratory disease*. Vol.1, pp.29-37, ISSN 1479-9723.

Neill, T.W.; Prouse, P. & Bhalla, A.K. (2005). Ankylosing spondylitis associated with osteoporosis and vertebral deformity, *Clinical Rheumatology*, Vol.13, pp.113-114, ISSN 1434-9949.

Neumann, D.A. (2002). Kinesiology of the musculoskeletal system, In: *Foundations for physical rehabilitation*, Mosby, pp. 288-300, ISBN 0815163495, London.

Norkin, C.C. & Levangie, P.K. (1992). *Joint structure and function; A comprehensive analysis*, 2nd edition, FA Davis, ISBN 9780803623620, Philadelphia.

Ottenbacher, K.J. (1986). *Evaluating clinical change: strategies for occupational and physical therapy*, Williams&Wilkins, ISBN 0-683-06659-5, Sydney.

Pryor, J.A.; Webber, B.A.; Bethune, D.; Howarth, A.; Potter, H.M. & Tagg, L. (2000) Physiotherapy techniques, In: *Physiotherapy for respiratory and cardiac problem*,. 3rd edition, Pryor, J.A., Prasad, S.A, (Eds). pp.165-167, Churchill livingstone. ISBN 9780080449852, Toronto.

Putt, M.T. & Paratz, J.D. (1996). The effect of stretching pectoralis major and anterior deltoid muscles on the restrictive component of chronic airflow limitation In: *Proceedings of the National Physiotherapy Conference*, Brisbane, Queensland, Australian Physiothrapy Association, Australia.

Reid, W.D. & Chung, F. (2004). Chest radiology In: *Clinical management notes and case histories in Cardiopulmonary physical therapy*. pp.31-36. Slack Incoporated, ISBN 1-55642-568-6, New Jersy.

Rodrigues, J. & Watchie, J. (2010). Cardiovascular and pulmonary physical therapy treatment, In: *Cardiovascular and pulmonary physical therapy, A clinical Manual*. Watchie, J (Ed), 2nd edition, pp. 319-322, Saunders, ISBN 978-0-7216-0646-0, Missouri.

Spence, H. (2008). Case study report: postural restoration: an effective physical therapy approach to patient treatment, *Technques in reginonal anesthesia and pain management*. Vol.12, pp.102-104, ISSN 1084208x.

Suesada, M.M.; Martins, M.A. & Carvalho, C.R.F. (2007). Effect of short-term hospitalization on functional capacity in patients not restricted to bed. *Americal Journal of Physical Medicine Rehabilitation*, Vol.86, pp.455-462, ISSN 1537-7385.

Vibekk, P. (1991) Chest mobilization and respiratory function, In: *Respiratory care*, Pryor, J.A, (Ed). pp.103-119, Churchill livingstone. ISBN 0-443-03611, Tokoyo.

Vines, D.L. (2010). Respiratory monitoring in the intensive care unit, In: *Clinical assessment in respiratory care*, Wilkins, R.L., Dexter, J.R., Heuer, A.J, (Eds). 6th edition. pp. 286-291, St. Louis, ISBN 978-1-4160-5923-3, Missouri.

West, J.B. (2003). *Pulmonary pathophysiology-the essential*, 6th edition, Lippincott Williams & Wilkins, ISBN-13: 978-0683307344 Baltimore.

Wetzel, J,L.; Lunsford, B.R.; Peterson, M.J. & Alvarez, S.E. (1995). Respiratory Rehabilitation of the patients with a spinal cord injury, In: *Cardiopulmonary rehabilitation*, 3rd ed, Irwin, S., Tecklin, J.S (Eds), p.596, Mosby, ISBN 0-8016-7926-5, Wiesbaden.

Wise, C.M.; Semble, E.L.& Dalton, C.B. (1992). Musculoskeletal chest wall syndromes in patients with noncardiac chest pain: a study of 100 patients, *Archives of Physical Medicine and Rehabilitation*, Vol.73, pp.147–149, ISSN 0003-9993

Woo, P.; Laxer, R.M. & Sherry, D.D. (2007). Scleroderma, In: *Pediatric rheumatology in clinical practice*, Springer, pp. 77-89, ISBN 978-1-84628-420-5, London.

9

A Multi-Targeted Antisense Oligonucleotide-Based Therapy Directed at Phosphodiesterases 4 and 7 for COPD

Rosanne Seguin and Nicolay Ferrari
Topigen Pharmaceuticals Inc.,
Part of the Pharmaxis Ltd. Group, Montréal, QC
Canada

1. Introduction

Recent drug development for chronic obstructive pulmonary disease (COPD) has focused on strategies aimed at reducing the underlying inflammation by selective inhibition of phosphodiesterases (PDE), specifically the PDE4 isoforms. The anti-inflammatory and bronchodilator activities of PDE4 inhibitors have been well documented (Giembycz &Field 2010), however their clinical development has been hampered by their low therapeutic ratio and dose-dependent systemic side effects. PXS TPI1100 is an inhaled drug candidate consisting of two modified antisense oligonucleotides (AON) directed at PDE isoforms 4B, 4D and 7A. PXS TPI1100 has been designed to reduce the recruitment and persistence of inflammatory cells in COPD through an unique mechanism of action and has the potential to be a novel, highly effective approach for this respiratory disease.

In this chapter, we will present the rationale for the design of PXS TPI1100 including a summary of the PDE families and the proposed role they play in regulating inflammation in the lung. Next we will present an overview of the discovery and selection process for the drug candidate, including a summary of the key results from pre-clinical pharmacology, both *in vitro* models as well as two *in vivo* models of neutrophilic inflammation: cigarette smoke mouse model and LPS challenge model. These results will be compared to the first-in-class PDE4 inhibitor, roflumilast (Daxas/Daliresp). We shall conclude with the expected development plan for PXS TPI1100 including the design of upcoming clinical study trials.

2. Chronic obstructive pulmonary disease

COPD is a respiratory disease of airway obstruction and lung damage and is sometimes called chronic bronchitis and/or emphysema. COPD kills millions of people each year and it is currently the fourth leading cause of death worldwide, with forecasts to be the third leading cause by 2020 (ref www.goldcopd.com). COPD, as defined by the Global Initiative for Chronic Lung Disease (GOLD) is *"a preventable and treatable disease with some extrapulmonary effects that may contribute to the severity in individual patients. Its pulmonary component is characterized by airflow limitation that is not fully reversible. The airflow limitation is usually progressive and associated with an abnormal inflammatory response of the lungs to noxious particles or gases"* (Gold 2009). Symptoms of COPD include chronic cough, excessive sputum production, wheeze, shortness of breath and chest tightness. The 4 stages of COPD, designated as Mild, Moderate, Severe and Very Severe, are defined according to lung function as assessed by spirometry, usually the post-bronchodilator ratio of forced expiratory volume in 1 second (FEV_1) to forced vital capacity (FVC). The cellular and molecular mechanisms that contribute to COPD pathogenesis remain incompletely understood yet it is believed that COPD is caused by underlying inflammation characterized by increased presence of neutrophils, macrophages and CD8+ T cells (Gold 2009). Products of neutrophils induce mucus hypersecretion and are implicated both in the generation of mucus metaplasia in chronic bronchitis and the destruction of lung tissue in emphysema. Macrophages are also sources of proteinases and antiproteinases in the lung, oxidative stress and mucus hypersecretion (Ward 2010). Exacerbations play a large role in the disease progression of COPD, and exacerbations become more frequent and more severe as COPD progresses (Hurst et al. 2010).

2.1 Traditional management of COPD

Currently, the only intervention known to influence the loss of lung function is smoking cessation (Gold 2009). Besides treating symptoms and improving quality of life, the treatment focus includes prevention of future exacerbations, reduction of mortality and prevention of disease progression. Treatment for COPD falls into two categories: those medications which relieve symptoms of airflow limitations and those medications which control the underlying inflammation. As such, the current gold standard of treatment for COPD patients involves a step-up paradigm commencing with short-acting bronchodilators (either short-acting β2 agonists or antimuscarinic agents), then adding on long-acting bronchodilators again either long-acting β2 agonists (LABA) or long acting muscarinics, (LAMA) followed by inclusion of inhaled corticosteroids (ICS). Lastly, long term oxygen and possible surgical treatments are final treatment options. Typically, the most common treatment involves ICS/LABA class of drugs, but can also include methylxanthines (bronchodilator) and leukotriene antagonists (anti-inflammatory) (Hurst et al. 2010). The majority of novel treatments for COPD forecasted to launch prior to 2018, are in fact minimally differentiated from current options, with either being improved dosing or combining therapies such as combinations of LABA/LAMA.

Another dilemma is that although highly effective in asthma, ICS have provided little therapeutic benefit in COPD (Barnes 2006). In patients with severe COPD, histological analysis of their peripheral airways have shown an intense inflammatory response, despite treatment with high doses of ICS, suggesting steroid resistance (Hogg et al. 2004). Combinations of ICS and LABA have been shown to be more effective at reducing COPD exacerbations (Calverley et al. 2007) but have not been shown to statistically decrease mortality (Calverley et al. 2007) (Tashkin et al. 2008). ICS use has been associated with osteoporosis, glaucoma, cataracts and skin thinning (Giembycz &Field 2010) and increased risk of pneumonia in patients with COPD (Ernst et al. 2007). Even with the current and immediate future medications, there are clear unmet needs for more effective anti-inflammatories in COPD both for reducing progression of the disease and reducing mortality.

2.2 Phosphodiesterases as targets for COPD

PDE4 is a member of the PDE family of enzymes whose function is to selectively catalyze the hydrolysis of cycle adenosine monophosphate (cAMP) and/or cyclic guanosine monophosphate (cGMP) (Bender &Beavo 2006). Second messengers perform intracellular signaling and cAMP is a key member. The level of cAMP can be regulated by its rate of degradation which is controlled by PDEs (Figure 1). As such, the regulation of PDEs is sophisticated and complex. This family currently includes 11 members (PDE1 to PDE11) of which there are multiple isoforms or splice variants. Several different PDEs can be expressed in a single cell type, and the localization of these PDEs within a cell regulates the local concentration of cAMP or cGMP. Besides being regulated through differential genetic expression, PDEs can be biochemically regulated by phosphorylation, binding of Ca2+/calmodulin and various protein-protein interactions (Bender &Beavo 2006). The PDEs with higher affinity for cAMP than cGMP include PDE3, PDE4, PDE7, PDE8 and PDE11 (similar affinities). These multiple isoforms and their differential expression across cell types

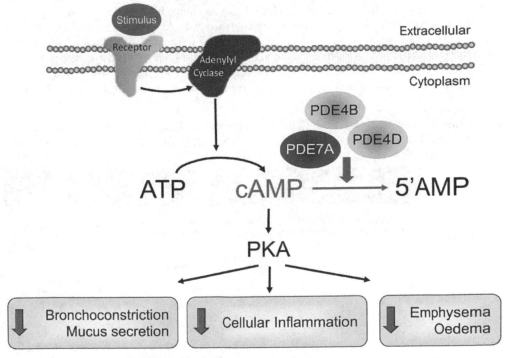

Fig. 1. Cartoon of the cAMP pathway, which is presumably activated upon binding of a stimuli to its receptor embedded in the cell membrane. Known components of this pathway include the calcium/calmodulin-activated adenylyl cyclase, the phosphodiesterase (PDE), and cAMP-dependent protein kinase (PKA) with its catalytic and regulatory subunits. Activation of PKA will lead to phosphorylation of cytoplasmic and nuclear targets. In the lung, inhibition of the PDE will lead to an elevation of the intracellular levels of cAMP resulting with a reduction of the bronchoconstriction, mucus secretion, cellular inflammation and in the long term decrease the emphysema/oedema.

are reasons PDEs are good drug targets as selective inhibition of a specific PDE isoform would limit nonspecific sides effects associated with broader PDE inhibition.

Another reason PDEs have been the focus of drug companies is based on the pharmacologic principle that a more rapid and larger percentage change in concentration is achieved through regulating the degradation of a second messenger than comparable regulation of the rates of synthesis (Bender &Beavo 2006). In most cells the levels of cAMP are between <1 to 10 μM which enables a competitive inhibitor to not need to compete with high levels of endogenous substrate to be effective, in contrast to many protein kinase inhibitors which need to have sufficient affinity to displace mM concentrations of ATP (Bender &Beavo 2006).

There are four PDE4 (A/B/C/D) genes which generate multiple variants as a result of splicing differences in their N termini (Bender &Beavo 2006). PDE4 isoforms, which are widely expressed in many tissues and cell types including the lung, have been shown to play a key role in macrophage and monocyte activation and functions, neutrophils infiltration and vasodilation (Table 1). There has been more information collated on PDE4 than other PDEs mostly from the work resulting from PDE4A, 4B and 4D knock out mice. In PDE4D knockout mice, their airways were shown to be refractory to cholinergic stimulation (Mehats et al. 2003) while PDE4B knockout mice were shown to have effects on immune cells (Jin &Conti 2002; Jin et al. 2005) and both genes were shown to be required for neutrophils recruitment in a model of lung injury in response to inhaled endotoxin (Ariga et al. 2004).

A new first-in class treatment, the PDE4 inhibitor Daxas/Daliresp (Nycomed), has recently been approved in Europe in 2010 and in the USA in 2011 for patients with severe COPD.

cAMP modulator	Structural Lung Cells			Inflammatory Cells		
	Lung Epithelium	Smooth Muscle	Epithelial Cells	Monocyte/ Macrophage	Neutrophils	T-Cells
PDE3	+	+	++	+++	+	+
PDE4	++	++	+++	++++	+++	++
PDE7	+++	+++	+++	+++	+	+
PXS TPI 1100	●	●	●	●	●	●

Table 1. Expression of different cAMP-modulating PDE isoforms in lung cells and inflammatory cells. PDE4 and PDE7 are highly expressed in lung structural cells as well as in inflammatory cells. Delivered to the lung, PXS TPI1100 can inhibit expression of PDE4 and PDE7 in both lung structural and inflammatory cells.

Daxas (3-cyclopropylmethoxy-4-difluoromethoxy-N-[3,5-di-chloropyrid-4-yl]-benzamide) is a once-a-day tablet, taken orally, whose principal action is to reduce inflammation. The clinical results from the six Phase III trials performed using Daxas will be reviewed below. Before, touting the benefits of PDE4 inhibitors in COPD, it is important to note that Daxas is not without its adverse events which include diarrhea, weight loss, nausea, headache and abdominal pain (Giembycz &Field 2010), which have been observed previously with other PDE4 inhibitor drugs (Down et al. 2006).

Like the PDE4 family, the PDE7 family, which consists of PDE7A and PDE7B, is highly selective for cAMP as a substrate (Bender &Beavo 2006). While the function of PDE7 has not been fully elucidated, PDE7 isoforms have been implicated in the activation of inflammatory cells (Li L et al. 1999), including T cells (Smith et al. 2003). PDE7A mRNA has been shown to be expressed in multiple tissues including the lung and inflammatory cells (Table 1) (Bloom &Beavo 1996) (Han et al. 1997) (Lugnier 2006). Inhibitors of PDE7 have shown to potentiate the effects of PDE4 inhibitors, suggesting that a combined PDE4:PDE7 inhibitor would be an effective drug.

3. PXS TPI1100: The drug

The relative lack of advancement and the slow pace of innovation to identify new drug products for COPD can be indicative of the complicated nature of this chronic diseases as well as a potential limited number of targets for conventional small molecule drugs and biologics. Moreover, the activity of cytokines, growth factors and chemokines depends on the interaction of these proteins with their cell surface receptors involving large protein-protein interactions or involving interactions between multiple sites on the protein, which could be particularly challenging to disrupt with small molecule inhibitors or biologics (Johnson et al. 2005). To side-step these complications, we have attempted to design an antisense oligonucleotide (AON) based therapy which functions by targeting RNA directly rather than the protein product.

3.1 Antisense oligonucleotides: An overview

Oligonucleotides (ODN) are short polymers of nucleotides that come in various forms, lengths and modifications which can be distinguished into two main groups based on two distinct mechanisms of action; ODN in the first group target RNA and those from the second group target proteins.

RNA-targeting ODN drugs are designed to bind to a specific sequence of a messenger RNA (mRNA) through Watson-Crick base-pairing interactions. Therefore, the site of action of this class of drug is not the protein itself, but rather "upstream" of it, the RNA coding for the protein. The principle of RNA-based therapy is the reduction in the level of a protein through hindrance of its translation. Archetypes of this class of ODN are AON and small interfering RNA (siRNA). AON drugs are single stranded, usually only approximately 20-bases long, which prevent translation of the target RNA via one of two mechanisms. The first mechanism involves the activation of the enzyme RNAse H, which cleaves the RNA moiety of the duplex formed by the binding of the AON drug to its target RNA leading to subsequent reduction in protein synthesis (Stein &Hausen 1969). The second mechanism involves a steric interaction of the AON with the target mRNA that prevents key maturation steps processes such as splicing and thus preventing translation (Crooke 2008). siRNA drugs share the same mechanism of action to AON, degradation of the protein encoding RNA. However, these drugs are distinct from AON molecules, as they comprise double stranded RNA (varying from 19 to 27 base pair long) (Wu et al. 1998) and induces silencing via the RNA-induced silencing complex (RISC), which is composed of several proteins, including specific RNA-degrading enzymes (Holen et al. 2003).

Similar to conventional small molecules drugs or biologics, the second group of ODN comprises molecules that target proteins directly. Two examples of this group include aptamers and immunostimulatory sequences (ISS). Aptamers comprise either DNA or RNA and typically have a longer chain length (ie, approximately 40 nucleotides) than other ODN. These agents have a specific 3D structure (Ellington &Szostak 1992; Jayasena 1999) that determines their ability to bind specifically to their protein target acting in a similar manner to conventional antibody therapies (Lee et al. 2006). ISS molecules are single stranded, which sequence is enriched with unmethylated cysteine and guanine motifs (CpG) motifs (Vollmer et al. 2004). ISS can mediate immunostimulatory effects following binding to TLR9, a key member of the innate immune system (Agrawal &Kandimalla 2007).

ODN drugs share a relatively common chemical composition that is based on naturally occurring RNA and DNA, and comprises the three elements of nucleotide bases, pentose sugars and linking phosphate groups. In the past decade, medicinal chemistry has allowed significant improvements in the drug-like properties of ODN including the potential to optimize the stability as well as the pharmacologic, pharmacokinetic and toxicologic properties of these molecules. In general, three types of modifications of ODN can be distinguished. The first type of modification, and the one most commonly used, is the replacement of the oxygen atoms of the naturally occurring phosphodiester bond by sulfur groups (phosphorothioate (PS) linkages) to confer stability to the drug molecule. Nucleotide analogs have also been incorporated. For example, adenosine has been replaced with 2-amino-2'-deoxydenosine, which improves binding of the drug to the target and minimizes the potential for bronchospasm and inflammation induced by adenosine (Vollmer et al. 2004). Finally, the sugar moiety can be modified; for example, the addition of a 2'-O-methoxyethyl group to the pentose sugar confers stability to the ODN and enhances binding affinity to the target mRNA (Ward 2010).

The AON constituents comprising PXS TPI1100 incorporate two modifications: a modified phosphate backbone and the incorporation of 2-amino-2'-deozyadenosine. These modifications were aimed at improving the binding affinity of the drug to its mRNA target, reduce the immunostimulatory effect of this class of drug, and improve the lung tolerability after administration by the pulmonary route. In vivo testing of these molecules by multiple dosing via intratracheal (i.t.) administration in mice demonstrated that the modified chemistry contained in the PXS TPI1100 sequences was far less immunostimulatory than the typical PS-containing AON. Repeated daily i.t. delivery of PS-containing AON at a dose of 2.5 mg/kg induced a 4-fold increase in the recruitment of total cells in bronchoalveolar lavage (BAL) compared to control mice (treated with vehicle) and lung tissue changes as assessed by the presence of moderate (grade 3) perivascular mixed cell infiltrate and severe (grade 4) alveolar inflammation. In contrast, in mice treated with the same dose of AON bearing the modified chemistry no difference in BAL cells (total cells as well as differential cells) as compared to the vehicle group were observed, nor were there any histopathological changes in the lung following administration of the modified AON demonstrating an overall improved lung tolerability.

3.2 Drug design

The drug candidate, PXS TPI1100, is a 1:1 mixture of two AON, one which targets two isoforms of PDE4 (4B and 4D) and the second AON targeting PDE7A (Fortin et al. 2008). The rationale for developing these new specific and multi-targeted AON is to provide a new class of anti-inflammatory agents that act more broadly on the underlying inflammatory-triad - recruitment, activation and potentiation of processes in chronic respiratory diseases and that is more potent than selective PDE4 inhibitors. Delivery directly to the site of action, the lung, will ensure local deposition of the drug and limited systemic exposure thus reducing potential side effects associated with the systemic delivery (e.g. oral delivery) of PDE4 inhibitors. Lastly, PXS TPI1100 consists of aerosolization of a simple aqueous solution, and does not require any specialized carriers.

AON drugs, while still early in development, possess properties that could be advantageous over classical small molecule drugs (Table 2). First, as a single mRNA strand can be translated into multiple copies of proteins (~5000 copies), there is a clear advantage of "upstream" targeting, that is targeting the mRNA rather than the protein (Popescu 2005). The "upstream" targeting approaching with AON can be achieved irrespectively of the location of the target protein, whether it is inside the cell or outside the cell. AON have the potential to amplify

Potential advantages	• High degree of specificity (primarily for RNA-targeted drugs)
	• Broad range of potential targets
	• Ability to modify the properties of the oligonucleotide through chemical modification
	• Ability to screen efficiently for off-target effects
	• Absence of hypersensitivity reactions
	• Relatively short development timelines
	• Relative ease of formulation for inhaled delivery
	• Relative ease of formulation of combination products
	• Relative stability of drug compound and product
Challenges	• Cellular uptake and intracellular release for larger oligonucleotides
	• Potential immunostimulatory effects
	• Oligonucleotide stability
	• Specific systemic toxicological findings
Potential advantages of application in lung disease	• Multi-targeting feasible
	• Direct delivery to the site of action in the lungs
	• Cellular uptake and release without additional carrier or formulation technologies
	• Low systemic exposure

Table 2. Advantages and challenges in the development of antisense oligonucleotides drug candidates.

potency as compared to small molecule drugs which target the protein directly. Furthermore, by targeting the mRNA this method avoids the complications of protein interactions and effects of phosphorylation which can be of concern for PDE inhibitors.

By its very nature, AON are designed to target a specific RNA sequence and this specificity lends an advantage over ICS. As comparison, corticosteroids which are believed to directly regulate between 10 to 100 genes per cell, with a further estimation of many other genes indirectly regulated through interaction of other transcription factors and coactivators by yet unclarified mechanisms (Barnes 2006). In contrast, the inherent specificity of AON for its target avoids the non-selective inhibition nature of steroids. However, AON, as all drugs, have the potential of causing unwanted toxicities or side effects, of which some of these unwanted toxicities can arise because of the inherent capacity of AON to hybridize to RNA. Such toxicities are termed hybridization-dependent and can be subdivided into effects caused by exaggerated pharmacology, i.e. inhibition of the intended target to a degree that produces deleterious effects, and hybridization-dependent effects on unintended RNA targets (off-targets) that happen to be completely or partially complementary to the AON sequence. For the former, with recent advances for the modifications of the AON chemistry to improve binding affinity, as well as improvements for more effective delivery systems, there could be potential risk in designing AON that are too effective. Correct dosing assessment would be imperative. With regard to off-target effects, the use of genomic information databases allows for identification of possible off targets early in the drug discovery process. Any potential off targets can then be monitored both during the preclinical development and safety assessment stage as well as in clinical studies if needed. Along with the hybridization-dependent toxicities, there are also hybridization-independent which are due to interactions between the AON and proteins. The majority of toxicities observed for AON tested to date are hybridization independent and result from AON chemistry or composition of the delivery system and such potential is assessed in animal toxicology studies (Levin et al. 2001).

A further advantage of AON is the common composition and chemical nature of AON allow for an ease in combining two or more AON for a multi-targeted drug, unlike typical combination therapies. Historically, combination therapies have resulted from combining two marketed drugs into a single drug product. In the respiratory space, the combination of a corticosteroid with a long acting β2-adrenergic receptor agonist has been effective at producing billion dollar drugs like Advair (fluticasone/salmeterol), and Symbicort (budesonide/formoterol). Each of the individual components of these drugs had undergone the development process as single entities which were then combined later for a final product. However, the current understanding of various disease systems would suggest the selection and development of drugs that contain at least 2 molecules directed against at least 2 targets from the beginning of the development process.

The rationale for developing these new specific and multi-targeted ODN inhibitors is to provide a new class of anti-inflammatory agents that act more broadly on the underlying inflammatory-triad - recruitment, activation and potentiation of processes in chronic respiratory diseases. Complex diseases require multiple approaches to circumvent the cellular signaling redundancy underlying inflammatory conditions. In an attempt to improve bronchoconstriction and airway hyperresponsiveness in respiratory diseases, drugs have been designed to modulate the immune response by targeting immune mediators such as cytokines, chemokines or their receptors. It is believed that in order to treat chronic inflammation a single drug directed against multiple targets and pathways would be better at arresting the progression of these respiratory diseases. However, to date there has been limited success with therapies targeting either a single cytokine, chemokine or their receptor highlighting the challenge in treating these complex inflammatory diseases by focusing on a single component or aspect of the inflammation process. Drugs acting on individual molecular targets usually exert unsatisfying therapeutic effects or have severe toxicity or undesired side effects when used in diseases of complicated causes such as in oncology or in inflammatory diseases. One approach to address such limited efficacy and toxicity has been by the development of novel therapies using a mixture of molecules. In oncology for example, a prevailing idea is that inhibiting both cancer cells and cells of the stroma supporting the tumor or blood vessels would gain better results in fighting this disease.

There is a fine balance between specificity and reduced toxicity that can be obtained by targeting more than one cytokine or chemokine or receptor in the immune response without the overwhelming suppression observed with corticosteroids. The era of designing "one target for one disease" has evolved such that the single-target therapy is fading in favor of a multi-targeted approach and the new generation therapies are selected on the basis of their ability to simultaneously inhibit or affect several targets. Through combining two or more molecules which individually have their own target into a single therapeutic product, it may be possible to generate a drug that is potentially more effective, in particular in those patients non-responding to the conventional therapies. In addition, the lower doses could results in less side effects than with broader therapies like corticosteroids. This approach is especially important because of the redundancy of inflammatory pathways indicates the need for AON against multiple genes in one product.

Lastly, PXS TPI1100 consists of aerosolization of a simple aqueous solution, and does not require any specialized carriers unlike many other AON therapies. Indeed, direct administration of low doses to the site of action by inhalation permits AON to efficiently reach and enter the target cells (Figure 2).

3.3 Preclinical pharmacology

In vitro pharmacology studies of the AON candidates of PXS TPI1100 were conducted in both human and animal cell cultures. Results in normal human bronchoepithelial (NHBE) primary cells and a lung epithelial cell line (A549) confirmed the efficacy of PXS TPI1100 at reducing PDE mRNA target knockdown, which is the proposed mechanism of action of the drug. Moreover, in NHBE cells, inhibition of the PDE4B, PDE4D and PDE7A with PXS TPI 1100 resulted with a synergistic effect on the inhibition of IL-8 secretion in response to a stimulus (a mixture of cytokines TNF-α, IL-1β and IFN-γ) compared to when cells were treated with each AON alone (Figure 3). These results and the lack of efficacy of rolipram (small molecule PDE4 inhibitor) on IL-8 confirmed the benefit of PDE4 and PDE7 inhibition. Besides IL-8, cells treated with PXS TPI1100 had an inhibition of the expression and release of other inflammatory mediators (e.g. MCP-1, MMPs). A second model used the lung epithelial cell line, A549, stimulated with the cytokine IL-1β, and again the inhibitory effect of PXS TPI1100 upon the induction of key inflammatory mediators (IL-8, MCP-1) in response to IL-1β was observed.

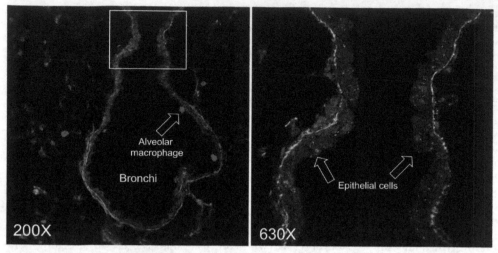

Fig. 2. Intracellular localization of PXS TPI1100 AON constituents in the lung of mice following cigarette smoke exposure. Mice exposed to cigarette smoke were treated intratracheally with a single dose of labelled PXS TPI1100 (a FITC-labeled AON against PDE4B/4D) and a Cy3-labeled AON against PDE7A. Images obtained using a confocal microscope (FITC in green, Cy3 in red and DAPI in blue). Magnification of 200X (left panel) and insert shown at 630X (right panel).

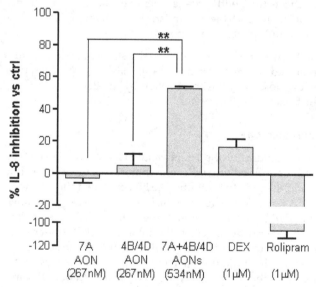

Fig. 3. Activity of PXS TPI1100 in NHBE cells. NHBE cells were treated with the PDE7A or the PDE4B/4D AON alone at indicated concentration or in combination prior to stimulation of the cells (mix of TNF-α, IL-1β and IFN-γ). Inhibition of the three PDE isoforms resulted with a synergistic effect (**p<0.05) on IL-8 secretion compared to each AON alone, and a more potent effect than rolipram or dexamethasone (DEX).

In two different *in vivo* models, PXS TPI1100 was shown to reduce the neutrophil influx in the BAL of mice either in response to cigarette smoke or to LPS challenge. Cigarette smoke exposure of laboratory animals reproduces many of the anatomic/physiologic lesions (neutrophilic inflammation, emphysema, small-airway remodeling and pulmonary hypertension) of human COPD (Wright et al. 2008) and has been used for the preclinical assessment of Daxas/Deliresp (Martorana et al. 2005). In this model, mice were exposed to cigarette smoke for 4 consecutive days and treated with PXS TPI1100 every other day (two treatments only) 3 h prior to cigarette smoke exposure. Following repeated smoke exposure, a significant increase (180-fold) recruitment of neutrophils in BAL collected the day after the last smoke exposure was observed compared to mice not exposed to smoke. The percentage of neutrophils in BAL also increased with smoke from 0.8% to 35%. When mice were treated with PXS TPI1100 at 0.1 or 0.4 mg/kg every other day, the smoke-induced neutrophil recruitment was significantly reduced (up to 52% inhibition p<0.01) when compared to mice treated with vehicle or a comparable dose of a control AON.

In the second model of acute lung inflammation, mice exposed to LPS (nasal instillation) had a strong inflammatory response with significant increase in neutrophils in BAL. PXS TPI1100 treatment at 1.2 mg/kg (1 h prior to LPS challenge) resulted in a 33% reduction of neutrophil recruitment induced by LPS (p<0.05) whereas treatment with the control AON had no effect.

The potency of PXS TPI1100 at reducing the smoke-induced or LPS-induced lung inflammation was compared to the PDE4 inhibitor roflumilast (Daxas). Roflumilast (5 mg/kg, p.o.) given daily 1 h prior to cigarette smoke exposure reduced neutrophil recruitment by only 25% (Fortin et al., 2009). In the LPS model, roflumilast, given once at a dose of 10 mg/kg (~10-fold more than PXS TPI1100) had no effect on the neutrophil influx, whereas at a higher dose of 100 mg/kg (~100-fold that of PXS TPI1100) it reduced neutrophil recruitment by 46% (p<0.05). This effective dose of roflumilast exceeds the current clinical dose for Daxas of 500 microgram per adult per day. PXS TPI1100 is continuing its pre-clinical development as a treatment for COPD.

PXS TPI1100 has not yet performed nonclinical drug depositions studies however, from tests with different AON that recognize the same PDE targets yet lacked the modified chemistry backbone we can extrapolate how PXS TPI1100 will behave following pulmonary delivery. In CD-1 mice, following 14 days of daily dosing with AON by inhalation, AON plasma concentrations were not detectable (< LLOQ of 5-10 ng/mL) at all time points for all dose levels. In the lungs, the AON concentrations were dose-related, and there was evidence of accumulation in lungs over the 14 days, based on the higher levels at 24 h after the last dose *vs.* 24 h after the first dose. The systemic exposure was extremely low with only small amounts of AON detectable in the kidneys and liver of high-dose mice (2.5 mg/kg/day), and the levels were similar following the first and last doses. In monkeys, following 14 days of inhalation of AON there were detectable levels of AON in plasma only in a few high-dose animals up to 1 h post dosing on Day 1 while samples from Day 14 were all <LLOQ (Guimond et al. 2008). In the lung of animals on the day after last drug exposure, the AON levels were approximately dose proportional. In kidney and liver, low levels of AON were quantified one day after the last dose and only in high dose animals, demonstrating that similar to mice, the systemic exposure was low. When AON were delivered by slow bolus intravenous (IV) administration in monkey, the highest plasma levels were measured immediately at the first time point after IV

injection (approximately 5 min) and these levels were greatly reduced by 4 h post-dose and near LLOQ by 24 h demonstrating the clearance of AON from the system.

The pharmacokinetics properties following pulmonary delivery has been well characterized (Templin et al. 2000; Ali et al. 2001; Guimond et al. 2008) and confers a significant advantage of AON over small molecule drugs. For example, orally-delivered Daxas/Daliresp has a bioavailabilty of 79% (David 2004) and with an elimination half-life of 14-18 h there is a greater opportunity for this drug to act upon PDE4 outside of the lung and for a long period of time. In comparison, PXS TPI1100 has reduced systemic bioavailability and based on results in mouse lung, the half-life of PXS TPI 1100 has been shown to be relatively short (<5h) suggesting a potentially safer drug that would work locally at the site of action in the lung.

3.4 Clinical experience

To date, PXS TPI1100 has not been dosed in human subjects, however, a review of the current literature on clinical study designs and using the Daxas/Daliresp background as guidance, the projected clinical path for PXS TPI1100 has been defined. Furthermore, reviewing its pharmacology profile, there are potential advantages for PXS TPI1100 which may be manifested in the clinic. In this section, we will first outline some general challenges facing COPD clinical study design, then capture some of the salient points from the Daxas/Daliresp experience in clinical study design.

3.4.1 Challenges in COPD clinical studies

Typically COPD clinical studies measure as a primary outcome lung function by spirometry, either through improvement in postbronchodilator FEV_1 or in cases where assessing the efficacy of nonbronchodilators is preferred, the measure is of the change from baseline in prebronchodilator FEV_1 (Giembycz &Field 2010). As a procedure for detection of airflow obstructions spirometry is a reliable, simple, non-invasive, safe, and non-expensive (Soriano et al. 2009). The test is relatively standardized with most COPD guidelines accepting the threshold to define a positive bronchodilation test as suggested by the Global Initiative for asthma (increase in FEV_1 larger than 12% and 200 mL from the prebronchodilator value) (Bateman et al. 2008) with the variation of suggesting minimum limits of 300 or 400 mL.

Besides the use of these spirometry measures, there have been attempts to determine a relevant easily accessible and rapid assessed biomarker as a measure of improvement. In preclinical pharmacology studies, animal models of neutrophil inflammation are routinely used for efficacy measures in an attempt to mimic the disease state in humans. It is known that in COPD patients the percentage of sputum neutrophils are increased with each GOLD stage, are also raised in COPD exacerbations (Caramori et al. 2003) (Papi et al. 2006), and that neutrophils are involved in the pathogenesis of emphysema through the secretion of proteases and elastases (Cowburn et al. 2008) (Sharafkhaneh et al. 2008). Taken together, these observations would suggest that sputum neutrophils have the potential to be a biomarker predictor of the degree of airflow obstruction, however the reality is far from clear. Reports with small cohorts of patients suggest a relationship between sputum neutrophils measures and FEV_1 (% predicted) (O'Donnell et al. 2004), however a larger cohort study by Singh et al. (Singh et al. 2010) demonstrated that this relationship is only weakly associated. A similar finding was shown with regard to sputum neutrophils measures and the relationship to health status as defined by the use of the St. Georges Respiratory Questionnaire (SGRQ) (Singh et al. 2010). Furthermore sputum neutrophil measures in the stable state were shown not be predictive of the future rate of exacerbations (Singh et al. 2010). Lastly, no association between sputum neutrophils measures and emphysema or systemic inflammation as measured by serum levels of IL-6, IL-8, C-reactive protein (CRP) and surfactant protein D was observed (Singh et al. 2010). In short, although there is a plausible assumption for the use of sputum neutrophils as a biomarker, there is little validity in using them in face of the current evidence.

In lieu of the identification and validation of a biomarker that could predict the rate of lung function decline in COPD, most COPD clinical trials attempt to measure relevant changes in exacerbations. Exacerbation frequency has been considered to be an important outcome parameter in COPD as it is associated with increase in mortality (Patil et al. 2003) (Fuso et al. 1995). Measuring exacerbations is not without its challenges. It is difficult among studies to find consensus on what is defined as an exacerbation and to gauge the severity of the exacerbation. Symptom-based definitions include use of diaries, while event-based definitions may refer to hospitalizations or use of antibiotics and/or steroids (Miravitlles et al. 2004). Although a systematic literature review of studies reporting exacerbation frequency in COPD patients showed the relationship between increased exacerbation frequency with decreasing lung function to be borderline significance (p=0.053) (Spencer et al. 2004), exacerbations are still considered to be an important parameter in COPD. Exacerbations are more likely to occur in winter and according to current recommendations (Cazzola et al. 2008) studies need to have at least a 12 month follow up to give reliable estimate of exacerbation frequency, which requires the planning of lengthy clinical trials.

The clinical program of PXS TPI1100 has not been initiated yet we expect its design can follow that of other PDE4 inhibitors. An initial Phase 2 study design does not test in COPD patients but rather in allergic asthmatic patients following inhaled allergen challenge (2009). Another AON drug, ASM8 designed specifically for asthma and as such has targets different from PXS TPI1100, has demonstrated clinical efficacy in this allergen challenge model (Gauvreau et al. 2008; Gauvreau 2010) clearly showing the potential for the AON approach. An advantage of this allergen challenge model is that the studies are generally brief in duration and the fall in FEV_1 is a well-recognized response as well as the incorporation of monitoring induced sputum allows for other inflammatory indicators to be measured.

PXS TPI1100 has an advantage in that the clinical studies performed by Daxas/Daliresp can be used as a guide, as the two drugs share a common target. As Daxas/Daliresp was breaking new ground many studies had to be performed and it is plausible to conclude that for other drugs in the same class fewer studies may be required. In all, six phase 3 clinical trials were undertaken with Daxas/Daliresp which have been excellently reviewed by Giembycz and Field (Giembycz &Field 2010). Key aspects of these trials that can be used for PXS TPI1100's clinical development include criteria for patient selection and parameters selected for primary and secondary outcomes. In the phase 3 study named RECORD, patients with moderate-to-severe COPD (postbronchodilator FEV_1 of 30% to 80% predicted and a FEV_1/FVC ratio of less than 70%) were randomized to receive either Daxas/Daliresp at 250 µg or 500 µg or placebo (2:2:1 ratio) for 24 weeks (Rabe et al. 2005). Results showed treated patients experienced improvement in postbronchodilator FEV_1 (Rabe et al. 2005) and a change in SGRQ but this change did not reach clinical significant threshold. Although direct comparisons between doses were not made, as it seemed that patients receiving the higher dose had better and earlier responses in most outcomes the daily dose of Daxas/Daliresp of 500 µg was then used in two subsequent identical trials (RATIO and OPUS). In these studies the patients had more severe COPD than in the RECORD study (postbronchodilator FEV_1 of 50% or less, FEV_1:FVC ratio of 0.7 or less, or FEV_1 reversibility of 5% or less). Although completed, the results from the OPUS trial have not been published, however results from the RATIO study showed an improvement for the change from baseline for post bronchodilator FEV_1, yet again no effect on the SGRQ (Calverley et al. 2007). A post-hoc analysis of a subgroup of patients with GOLD stage IV disease in the RECORD study showed a significant effect on reduction of exacerbation frequency (Calverley et al. 2007) which then led to the design of two identical studies AURA and HERMES where patients had a diagnosis of clinical COPD (confirmed by postbronchodilator FEV_1/FVC of at least 70%, and a FEV_1 at least 50% of predicted), had symptoms of chronic bronchitis and a history of exacerbations. Patients experienced an improvement in pre- and postbronchodilator FEV_1 and a reduction in exacerbation rate (Calverley et al. 2009) which were independent of LABA use, but no differences in mortality or C-reactive protein levels.

Taken together, the Daxas/Daliresp studies clearly show effects in patients with GOLD stage IV disease, with focus on measuring flow rates and exacerbation reduction as parameter outcomes. The clinical program for PXS TPI1100 can use this information in designing studies so as to sharply define the patient population at the onset and include the key primary outcomes as success measures.

As ICS and LABA have been shown to be more effective at improving lung function, health status and reducing COPD exacerbations when combined than when used individually (Calverley et al. 2007) the effect of combining Daxas/Daliresp with either the long-acting β2-agonist salmeterol (EOS study) or the long-acting inhaled antimuscarinic tiotroprium (HELIOS study) was studied in patients with less severely reduced lung function as compared to the previous studies. Results showed that the pre- and postbronchodilator FEV_1 improved in patients treated with Daxas/Daliresp versus placebo when combined with either LABA or LAMA (Fabbri et al. 2009). PXS TPI1100 can be expected to also function in combination with LABA, similar to that demonstrated by Daxas/Daliresp and could potentially replace ICS.

As with any drug, adverse events to Daxas/Daliresp were reported which included weight loss, diarrhea, nausea, headache, influenza and nasopharyngitis as well as certain cancers such as lung and prostate (Giembycz &Field 2010). There was a greater risk of discontinuation of therapy within the first 12 weeks of treatment for those patients taking Daxas/Daliresp than placebo although by the end of the studies, similar numbers of patients withdrew in both groups. In the Daxas/Daliresp treated groups, the most common reason for withdrawal were the gastrointestinal adverse events or headache (Giembycz &Field 2010).

There are aspects of PXS TPI1100 which may lend itself advantages over Daxas/Daliresp. Firstly, as PXS TPI1100 is administered via inhalation, it is delivered directly to the intended site of action of the lung (Ali et al. 2001; Duan et al. 2005; Gauvreau et al. 2008; Guimond et al. 2008) where the drug can enter target cells directly (Zhang et al. 2004; Griesenbach et al. 2006) thus potentially reducing total dose as compared to orally-available treatments. A further advantage of pulmonary administration of AON is that they are principally metabolized in the lung with very limited systemic delivery after inhalation (Templin et al. 2000; Ali et al. 2001; Guimond et al. 2008) which leads to reduced systemic bioavailability of the drug. In comparison to Daxas/Daliresp, which is delivered orally and has a high level of bioavailability, the projected low systemic bioavailability of PXS TPI1100 may limit adverse events associated with PDE4 inhibitors, namely the gastrointestinal and neurological side effects. Another consideration is the projected brief half-life of PXS TPI1100. Based on the mouse lung, the half-life of PXS TPI1100 has been shown to be relatively short (<5h), although it is reassuring that this short tissue half-life does not appear to affect the efficacy of the drug as every-other day dosing of PXS TPI1100 in the smoking mouse model was highly effective. Reconciling the short half-life with longer term efficacy may be a reflection of the mechanism of action of the drug, suggesting that inhibition of PDE mRNA has longer term consequences on downstream effects including limitation of inflammatory responses.

Besides a projected favorable safety profile resulting from low systemic bioavailability, PXS TPI1100 can be expected to avoid the toxicity associated with the broader approach of anti-inflammatories such as ICS by specifically targeting PDE.

4. Conclusions

PXS TPI1100 faces challenges, in part of being the first respirable antisense drug product in COPD. As COPD is a chronic disease, it can be expected that patients will be dosed for years. The long-term effects of this drug class have never before been studied. In addition, in pulmonary/respiratory diseases, there is a risk that administration of therapeutic nucleic acids may lead to immune stimulation, inflammation and possibly hypersensitivity and bronchoconstriction of the airways. Except for the latter, these risks are not specific to the lung as they have been observed with other routes of administration. As with any novel inhaled medication, local tolerability and the absence of long-term effects following chronic dosing will require careful evaluation as drug candidate progresses through the later stages of development. The publicly available toxicological data on inhaled AON are not extensive (Guimond et al. 2008), and therefore deriving definitive conclusions on toxicology at this time is not possible. The phase 2a studies that have been performed until now have not shown any of this potential toxicity but longer term studies are needed to confirm these results. Furthermore, to date AON have been delivered via inhalation of a nebulisate to asthma patients (Gauvreau et al. 2008; Gauvreau 2010), but not to COPD patients who have severely decreased FEV_1. How well this patient cohort inhales the nebulisate would need to be determined. The range of delivery devices (including newer portable soft-mist inhalers) have increased and permit liquid aerosols to be targeted more effectively to the specific airways of interest (upper or lower airways), improve ease of use by patients and would be expected to improve compliance to therapy. In contrast, the particle processing and formulation of AON for delivery in dry powder inhalers or pressurized metered dose inhalers, which are most commonly used by COPD patients has, however, proven to be significantly more challenging than that of liquid aerosols.

Another challenge facing PXS TPI1100 is the selection of its targets PDE4B/D and PDE7A. While the success of Daxas/Daliresp demonstrates the effectiveness of targeting PDE4 in COPD, to date there is less corroborative clinical evidence for the efficacy of targeting PDE7A isoform. The success or failure of a specific drug development program is determined by a range of different factors, which includes the clinical relevance of the selected drug target.

One early pioneer in the respiratory field was the AON drug EPI 2010 (Epigenesis) targeting the promoter region of the adenosine A1 receptor. Although demonstrating efficacy *in vitro* and in animal models (Ball et al. 2004), EPI 2010 failed in later clinical studies to demonstrate efficacy to improve lung function in asthmatics. With the more recent understanding of the role the different adenosine receptors have in asthma (Brown et al. 2008), it could be argued that the absence of clinical efficacy for EPI 2010 could either be a result of targeting the wrong adenosine receptor or perhaps the need to combine it with other adenosine receptor inhibitors. Similarly, early preclinical efficacy and effect on biomarkers in a phase 1 study with AIR-645 (AON targeting IL-4/IL-13Rα Altair/Isis) met with apparent insufficient efficacy on lung function in phase 2 study (personal communication). This may perhaps be attributed to the target selection as other non-ODN drugs targeting these receptors have also had limited success in clinical trials. As mentioned, although few PDE7 inhibitors have been tested in clinical studies, our preclinical pharmacology results indicate a clear benefit in targeting this PDE isoform along with the PDE4. There is growing acceptance that multi-targeted approaches may provide significant therapeutic advantages, as demonstrated by the issuance of new guidance on drug combinations by the Food and Drug Administration.

There is a clear need for innovative products with novel mechanisms of action to complement today's inhaled products particularly for severe patients who seem resistant to current therapeutic interventions. In spite of many attempts, success in these respiratory indications has been modest, at most. This may reflect the challenge of delivering the therapies to the site of action (lung) or more importantly the complexity of these diseases. PXS TPI1100 belongs to a new class of therapeutics that is poised to expand in the upcoming decades because of its advantages, especially with lung administration. Outstanding challenges for PXS TPI1100 remain the need to establish long term safety and tolerability data as well as commence clinical efficacy. The future remains very promising for this novel drug.

5. Acknowledgements

The authors wish to thank Drs. Ian McDonald, Wolfgang Jarolimek and Gary Phillips for critical review of the manuscript.

6. References

(2009). Study To Evaluate GSK256066 In Subjects With Mild Bronchial Asthma.

Agrawal, S. and Kandimalla, E. R. (2007). Synthetic agonists of Toll-like receptors 7, 8 and 9 *Biochem. Soci. Trans.* Vol.35 No.(6): pp.1461-1467

Ali, S., Leonard, S. A., Kukoly, C. A., James Metzger, W., Wooles, W. R., McGinty, J. F., Tanaka, M., Sandrasagra, A. and Nyce, J. W. (2001). Absorption, Distribution, Metabolism, and Excretion of a Respirable Antisense Oligonucleotide for Asthma *Am. J. Respir. Crit. Care Med.* Vol.163 No.(4): pp.989-993

Ariga, M., Neitzert, B., Nakae, S., Mottin, G., Bertrand, C., Pruniaux, M. P., Jin, S. L. C. and Conti, M. (2004). Nonredundant Function of Phosphodiesterases 4D and 4B in Neutrophil Recruitment to the Site of Inflammation *J Immunol* Vol.173 7531-7538

Ball, H. A., Van Scott, M. R. and Robinson, C. B. (2004). Sense and antisense: therapeutic potential of oligonucleotides and interference RNA in asthma and allergic disorders *Clin Rev Allergy Immunol* Vol.27 No.(3): pp.207-217

Barnes, P. J. (2006). How corticosteroids control inflammation: Quintiles Prize Lecture 2005 *Br J Pharmacol* Vol.148 No.(3): pp.245-254

Bateman, E. D., Hurd, S. S., Barnes, P. J., Bousquet, J., Drazen, J. M., FitzGerald, M., Gibson, P., Ohta, K., O'Byrne, P., Pedersen, S. E., Pizzichini, E., Sullivan, S. D., Wenzel, S. E. and Zar, H. J. (2008). Global strategy for asthma management and prevention: GINA executive summary *Eur. Respir. J.* Vol.31 No.(1): pp.143-178

Bender, A. T. and Beavo, J. A. (2006). Cyclic nucleotide phosphodiesterases: molecular regulation to clinical use *Pharmacol Rev* Vol.58 No.(3): pp.488-520

Bloom, T. J. and Beavo, J. A. (1996). Identification and tissue-specific expression of PDE7 phosphodiesterase splice variants *Proc Natl Acad Sci U S A* Vol.93 No.(24): pp.14188-14192

Brown, R. A., Spina, D. and Page, C. P. (2008). Adenosine receptors and asthma *Br J Pharmacol* Vol.153 Suppl 1 S446-456

Calverley, P. M., Anderson, J. A., Celli, B., Ferguson, G. T., Jenkins, C., Jones, P. W., Yates, J. C. and Vestbo, J. (2007). Salmeterol and fluticasone propionate and survival in chronic obstructive pulmonary disease *N Engl J Med* Vol.356 No.(8): pp.775-789

Calverley, P. M., Rabe, K. F., Goehring, U. M., Kristiansen, S., Fabbri, L. M. and Martinez, F. J. (2009). Roflumilast in symptomatic chronic obstructive pulmonary disease: two randomised clinical trials *Lancet* Vol.374 No.(9691): pp.685-694

Calverley, P. M. A., Sanchez-Toril, F., McIvor, A., Teichmann, P., Bredenbroeker, D. and Fabbri, L. M. (2007). Effect of One Year Treatment with Roflumilast in Severe Chronic Obstructive Pulmonary Disease *Am. J. Respir. Crit. Care Med.* Vol.200610-201563OC

Caramori, G., Romagnoli, M., Casolari, P., Bellettato, C., Casoni, G., Boschetto, P., Chung, K. F., Barnes, P. J., Adcock, I. M., Ciaccia, A., Fabbri, L. M. and Papi, A. (2003). Nuclear localisation of p65 in sputum macrophages but not in sputum neutrophils during COPD exacerbations *Thorax* Vol.58 No.(4): pp.348-351

Cazzola, M., MacNee, W., Martinez, F. J., Rabe, K. F., Franciosi, L. G., Barnes, P. J., Brusasco, V., Burge, P. S., Calverley, P. M. A., Celli, B. R., Jones, P. W., Mahler, D. A., Make, B., Miravitlles, M., Page, C. P., Palange, P., Parr, D., Pistolesi, M., Rennard, S. I., Rutten-van Molken, M. P., Stockley, R., Sullivan, S. D., Wedzicha, J. A., Wouters, E. F. and on behalf of the American Thoracic Society/European Respiratory Society Task Force on outcomes of, C. (2008). Outcomes for COPD pharmacological trials: from lung function to biomarkers *Eur Respir J* Vol.31 No.(2): pp.416-469

Cowburn, A. S., Condliffe, A. M., Farahi, N., Summers, C. and Chilvers, E. R. (2008). Advances in neutrophil biology: clinical implications *Chest* Vol.134 606-612 0012-3692 (Print)

Crooke, S. T., Ed. (2008). *Antisense Drug Technology: Principles, Strategies and Applications*, CRC Press, Boca Raton FL

David, M., Zech. K., Seiberling, M., Weimar, C. and Bethke, TD. (2004). Roflumilast, a novel, oral, selective PDE4 inhibitor, shows high absolute bioavailabilty. *Journal of Allergy and Clinical Immunology* Vol.113 No.(suppl 2): pp.S220-221

Down, G., Siederer, S., Lim, S. and Daley-Yates, P. (2006). Clinical pharmacology of Cilomilast *Clin Pharmacokinet* Vol.45 No.(3): pp.217-233

Duan, W., Chan, J. H., McKay, K., Crosby, J. R., Choo, H. H., Leung, B. P., Karras, J. G. and Wong, W. S. (2005). Inhaled p38alpha mitogen-activated protein kinase antisense oligonucleotide attenuates asthma in mice *Am. J. Respir. Crit. Care Med.* Vol.171 571-578 1073-449X (Print)

Ellington, A. D. and Szostak, J. W. (1992). Selection in vitro of single-stranded DNA molecules that fold into specific ligand-binding structures *Nature* Vol.355 No.(6363): pp.850-852

Ernst, P., Gonzalez, A. V., Brassard, P. and Suissa, S. (2007). Inhaled corticosteroid use in chronic obstructive pulmonary disease and the risk of hospitalization for pneumonia *Am J Respir Crit Care Med* Vol.176 No.(2): pp.162-166

Fabbri, L. M., Calverley, P. M., Izquierdo-Alonso, J. L., Bundschuh, D. S., Brose, M., Martinez, F. J. and Rabe, K. F. (2009). Roflumilast in moderate-to-severe chronic obstructive pulmonary disease treated with longacting bronchodilators: two randomised clinical trials *Lancet* Vol.374 No.(9691): pp.695-703

Fortin, M., Higgins, M., Aubé, P., Séguin, S., Moktefi, K., Paquet, L. and Ferrari, N. (2008). TPI 1100: An inhaled antisense oligonucleotide (AON) against phosphodiesterase (PDE) 4 and 7 with significant anti-inflammatory effects in a mouse model for COPD [abstract]. Am. J. Respir. Crit. Care Med. 177: A653.

Fuso, L., Incalzi, R. A., Pistelli, R., Muzzolon, R., Valente, S., Pagliari, G., Gliozzi, F. and Ciappi, G. (1995). Predicting mortality of patients hospitalized for acutely exacerbated chronic obstructive pulmonary disease *Am J Med* Vol.98 No.(3): pp.272-277

Gauvreau, G. M., Boulet, L. P., Cockcroft, D. W., Baatjes, A., Cote, J., Deschesnes, F., Davis, B., Strinich, T., Howie, K., Duong, M., Watson, R. M., Renzi, P. M. and O'Byrne, P. M. (2008). Antisense Therapy against CCR3 and the Common Beta Chain Attenuates Allergen-induced Eosinophilic Responses *Am. J. Respir. Crit. Care Med.* Vol.177 952-958

Gauvreau, G. M., Pageau, R., Seguin, R., Carballo, D., D'Anjou, H., Campbell, H., Watson, R., Parry-Billings, M., Killian, K., and Renzi, P.M. (2010). Efficacy of increasing doses of TPI ASM8 on allergen inhalation challenges in asthmatics. *American Thoracic Society*New Orleans

Giembycz, M. A. and Field, S. K. (2010). Roflumilast: first phosphodiesterase 4 inhibitor approved for treatment of COPD. *Drug Des. Devel. Ther.* Vol.4 147-158

Gold, P. M. (2009). The 2007 GOLD Guidelines: a comprehensive care framework *Respir Care* Vol.54 No.(8): pp.1040-1049

Griesenbach, U., Kitson, C., Escudero Garcia, S., Farley, R., Singh, C., Somerton, L., Painter, H., Smith, R. L., Gill, D. R., Hyde, S. C., Chow, Y. H., Hu, J., Gray, M., Edbrooke, M., Ogilvie, V., MacGregor, G., Scheule, R. K., Cheng, S. H., Caplen, N. J. and Alton, E. W. (2006). Inefficient cationic lipid-mediated siRNA and antisense oligonucleotide transfer to airway epithelial cells in vivo *Respir. Res.* Vol.7 26 1465-993X (Electronic)

Guimond, A., Viau, E., Aube, P., Renzi, P. M., Paquet, L. and Ferrari, N. (2008). Advantageous toxicity profile of inhaled antisense oligonucleotides following chronic dosing in non-human primates *Pulm. Pharmacol. Ther.* Vol.21 845-854 1094-5539 (Print)

Han, P., Zhu, X. and Michaeli, T. (1997). Alternative splicing of the high affinity cAMP-specific phosphodiesterase (PDE7A) mRNA in human skeletal muscle and heart *J Biol Chem* Vol.272 No.(26): pp.16152-16157

Hogg, J. C., Chu, F., Utokaparch, S., Woods, R., Elliott, W. M., Buzatu, L., Cherniack, R. M., Rogers, R. M., Sciurba, F. C., Coxson, H. O. and Pare, P. D. (2004). The nature of small-airway obstruction in chronic obstructive pulmonary disease *N Engl J Med* Vol.350 No.(26): pp.2645-2653

Holen, T., Amarzguioui, M., Babaie, E. and Prydz, H. (2003). Similar behaviour of single-strand and double-strand siRNAs suggests they act through a common RNAi pathway *Nucleic Acids Res.* Vol.31 No.(9): pp.2401-2407

Hurst, J. R., Vestbo, J., Anzueto, A., Locantore, N., Mullerova, H., Tal-Singer, R., Miller, B., Lomas, D. A., Agusti, A., Macnee, W., Calverley, P., Rennard, S., Wouters, E. F. and Wedzicha, J. A. (2010). Susceptibility to exacerbation in chronic obstructive pulmonary disease *N Engl J Med* Vol.363 No.(12): pp.1128-1138

Jayasena, S. D. (1999). Aptamers: An Emerging Class of Molecules That Rival Antibodies in Diagnostics *Clin. Chem.* Vol.45 No.(9): pp.1628-1650

Jin, S. L. C. and Conti, M. (2002). Induction of the cyclic nucleotide phosphodiesterase PDE4B is essential for LPS-activated TNF-alpha responses *PNAS* Vol.99 No.(11): pp.7628-7633

Jin, S. L. C., Lan, L., Zoudilova, M. and Conti, M. (2005). Specific Role of Phosphodiesterase 4B in Lipopolysaccharide-Induced Signaling in Mouse Macrophages *J Immunol* Vol.175 1523-1531

Johnson, Z., Schwarz, M., Power, C. A., Wells, T. N. C. and Proudfoot, A. E. I. (2005). Multi-faceted strategies to combat disease by interference with the chemokine system *Trends Immunol.* Vol.26 No.(5): pp.268-274

Lee, J. F., Stovall, G. M. and Ellington, A. D. (2006). Aptamer therapeutics advance *Curr. Opin. Chem. Biol.* Vol.10 No.(3): pp.282-289

Levin, A. A., Henry, S. P., Monteith, D. K. and Templin, M. (2001). Toxicity of antisense oligonucleotides. Antisense Drug Technology: Principles, Strategies, and Applications S. T. Crooke. New York, Marcel Dekker, Inc.: 201-267.

Li L, Yee C and JA., B. (1999). CD3- and CD28-dependent induction of PDE7 required for T cell activation. *Science.* Vol.283 No.(5403): pp.848-851

Lugnier, C. (2006). Cyclic nucleotide phosphodiesterase (PDE) superfamily: A new target for the development of specific therapeutic agents *Pharmacology & Therapeutics* Vol.109 No.(3): pp.366-398

Martorana, P. A., Beume, R., Lucattelli, M., Wollin, L. and Lungarella, G. (2005). Roflumilast Fully Prevents Emphysema in Mice Chronically Exposed to Cigarette Smoke *Am. J. Respir. Crit. Care Med.* Vol.172 No.(7): pp.848-853

Mehats, C., Jin, S. L. C., Wahlstrom, J. A. N., Law, E., Umetsu, D. T. and Conti, M. (2003). PDE4D plays a critical role in the control of airway smooth muscle contraction *FASEB J.* Vol.17 No.(13): pp.1831-1841

Miravitlles, M., Ferrer, M., Pont, A., Zalacain, R., Alvarez-Sala, J. L., Masa, F., Verea, H., Murio, C., Ros, F. and Vidal, R. (2004). Effect of exacerbations on quality of life in patients with chronic obstructive pulmonary disease: a 2 year follow up study *Thorax* Vol.59 No.(5): pp.387-395

O'Donnell, R. A., Peebles, C., Ward, J. A., Daraker, A., Angco, G., Broberg, P., Pierrou, S., Lund, J., Holgate, S. T., Davies, D. E., Delany, D. J., Wilson, S. J. and Djukanovic, R. (2004). Relationship between peripheral airway dysfunction, airway obstruction, and neutrophilic inflammation in COPD *Thorax* Vol.59 No.(10): pp.837-842

Papi, A., Bellettato, C. M., Braccioni, F., Romagnoli, M., Casolari, P., Caramori, G., Fabbri, L. M. and Johnston, S. L. (2006). Infections and Airway Inflammation in Chronic Obstructive Pulmonary Disease Severe Exacerbations *Am. J. Respir. Crit. Care Med.* Vol.173 No.(10): pp.1114-1121

Patil, S. P., Krishnan, J. A., Lechtzin, N. and Diette, G. B. (2003). In-hospital mortality following acute exacerbations of chronic obstructive pulmonary disease *Arch Intern Med* Vol.163 No.(10): pp.1180-1186

Popescu, F.-D. (2005). Antisense- and RNA interference-based therapeutic strategies in allergy *J. Cell. Mol. Med.* Vol.9 No.(4): pp.840-853

Rabe, K. F., Bateman, E. D., O'Donnell, D., Witte, S., Bredenbroker, D. and Bethke, T. D. (2005). Roflumilast-an oral anti-inflammatory treatment for chronic obstructive pulmonary disease: a randomised controlled trial *Lancet* Vol.366 563-571 1474-547X (Electronic)

Sharafkhaneh, A., Hanania, N. A. and Kim, V. (2008). Pathogenesis of emphysema: from the bench to the bedside *Proc Am Thorac Soc* Vol.5 No.(4): pp.475-477

Singh, D., Edwards, L., Tal-Singer, R. and Rennard, S. (2010). Sputum neutrophils as a biomarker in COPD: findings from the ECLIPSE study *Respir Res* Vol.11 77

Smith, S. J., Brookes-Fazakerley, S., Donnelly, L. E., Barnes, P. J., Barnette, M. S. and Giembycz, M. A. (2003). Ubiquitous expression of phosphodiesterase 7A in human proinflammatory and immune cells *Am. J. Physiol. Lung Cell Mol. Physiol.* Vol.284 L279-289

Soriano, J. B., Zielinski, J. and Price, D. (2009). Screening for and early detection of chronic obstructive pulmonary disease *Lancet* Vol.374 No.(9691): pp.721-732

Spencer, S., Calverley, P. M., Burge, P. S. and Jones, P. W. (2004). Impact of preventing exacerbations on deterioration of health status in COPD *Eur Respir J* Vol.23 No.(5): pp.698-702

Stein, H. and Hausen, P. (1969). Enzyme from calf thymus degrading the RNA moiety of DNA-RNA Hybrids: effect on DNA-dependent RNA polymerase *Science* Vol.166 No.(903): pp.393-395

Tashkin, D. P., Celli, B., Senn, S., Burkhart, D., Kesten, S., Menjoge, S. and Decramer, M. (2008). A 4-year trial of tiotropium in chronic obstructive pulmonary disease *N Engl J Med* Vol.359 No.(15): pp.1543-1554

Templin, M., Levin, A., Graham, M., Aberg, P., Axelsson, B., Butler, M., Geary, R. and Bennett, C. (2000). Pharmacokinetic and toxicity profile of a phosphorothioate oligonucleotide following inhalation delivery to lung in mice. *Antisense Nucleic Acid Drug Dev.* Vol.10 No.(5): pp.359-368

Vollmer, J., Weeratna, R., Payette, P., Jurk, M., Schetter, C., Laucht, M., Wader, T., Tluk, S., Liu, M., Davis, H. L. and Krieg, A. M. (2004). Characterization of three CpG oligodeoxynucleotide classes with distinct immunostimulatory activities *Eur. J. Immunol.* Vol.34 No.(1): pp.251-262 1521-4141

Ward, P. A. (2010). Oxidative stress: acute and progressive lung injury *Annals of the New York Academy of Sciences* Vol.1203 No.(1): pp.53-59

Wright, J. L., Cosio, M. G. and Churg, A. (2008). Animal Models of Chronic Obstructive Pulmonary Disease *Am J Physiol Lung Cell Mol Physiol* Vol.90200.92008

Wu, H., MacLeod, A. R., Lima, W. F. and Crooke, S. T. (1998). Identification and partial purification of human double strand RNase activity. A novel terminating mechanism for oligoribonucleotide antisense drugs *J. Biol. Chem.* Vol.273 No.(5): pp.2532-2542

Zhang, X., Shan, P., Jiang, D., Noble, P. W., Abraham, N. G., Kappas, A. and Lee, P. J. (2004). Small Interfering RNA Targeting Heme Oxygenase-1 Enhances Ischemia-Reperfusion-induced Lung Apoptosis *J. Biol. Chem.* Vol.279 No.(11): pp.10677-10684

10

Cell Therapy in Chronic Obstructive Pulmonary Disease: State of the Art and Perspectives

João Tadeu Ribeiro-Paes, Talita Stessuk and Rodrigo de las Heras Kozma
Laboratory of Genetics and Cell Therapy, GenTe Cel, Department of Biological Sciences,
University of the State of São Paulo – UNESP, Campus Assis
Brazil

1. Introduction

The pulmonary diseases of obstructive character have high prevalence in the human population and has been subject of several clinical and experimental studies in order to seek a wider understanding of their pathogeny, physiopathology and, especially, the establishment of more rational ways for their treatment. Accordingly, this great effort has led to an extraordinary widening in the concepts of obstructive diseases in the last years, involving the integration of mechanical factors, inflammatory agents, autonomic regulation of airways and environmental aspects.

The COPD may be understood as a pathologic condition in which a non-reversible and limited gas exchange occurs. There are two clinical entities that constitute the COPD: chronic bronchitis and emphysema. Within the COPD spectrum, the main characteristic of pulmonary emphysema is air flow blockage and progressive dyspnea, arising out of the impairment of alveolar walls and increase of air spaces distal to terminal bronchiole, without significant pulmonary fibrosis (Barnes et al., 2003; GOLD, 2009; Oliveira et al., 2000).

The oxidative damage to which lungs are submitted to, as well as the inflammation occurring as a response to irritant agents, such as those coming from air pollution and cigarette smoke, contributes to the induction of the pulmonary degeneration (Lee et al., 2011). Therefore, it may be concluded that chief characteristic of COPD is the acceleration of functional and morphologic loss, with limitation of gas exchanges, resulting in progressive dyspnea, disability and premature death.

Therefore, the development and progression of the pathology are resulting from the interaction of genetic and environmental factors (Ribeiro-Paes et al., 2009). About 1-3% of cases of emphysema are generated by enzyme α1-antitrypsin deficiency, that characterizes a genetic abnormality as an inheritance of autossomal recessive pattern. The other risk factors include: age, infections, as well as social and economic factors (Mannino & Buist, 2007).

Smoking, however, has been established as the major cause related with COPD, resulting for active or passive exposure to the cigarette smoke, and corresponds to 15-20% of cases of pulmonary emphysema (Ribeiro-Paes et al., 2009). The cigarette smoke in their gas and particle stages has a significant quantity of oxidant substances. A high number of particles and oxidant agents are contained in cigarette smoke. Oxidant agents are capable of reducing the effect of the anti-protease system through the oxidation of the active site of those enzymes and leading to a direct injury to the extracellular matrix (Barnes 2000; Barnes et al., 2003; Bast et al., 1991; Rufino & Lapa e Silva, 2006).

The Global Initiative for Chronic Obstructive Lung Disease (GOLD, 2009) has pointed out COPD as a serious public health issue. The pathology is considered the fifth largest cause of death worldwide, and has 210 million patients, with 80 million already in the moderate and/or serious stage of the disease. Estimates put it at the third ranking of cause of death in 2020 (GOLD, 2009; WHO, 2008). Moreover, faced with the ageing of world population, the economic burden of COPD should represent a significant parcel of the future global investments in health (Mannino & Buist, 2007).

Several clinical strategies, associated with the pulmonary rehabilitation techniques have contributed to the extension and improvement of the quality of life of emphysema patients. Notwithstanding the significant advances resulting from the introduction of new therapeutic approaches and rehabilitation, there has not been any efficient form of treatment up to now, other than the one in the palliative scope. The surgery treatment entails highly complex procedures and, in the specific case of lung transplant, a shortage of donors. By taking these aspects into account, experimental models have been proposed, in order to advance the knowledge about the physiopathological processes and new therapeutic approaches to the pulmonary emphysema (Gross et al., 1965; Hele, 2002; Mahadeva & Shapiro, 2002; Martorana et al., 1989; Nikula et al., 2000; Ribeiro-Paes et al., 2009).

2. Experimental models in COPD

Experimental models represent an important tool, since they enable the broadening of knowledge about COPD physiopathology, besides allowing the application of new therapeutic approaches.

The methodology of papain intratracheal instillation, proposed by Gross and coworkers in 1965, represented an original model for pulmonary emphysema induction. Starting from the proposition of this pioneer methodology, a series of studies were conducted, which led to the development of the models of induced pulmonary emphysema by the instillation of other proteases. (Pushpakom *et al.*, 1970; Fusco *et al.*, 2002).

The use of proteolytic enzymes, chiefly of porcine pancreatic elastase (PPE) for the generation of DPOC in an animal model is a widely employed methodology for the conduction of experimental studies, since it is mainly a simple and fast method and produces physiopathological effects similar to the human disease (March, 2000; Shapiro, 2000). The experimental models of pulmonary emphysema induced by proteases instillation have not reproduced precisely the mechanisms of alveolar destruction ensuing the inhaling of smoke and other toxic particles, and, therefore, they do not mimic exactly the sequence of pathological events that occur in the disease in humans (Cendron, 1007).

The use of animal models of cigarette-smoke-induced emphysema means seeking an accuracy in experimental models to match the human, chiefly with respect to the physiopathological mechanisms involved in the formation of the emphysema. Up to the beginning of the 80's decade, the studies involving induced pulmonary emphysema in animals by exposure to cigarette smoke were scarce and their reliability questioned (March, 2000). In 1981, Huber and coworkers proposed a study based on the model of induced emphysema through exposure to cigarette smoke. Some achieved results in the study, with respect to morphometric and physiological aspects provided the basis for the ensuing research. According to the report from the First Siena International Conference on Animal Models of COPD held at the University of Siena in 2001, the induced lesions with the use of this model are similar to those observed in emphysematous humans, highlighting the importance of the stimulus through cigarette smoke in COPD experimental models. (Hele, 2001).

At our laboratory, a new apparatus (Figure 1) for induced emphysema through exposure to cigarette smoke is under test. The present device has a series of innovations when compared to the already existing inhaling models, such as the fact that the animals are contained inside acrylic containers making up the device, while in other cages the animals stay freed. Another important aspect worth highlighting relates to the smoke, which is pumped inside the box. In the device created by our team, the smoke pumped into the box interior comes from puffing on the cigarette; therefore, the situation of an active smoking human is mimicked. This apparatus is expected to lead to a model which mimics, as close as possible, the human pathology and, accordingly, which can be applied to research projects oriented to the analysis of physiopathological processes and to the development of new therapies in chronic degenerative pulmonary diseases.

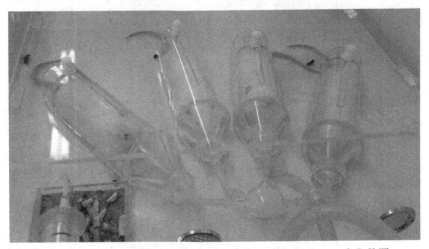

Fig. 1. Apparatus created by the team of the Laboratory of Genetics and Cell Therapy – GenTe Cel to induce emphysema by cigarette smoke.

Notwithstanding the challenges involved in some parameters related to the cigarette-smoke-induced emphysema models, mainly with respect to the age of the animals, exposure time and reproducibility difficulty due to the required resources and time, this is a promising approach to turning animal models closer to the human, chiefly in relation to the physiopathological processes featured in the human pulmonary emphysema (March, 2000).

Currently, the creation and use of genetic models is a very important tool for DPOC study, since the strains mimic a series of aspects related to the human disease, mainly with respect to the α_1-antitrypsin deficiency (March, et al., 2000). At present, several mice strains are known to have natural or laboratory-induced mutations (gene targeting), which generate abnormal conditions in the animal development and are completed with the spontaneous arise of DPOC (March, 2000; Shapiro, 2000). Other methodological approaches to emphysema induction entail animal models with genetic modifications. Martorana et al. (1995), showed the installation and development of pulmonary emphysema in Tight skin transgenic mice, which show mutation in the fibrillin-1 gene, a protein related to the elastic fibers assembly making up the pulmonary tissue (Kietly, 1998).

The Table 1 shows some advantagens and disadvantages of the main animal models of induction of COPD.

Experimental model of COPD	Advantages	Disadvantages	References
Protease-induced Emphysema	- Simple method, easy to apply, quick results, high reproducibility - Morphological features similar to human disease	- Lack of inflammatory constituents - Physiological process is different from human	March et al. (2000)
Genetic models	- Reproduction of human pathology, mainly in relation to deficiency of α_1-antitripsin - Demonstrate the role of proteases in the development of the disease	- The aspects of pathology are reproduced just individually - Need for further studies with respect to inflammatory mechanisms	Shapiro (2000) Fujita and Nakanishi (2007)
Smoke cigarette	- Reproduction of aspects related to the inflammatory processes of COPD - Changes in the airways similar to the human disease	- Long time to onset of symptoms - Time of exposure highly variable	Zheng et al. (2009)

Table 1. Comparison of the main experimental models of COPD.

Taking into account these aspects, is evident the great importance of experimental models of COPD, even though none of them entirely mimic all the features making up the human disease. The use of these models affords the broadening of knowledge, especially related to the physiopathology. The achieved results in animal models may be the grounds for the development of new therapeutic alternatives with the ensuing impact on the survival and improvement of the quality of life of COPD patients.

3. Stem cells and cell therapy: The rationale for use in the lung

The employment of cells for treating diseases is an ancient therapeutic practice, which dates back to the transfusion of whole blood or platelet concentrate in different acute or chronic clinical conditions. The first hematopoietic stem cells (HSC) transplantations were made according to the works of Till and Mculloch in 1961, on the response of mice with the bone marrow transplanted after lesion by ionizing radiation. Since then, new ranges and possibilities of use of other tissues according to the experimental model adopted by the authors have arisen.

The potential of differentiation of stem cells (SC), i.e., the wide range of options of commitments available for the cell (Smith, 2006), has aroused a growing and great interest, bearing in view the employment in the therapy of several types of degenerative diseases and in tissue bioengineering (Atala, 2008). According to The National Institutes of Health (NIH), SC can be defined as cells able to divide for indefinite time *in vitro* and to give origin to specialized cells. Melton and Cowan (2004) proposed a working definition of SC: "a clonal self-renewable entity which is multipotent and can generate several types of differentiated cells." Notwithstanding the concept variation, SC have two basic characteristic aspects: self-renewal, in order to maintain the pool of undifferentiated cells for tissue replacement, remodeling, and repair, as well as the differentiation into at least one mature cell type. These inherent properties for SC are afforded through particular asymmetric divisions, where undifferentiated cells are originated, or, alternatively, differentiation into specialized cells (Figure 2).

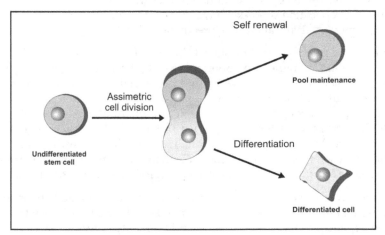

Fig. 2. Assimetric SC division. An undifferentiated SC under microenvironment stimulation start assimetric divisions producing two distinct daughter cells. One cell, undifferentiated, maintain the SC pool. In contrast, the differentiated cell acquires a new mature and specialized phenotype.

Considering their origin, SC are classified in three general types: embryonic stem cells (ESC), germinative stem cells (GSC), and adult or tissue-specific stem cells (ASC). The ESC are derived from the inner cell mass of the blastocyst, capable to generate any differentiated cellular type of the three primary germ layers (ectoderm, mesoderm and endoderm), as well as the GSC originated from the gonadal crest (Geijsen et al., 2004). On the other hand, ASC are undifferentiated cells, found in differentiated cell types in a tissue where they can renew themselves for long periods of time, and can differentiate to yield specialized cell types of the host tissue. By and large, ESC maintains the undifferentiated stage for a long period of time without losing their differentiation potential (Draper et al., 2004). Moreover, the ASC have a limited number of generations, and at each division there is loss of response to differentiation signals (Jiang et al., 2002).

The knowledge that undifferentiated cells exist in the bone marrow has been verified since the 40's decade; by the way, the blood progenitors are the first well characterized SC. Both in humans and in animal models, the literature reports consistent data with evidence for the existence of stained SC from the bone marrow in lungs after bone marrow transplant (Bittmann et al ., 2001; Kotton et al., 2001; Krause et al., 2001; Lama et al., 2007; Ribeiro_Paes et al., 2009; Schrepfer et al., 2007; Suratt et al., 2003; Yamada et al., 2004). At different experimental situations, these and others classical works have shown evidence for the migration of SC to the lung and have provided the theoretical reference which gives grounds for the idea of employing cell therapy in the regeneration of pulmonary tissue.

The experimental evidence of migration of SC from the bone marrow to the lungs was pioneering described in the work of Pereira et al. in 1995. Authors cultured murine cells expressing a collagen human gene and injected the expanded mesenchymal precursor cells into irradiated mice. The presence of transplanted cells in recipient animals for a period of up to 5 months was showed by PCR *in* situ assay. There was incorporation into the pulmonary tissue, where the cells disseminated through the mesenchymal parenchyma and could continue the replication process *in* vivo. Therefore, bone marrow cells can migrate and populate the pulmonary tissue and act as precursors of local cells.

Experimental animal models and clinical trials in regenerative tissue therapy by intravenous (IV) SC or BMMC infusion indicate a "pulmonary first-pass effect" as proposed by Fischer et al. 2009. The lungs act as a barrier, where administered cells are preferentially attracted and retained. Cell size and adhesion receptors of the stem and progenitors cells IV infused can determine this effect through pulmonary microvastulature (Fischer et al., 2009). Five minutes after labeled MSC IV infusion was verified, in animal model, a significant greater bioluminicensce signal in the lungs, in relation to several other organs, such as heart, spleen, liver and kidney. Therefore, the mean size of injected cells larger than the caliber of lung capillaries provides an efficient and fast cell trapping in lungs (Schrepfer et al., 2007).

Interesting works found on literature indicate the initial migration and chimerism in lungs after cell transplantation. Krause et al. (2001) transplanted male mice cells into females with bone marrow depleted by ionizing radiation and tracked the presence of Y chromosome in gastrointestinal tract, liver, lung and skin. It was verified co-staining of pneumocytes type II and Y chromosome in bronchi and alveoli showed by FISH assay (Y chromosome and surfactant B mRNA staining) and immunohistochemistry (anti-cytokeratin antibodies for the detection of epithelial cells). However, authors proposed that the significant damage to the lungs, arising out of the radiation, provided high levels of incorporation in the alveolar tissue.

In the same year, Kotton *et al.* (2001) IV infused Lac-Z stained cells of transgenic mice into recipient wild animals, which underwent pulmonary lesion by intratracheal instillation of bleomycin. There was typical staining of lac-Z expression (Incubation in medium containing X-gal), with statistically significant increase in the animals sustaining lesion with bleomycin. The grafted cells showed evidence for morphologic and molecular phenotype of pneumocytes type I. So, cultured or fresh aspirates of bone marrow cells can express pulmonary markers. Thereby, these cells could represent a potential therapy in extensive alveolar degeneration.

An elegant experimental model of suppression of bone marrow and later lesion with bleomycin was elaborated by Rojas *et al.*, (2005). The authors obtained full survival index and protective effect in mice which underwent MSC transplantation. The immunohistochemistry analysis of the pulmonary tissue of the animals with suppression of bone marrow disclosed, when compared to group without suppression, that the transplanted cells (GFP+) were present in the organ and in a large number, even 14 days after the administration of bleomycin.

As in the animal models, cell migration and chimerism were also observed in human patients who received, for different reasons, bone marrow allogeneic transplant, as in the models of animal studies. Suratt et al. (2003), in a pioneer work, showed pulmonary chimerism upon the incorporation of cells with Y chromosome in women receiving HSC allogeneic transplant from male donors. Another study, 7 patients who underwent pulmonary transplant between (donor and recipient) individuals of opposite sexes showed, by means of different assays of histochemistry staining and molecular analysis (RT-PCR), the presence of mesenchymal stem cells (MSC) in lungs of recipients with cytogenetic expression of the sex of donor. In a period of up to 11 and a half years after the transplant was verified donor cells in the recipient patients (Lama et al., 2007).

Nevertheless, the SC migration to the lungs can be overestimated and, therefore, they are allegedly present at a much lower rate with a questionable clinical meaning. So, the results obtained and reported have been evaluated more carefully by some authors, who challenge the accuracy of the employed detection techniques. For example, after transplanting MSC GFP+ in mice which had previously received an LPS intraperitoneal injection, Xu et al. (2008) did not find, in the immunohistochemistry analysis of the pulmonary tissue conducted 14 days after the transplant, circumstantial evidence for a significant presence of cells with positive sign of GFP. However, although the authors did not find evidence for an actual integration of MSC to the pulmonary tissue and the presence of cells with the pulmonary phenotype, there was demonstration that the SC transplant afforded a decrease in the lungs inflammation and edema induced by the LPS. There are, accordingly these results, the indication that the action mechanism of cells would be mediated by paracrine factors that stimulate tissue regeneration rather than cell engraftment into lungs (Huh et al., 2011).

More recently, Katsha and collaborators (2011) reported a significant improvement resulting from the use of MSC from the murine bone marrow for the repair and regeneration of the pulmonary parenchyma, in an elastase-induced experimental model of emphysema. The authors suggest in the same study the importance of paracrine factors derived from MSC as the regenerative mechanism operating in the pulmonary parenchyma.

Notwithstanding the diversity of used methodologies, in human patients and animal models, has been proposed that ASC from several tissue sources can migrate and populate injured areas in the lung. It is propounded that the regenerative property of SC involves cellular migration to the site of tissue damage and probable promotion of functional and structural organ repair. This mobilization process (homing) is related to liberation of chemotactic mediators by injured organ (Chen et al., 2011).

4. Use of stem cells in chronic obstructive pulmonary disease: Experimental basis

In lungs, affected by chronic inflammation, there is intense production of molecules that signal and can recruit SC (endogenous and transplanted) capable of tissue reconstruction (Rojas *et al.*, 2005). In this context, the rationale for cell therapy in COPD comprehends the ability of SC homing toward injured pulmonary tissue, allowing repair of the lung parenchyma and probable clinical efficacy.

Two groups of Japanese researchers reported in 2004 the first consistent results of pulmonary regeneration in an experimental mouse model (C57BL/6 strain) of lesion and later infusion of SC from bone marrow. The mice were submitted to lipopolysaccharide (LPS) intranasal treatment after irradiation. An experimental group received bone marrow-derived progenitor cells transplant from transgenic mice donors expressing GFP. There was protection of the lungs against the lesion of the emphysematous type in the animals transplanted with BMMC. It was also detection of stained cells (endothelial and epithelial) only in the recipient animals in which the induced pulmonary lesion (Yamada et al, 2004).

In a model of elastase-induced pulmonary emphysema, Ishizawa et al. (2004) reported that the treatment with retinoic acid or granulocyte colony-stimulating factor (G-CSF) led to the alveolar regeneration and the treatment, concurrently with both factors, resulted in an additive effect. There was BMC mobilization to injured alveoli by retinoic acid and G-CSF besides regeneration process.

Several authors around the world reported experimental and interesting results with cell therapy in animal models of COPD. Some of these works are shortly described in the Table 2.

At our laboratory, several research projects have been directed for the study of morphologic and functional pulmonary recovery after the treatment with ASC in mice with experimentally-induced COPD. Our model basically consists of the induction of emphysema by intranasal instillation of papain or elastase and later treatment with BMMC or MSC pool originated from the bone marrow (Figure 3).

Female mice of the C57BL/6 act as recipients. Transgenic male mice (with C57BL/6 background), which express the green fluorescent protein (GFP) are used as donors of BMMC and MSC for the purpose of cellular tracking and validation of the post transplant chimerism.

The achieved results both in quality and in quantity have shown the regeneration of the pulmonary tissue in animals with emphysema and treated with BMMC pool or MSC (Figure 4).

Animal	COPD induction	Stem cell type / source	Therapeutic effects	Probable action mechanism	Reference
Rabbit	Elastase	BMMC	Improves pulmonary function, decreases airspace enlargement	-	Yuhgetsu et al., 2006
Rat	Papain Co-60	MSC / bone marrow	Improves alveolar parameters (mean alveoli area and linear interval)	Inhibition of the apoptosis of alveolar cell wall	Liu et al., 2008
Rat	Cigarette smoke for 6 months	BMC MSC Conditioned medium of MSC/bone marrow	Attenuates cigarette induced emphysema, restores the increased Lm, increase pulmonary microvastulature,	Paracrine effects	Huh et al., 2011
Sheep	Elastase	MSC/ lung	Increases tissue mass, lung perfusion, cellularity and ECM content.	Paracrine effects	Ingenito et al., 2011
Mice	Cigarette smoke for 6 months	Human or murine MSC / cell-free contidioned medium adipose tissue	Decreases inflammation and airspace enlargement, prevents cigarette-induced weight loss, restores cigarette-induced BM dysfunction	Paracrine effects	Schweitzer et al., 2011
Mice	Elastase	MSC / bone marrow	Ameliorates alveolar structure, restores increased Lm and destructive index	Paracrine factors	Katsha et al., 2011

Table 2. Experimental animal models of cell therapy for COPD.

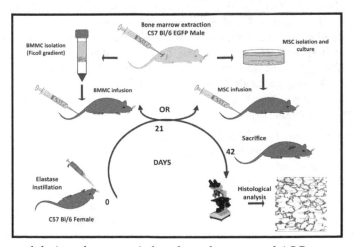

Fig. 3. Experimental design of protease-induced emphysema and ASC treatment.

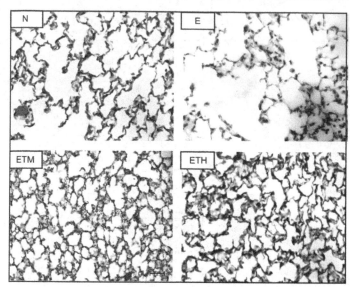

Fig. 4. Pulmonary tissue from female mice C57Bl/6 in representative histological cuts. Hematoxylin and eosin staining. Groups: N - no treatment, E - instillation of elastase only, ETM - instillation of elastase and MSC transplant and ETH - instillation of elastase and infusion of BMMC. Original magnification 200 x.

The regeneration of the pulmonary tissue, expressed in a quantitative way as the measurement of the mean linear intercept (Lm), had a significant statistical difference between animals treated with ASC and controls.

In accordance with the data showed in Figure 5, there is a statistically significant difference between E group, treated with elastase only, and N group, with no treatment, which shows evidence for the efficacy of elastase via intranasal administration in the induction of pulmonary emphysema. Between groups treated only with elastase (E) and treated with elastase and growth medium (EME) there is no statistically significant difference, which suggests the inability of the infusion vehicle in the regeneration of the pulmonary parenchyma. Furthermore, the experimental groups, treated with HSC or MSC have not shown statistically significant difference in comparison with N group, with no treatment. It is worth noting that groups treated with HSC and MSC have not turned out significant difference, which shows the therapeutic equivalence between the two stem strains originated from the bone marrow.

The comparison between the achieved values of Lm equivalent to the groups undergoing the elastase instillation (E) and treated with DMEM (EME), as well as the groups with experimentally-induced emphysema and treated with HSC or MSC has shown statistically significant difference, according to Figure 5 ($p > 0.05$).

Accordingly, it is possible that MSC and BMMC hold a potential role to deliver the required cellular strain diversity during the tissue regeneration process, possibly by paracrine mechanisms (Katsha et al, 2011) and to check, in a significant and effective way, the repair of the lesion in the pulmonary tissue.

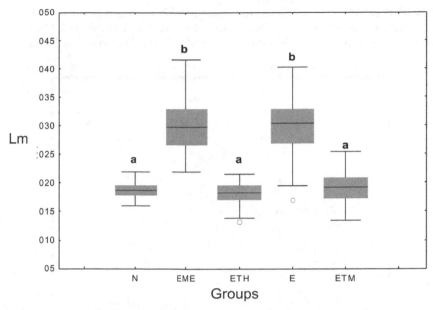

Fig. 5. Mean linear intercept (Lm) of the animals in the control and treated groups. N Group - no treatment, EME - instillation of elastase and infusion of DMEM growth medium, ETH - instillation of elastase and infusion of BMMC, E - instillation of elastase only, ETM - instillation of elastase and MSC transplant. Medians followed by the same letter indicate no significant difference (p>0,05).

As it can apprehended from the literature, there is a consistent set of results generated by several laboratories, including those achieved by our research group, which supplied the experimental basis and afforded the cell therapy application by our group in COPD patients.

5. Clinical application: Cell therapy as a new therapeutic approach for COPD

Due to the high prevalence and significant economic and social impact caused by COPD, there are, as already presented, several researches in cell therapy, described in animal models, which sustain the use of ASC in human patients with COPD.

The results arising out of the basic research in animal models of COPD cell therapy, at our laboratory, have shown regeneration of the pulmonary parenchyma both in the qualitative and in the quantitative forms, as demonstrated by the histological analyses and by the measurement of the Lm. These results were the grounds for the preparation of a research project submitted to the National Committee of Ethics in Research (CONEP-Brazil) in April 2008. The clinical protocol was approved in April 2009 (registration n° 14764, CONEP 233/2009) and, on May 11th, 2009, the first patient, with CPOD in advanced stage, was submitted to BMMC pool infusion (Ribeiro-Paes et al., 2011).

This first work corresponds to a phase 1 clinical screening for the evaluation of safety concerning SC infusion in COPD patients and it was registered with Clinical Trials – NIH – USA (NTC01110252). The experimental outlining consists, basically, of the autologous transplant of Bone Marrow Mononuclear Cells (BMMC) pool in patients with COPD in advanced stage, higher than 3 according to the Modified Medical Research Council (MRC) Dyspnea Scale Score (Curley, 1997; Mahler & Wells, 1988). The study design is shown in Figure 6.

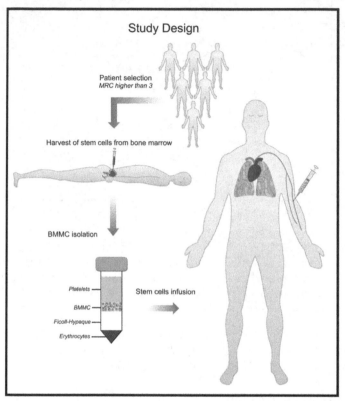

Fig. 6. Clinical protocol adopted for cell therapy in patients with advanced pulmonary emphysema (Ribeiro-Paes et al., 2011).

In the pre-procedure period, the selected patients were submitted to a full pulmonary and cardiac evaluation. Routine laboratory tests were also performed and the Dyspnea Scale Score test, modified according to the British MRC, was also conducted.The selection criteria is presented below.

Inclusion criteria: 1) age between 40 and 76 years; 2) severe obstructive pulmonary disease; 3) ineffective clinical treatment; 4) limited life expectancy; 4) limitation in daily physical activities; 5) possibility of pulmonary rehabilitation physiotherapy; 6) acceptable nutritional condition; 7) acceptable cardiac function; 8) no tobacco use for at least six months; 9) satisfactory psychosocial and emotional profile and family support and 10) Dyspnea Scale Score greater than 3.

Exclusion criteria: 1) active pulmonary or extra-pulmonary infection; 2) serious coronaropathy and/or ventricular dysfunction; 3) significant renal illness and/or hepatitis;

4) detected immunosuppressive illnesses, including HIV; 5) hepatitis B or C; 6) smoking habit; 7) carrier of known neoplasies; 8) pregnancy; 9) noncompliance with established medical protocol; 10) psychosocial problems, including drug or alcohol abuse; 11) lack of family support. After the selection, the participants received written and verbal information explaining the study and written consent was obtained from all participants before the beginning of the procedure.

After a thorough clinical evaluation, bone marrow of the voluntary patients was collected, processed and the BMMC pool achieved after isolation in Ficoll density gradient. The infusion of the achieved mononuclear fraction was made by peripheral IV (brachial medial) way and the clinical evolution of patients after the transplant has been monitored until the present date by the conduction of pulmonary function tests.

The use of BMMC pool for cell therapy in COPD patients has shown to be quite safe. No intercurrent disease occurred that could put the research's voluntary subjects in clinically serious situations or long lasting discomfort.

All the voluntary subjects of the research had some kind of clinical improvement. The spirometry tests showed a very slight improvement, as shown in Figure 7. The VEF 1 showed an improvement in all patients after thirty days.

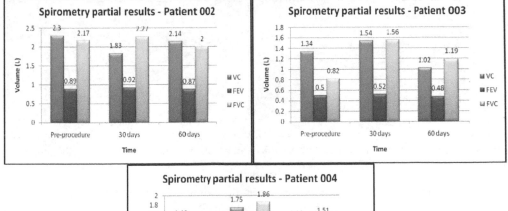

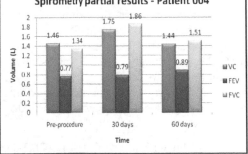

Fig. 7. Spirometry absolute values from 3 research patients included in clinical protocol and submitted to autologous BMMC transplantation.

Likewise, the increase in the CVF and CV parameters occurred in all patients after 30 days had lapsed from the procedure (Figure 7). However, after this period, there was a decrease in CVF; in spite of this fact, an important aspect is that the functional parameters remained always higher than the ones found before the procedure.

An interesting information turned out in the long term results, approximately 2 years of clinical monitoring. The spirometry parameters along the post transplantation period, by and large, maintain a certain regularity and similarity to those found before the procedure. One of the research subject disclosed a significant increase in the forced vital capacity, after 1 year and 3 months of treatment (Figure 8); The analysis of this parameter suggests a proximity to normality and reduction of the severity of the disease.

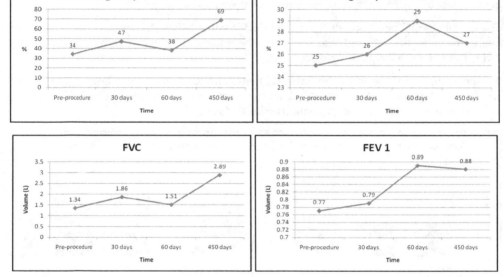

Fig. 8. Percentage of predicted and absolute values from a patient spirometry until 1 year and 3 months after BMMC autologous transplant.

The results from this clinical protocol show the procedure should be conducted at an earlier stage, that is, at a less advanced stage of the pathology. As mentioned, the laboratorial analysis, confirmed by clinical response, has reported a significant improvement in all patients, chiefly in the first 30 days after the procedure was carried out. After this period, laboratory tests displayed a tendency to decrease; however they did not drop to the base values obtained before the BMMC therapy treatment. These results advance the possibility that cell therapy may be applied in repeated doses from time to time for the purpose of stimulating pulmonary regeneration.

Another protocol under registration with Clinical Trials (NTC00683722) corresponds to a multicenter, double-blind, placebo controlled phase II study for patients with moderate to severe COPD. The clinical protocol, sponsored by Osiris Therapeutics Inc. (Columbia, MD), concerns the employment of *ex vivo* cultured adult human SC (PROCHYMAL) in the treatment of pulmonary emphysema. The purpose comprehends the evaluation of safety and efficacy of MSC multiple infusion.

As proposed by Osiris Therapeutics "Preclinical and clinical data suggest that Prochymal's unique mechanism of action may provide a first-in-class treatment option with the ability to reverse the underlying disease". However, there is no publication to date reporting the results arising out of the screening made in 62 patients. By virtue of the lack of results from the use of PROCHYMAL cell therapy in COPD, it is not possible to check and uphold the effect of regression of chronic inflammation in lungs as a response to the MSC treatment. Therefore, no critical evaluation may be made about the results of the protocol proposed by Osiris Therapeutics.

More recently, a phase 1 clinical study sponsored by Leiden University Medical Center (Leiden, Netherlands) was registered with Clinical Trials.gov (NCT01306513). The clinical protocol consists of the autologous transplant of bone-marrow-derived MSC in patients with COPD (MRC 3) before the surgery to reduce pulmonary volume. The purpose of the work, still in progress, is the evaluation of the cell therapy safety, as well as the feasibility of cultivating MSC.

The results achieved by our group, as well as the registration of clinical protocols concerning cellular therapy by other research centers, have led to the opening of new strategies of therapeutic investigation. Thus, it is possible to establish ew perspectives in regard to the formulation of cell therapy experimental designs which will be surely incorporated into future research projects for the purpose of optimizing the clinical effect and the quality of life of COPD patients.

6. Perspectives and challenges

COPD represents a serious public health problem, which, according to the latest projections of the World Health Organization, should gradually change for the worse in the coming years, with a great impact on the economy, on a global scale.

The incorporation of new drugs having more effectiveness and longer effect unquestionably has contributed to the improvement in quality of life of the patients; however, up to now, no significant change in the natural history of the disease has been achieved. In this context, cell therapy turns out as a potentially promising treatment option, which, perhaps, may represent a change of paradigm in therapeutics and in the natural course of the disease.

The results achieved at our laboratory and by several other coworkers, at different research centers, have shown a morphological recovery of the pulmonary parenchyma in animals with experimentally-induced emphysema by the employment of proteases and/or cigarette smoke. From said results, a pioneer treatment with BMMC pool was administered for patients with emphysema in advanced stage. It is a project in an initial phase and the sample of treated patients is still small, which limit the analyses from the statistical point of view. At our research center, a new project will soon start. It will comprehend a larger sample (about 40 patients) and the employment of a new methodology, which the use of MSC.

Notwithstanding the statistical limitations, the pioneer publication of the results by our research group (Ribeiro-Paes et al., 2011), has afforded the preparation of some logical inferences and methodological suggestions which will be incorporated into future projects. The use of MSC obtained from adipose tissue has disclosed a highly promising future perspective. Furthermore, the feasibility of establishing a protocol with repeated SC infusions should also be taken into account, just like in chronic treatments with drugs.

There are, finally, a series of questions and possibilities that arise from this pioneering studies and results obtained in our laboratory. The sample of treated patients is still small. There is, indeed, in these beginnings of research, far more doubts than certainties. Also, extreme caution should be exercised so as not to arouse false expectations and unrealistic hopes in COPD patients. Only the first trials have been carried out. We do not know exactly how this story is going to unfold. However, the first steps of a long and challenging journey have been taken, but surely it looks potentially promising, in therapeutic terms. For our group, it means a very stimulating journey of research and work.

7. References

Atala, A. (2000). Advances in tissue and organ replacement. *Current Stem Cell Research & Therapy*, Vol.3, No.1, (January 2000), pp. 21-31, ISSN 1574-888X

Barnes, P. (2000). Chronic obstructive pulmonary disease. *The New England Journal of Medicine*, Vol.343, No.4, (July 2000), pp. 269-280, ISSN 1533-4406

Barnes, P.; Shapiro, S. & Pauwels, R. (2003). Chronic obstructive pulmonary disease: molecular and celular mechanisms. *The European Respiratory Journal*, Vol.22, No.4, (October 2003), pp. 672-688, ISSN 0903-1936

Bast, A.; Haenen, G. & Doelman, C. (1991). Oxidants and antioxidants: state of the art. *The American Journal of Medicine*, Vol.91, No.3C, (September 1991), pp. 2S-3S, ISSN: 0002- 9343

Bittmann, I.; Dose, T.; Baretton, G.; Muller, C.; Schwaiblmar Lohrs, I.; Kur, F. & Lohrs, U. (2001). Cellular chimerism of the lung after transplantation. An interphase cytogenetic study. *American Journal of Clinical Pathology*, Vol.115, No.4, (April 2001), pp. 525-533, ISSN: 0002-9173

Cendon, S.; Battlehner, C.; Lorenzi-Filho, G.; Dohlnikoff, M.; Pereira, P.; Conceição, G.; Beppu, O. & Saldiva, P. (1997). Pulmonary emphysema induced by passive smoking: an experimental study in rats. *Brazilian Journal of Medical and Biological Research*, Vol.30, No.10, (October 1997), pp. 1241-1247, ISSN 1678-4510

Chen, F-M.; Wu, L-A.; Zhang, M.; Zhang, R. & Sun, H. (2011). Homing of endogenous stem/progenitors cells for *in situ* tissue regeneration: Promises, strategies and translational perspectives. *Biomaterials*, Vol.32, No.12, (April 2011), pp. 3189-3209, ISSN: 0142-9612

Curley, F.(1997). Dyspnea, In: Diagnosis and Treatment of Symptoms of the Respiratory Tract, Irwin, R.; Curley, F.; Grossman, R, (Ed), pp.56-115, Future Publishing, ISBN 978-0879936570, Armonk, NY

Draper, J.; Smith, K.; Gokhale, P.; Moore, H.; Maltby, E.; Johnson, J.; Meisner, L.;Zwaka, P.; Thomsom, J. &Andrews, P. (2004). Recurrent gain of chromosomes 17q and 12 in cultured human embryonic stem cells. *Nature Biotechnology*, Vol.22, No.1, (January 2004), pp.53-54, ISSN : 1087-0156

Fischer, U.; Harting, M.; Jimenez, F.; Monzon-Posadas, W.; Xue, H.; Savitz, S.; Laine, G. & Cox, C. (2009). Pulmonary passage is a major obstacle for intravenous stem cell delivery: the pulmonary first-pass effect. *Stem Cells and Development*, Vol.18, No.5, (June 2009), pp. 683-692, ISSN: 1557-8534

Fujita, M. & Nakanishi, Y. (2007). The pathogenesis of COPD: Lessons learned from in vivo animal models. *Medical Science Monitor*, Vol.13, No.2, (February 2007), pp. 19-24, ISSN: 1234-1010

Fusco, L.; Pêgo-Fernandes, P.; Xavier, A.; Pazetti, R; Rivero, D.; Capelozzi, V. & Jatene, F. (2002). Modelo experimental de enfisema pulmonar em ratos induzido por papaína. *Jornal de Pneumologia*, Vol.28, No.1, (January 2002), pp.1-7, ISSN 1806-3713

Geijsen, N.; Horoschak, M.; Kim, K.; Gribnau, J.;Eggan, K. & Daley, G. (2004). Derivation of embryonic germ cells and male gametes from embryonic stem cells. *Nature*, Vol.427, No.6970, (January 2004), pp. 148-154, ISSN: 1476-4687

GOLD – Global Initiative for Chronic Obstructive Lung Disease. (2009). Global Strategy for the Dagnosis, Management, and Prevention of Chronic Obstructive Pulmonary Disease, Executive Sumary

Gross, P.; Pfitzer, E.; Tolker, M.; Babyak, M. & Kaschak, M. (1965). Experimental emphysema: its production with papain in normal and silicotic rats. *Archives of Environmental Health*, Vol.11, (July 1965), pp. 50-58, ISSN 0003-9896

Hele, D. (2002). First Siena International Conference on animal models of chronic obstructive pulmonary disease, Certosa di Pontignano.Universidade of Siena, Italy, September 30-October 2, 2001. Respiratory Research, Vol.3, No.12, (November 2001) ISSN: 1465- 9921

Huh, J.; Kim, S-Y.; Lee, J.; Lee, J.; Ta, Q.; Kim, M.; Oh, Y.; Lee, Y. & Lee, S. (2011). Bone marrow cells repair cigarette smoke-induced emphysema in rats. *American Journal of Physiology. Lung Cellular and Molecular Physiology*, (Epub ahead of print). ISSN: 1522-1504

Ingenito, E.; Tsai, L.; Murthy, S.; Tyagi, S.; Mazan, M. & Hoffman, A. (2011). Autologous lung-derived msenchymal stem cell transplantation in experimental emphysema. *Cell Transplantation*, (Epub ahead of print). ISSN: 0963-6897

Ishizawa, K.: Kubo, H.; Yamada, M.; Kobayashi, S.; Numasaki, M.; Ueda, S.; Suzuki, T. & Sasaki, H. (2004). Bone marrow-derived cells contribute to lung regeneration after elastase-induced pulmonary emphysema. *FEBS Letters*, Vol.556, No.1-3, (January 2004), pp. 249-252, ISSN: 0014-5793

Jiang, Y.; Jahagirdar, B.; Reinhardt, R.; Schwartz, R.; Keene, C.; Ortiz-Gonzalez, X.; Reyes, M.; Lenvik, T.; Lund, T.; Blackstad, M.; Du, J.; Aldrich, S.; Lisberg, A.; Low, W.; Largaespada, D. & Verfaille, C. (2002). Pluripotency of mesenchimal stem cells derived from adult marrow. *Nature,* Vol.418, No.6893, (July 2002), pp. 41-49, ISSN: 1476-4687

Katsha, A.; Ohkouchi, S.; Xin, H.; Kanehira, M.; Sun, R.; Nukiwa, T. & Saijo, Y. (2011). Paracrine Factors of Multipotent Stromal Cells Ameliorate Lung Injury in an Elastase-induced Emphysema Model.*The American Society of Gene & Cell Therapy*, Vol.19, No.1, (September 2010), pp. 196–203, ISSN:1525-0016

Kielty, C.; Raghunath, M.; Siracusa, L.; Sherratt, M.; Peters, R.; Shuttleworth, C. & Jimenez, S. (1998). The tight skin mouse: Demonstration of mutant .brillin-1 production and assembly into abnormal microfibrils. *The Journal of Cell Biology*, Vol.140, No.5, (March 1998), pp. 1159–1166, ISSN: 1540-8140

Kotton, D.; Ma, B.; Cardoso, W.; Sanderson, E.; Summer, R.; Williams, M. & Fine, A. (2001). Bone marrow-derived cells as progenitors of lung alveolar epithelium. *Development*, Vol.128, No.24, (December 2001), pp. 5181-5188, ISSN: 1098-2795

Krause, D.; Theise, N.; Collector, M.; Henegariu, O.; Hwang, S.; Gardner, R.; Neutzel, S. & Sharkis, J. (2001). Multi-organ, multi-linage enfragment by a single bone marrow-derived stem cell. *Cell*, Vol.105, No.3, (May 2001), pp. 369-377, ISSN 1097-2765

Lama, V.; Smith, L.; Badri, L.; Flint, A.; Andrei, A-C.; Murray, S.; Wang, Z.; Liao, H.; Toews, G.; Krebsbach, P.; Potere-Golde, M.; Pinsky, D.; Martinez, F. & Thannickal, V. (2007). Evidence for tissue-resident mesenchymal stem cells in human adult lung from studies of transplanted allografts. *The Journal of Clinical Investigation*, Vol. 117, No.4, (Abril 2007), pp. 989-996, ISSN: 0021-9738

Lee, J., Sandford, A., Man, P.,.(2011). Is the aging process accelerated in chronic obstructive pulmonary disease? .*Current Opinion in Pulmonary Medicine*, Vol.17, pp. 90-97, ISSN: 1531-6971

Liu, H., Zhen, G., Zhang, Z., Zhang, H., Cao, Y., Wang, T., Gu, N. & Xu, Y. (2008). Effects of bone marrow mesenchymal stem cells transplantation on the apoptosis of alveolar wall cells in papain and Co60-induced pulmonary emphysema rats. *Chinese Journal of Applied Physiology*, Vol.24, No.2, (May 2008), pp.210-214, ISSN: 1000-6834

Mahadeva, R. & Shapiro S. (2002). Chronic obstrutive pulmonary disease: Experimental animal models of pulmonary emphysema. *Thorax*, Vol.57, pp.908-914, ISSN: 1468-3296

Mahler D. & Wells C. (1988). Evaluation of clinical methods for rating dyspnea. *Chest*, Vol.93, No.3, pp.580–586, ISSN: 0012-3692

Mannino D. & Buist A. (2007). Global burden of COPD: risk factors, prevalence and future trends. *Lancet*, Vol.370, pp.765-773, ISSN: 0140-6736

March T., Green F., Hahn F. & Nikula K. (2000). Animal models of emphysema and their relevance to studies of particle-induced disease. *Inhalation Toxicology*, Vol.12(Supplement 4), pp.155-187, ISSN: 1091-7691

Martorana, P., Even, P., Gardi, C. & Lungarella, G. (1989). A 16-Month Study of Development of genetic emphysema in Tight-skin mice. *The American Review of Respiratory Disease*, Vol.139, No.1, (January 1989), pp. 226-232, ISSN: 0003-0805

Martorana, P., Cassella, A. & Lungarella, G. (1995). Animal model of human disease. Genetic deficiency in α-1 proteinase inhibitor (α-1 PI) associated with emphysema. *Journal of Comarative Pathology*, Vol.27, No.4, pp. 3–6, ISSN: 0021-9975

Melton, D. & Cowan, C. (2004). "Stemness": Definitions, criteria, and standards, In: Handbo of Stem Cells Adult and Fetal Stem Cells, Lanza, R. (Ed), pp.xxv-xxxi, Elsevier/Academic Press, ISBN 0-12-436644, New York

NIH - Stem Cells: Scientific Progress and Future Research Directions. Department of Health and Human Services. June 2001. </info/scireport/2001report>.

Nikula K., March, T., Seagrave, J., Finch, G., Barr, E., Ménache, M., Hahn, F. & Hobbs, C. (2000). A mouse model of cigarette smoke-induced emphysema. *Chest*, Vol.117, No.5, (April 2006), pp. 246S-247S, ISSN:0012-3692

Oliveira, J., Jardim, J. & Rufino, R. (2000) I Consenso Brasileiro de Doença Pulmonar Obstrutiva Crônica (DPOC) *Jornal de Pneumologia*, Vol.26 No.1, (April 2000), pp. S1-S3, ISSN 1806-3713

Pereira, R., Halford, K., O'Hara, M., Leeper, D., Sokolov, B., Pollard, M., Bagasra, O. & Prockop D. (1995). Cultured adherent cells from marrow can serve as long-lasting precursor cells for bone, cartilage, and lung in irradiated mice. *Proceedings of The National Academy of Sciences of United States of America*, Vol.92, No.11, (May 1995), pp. 4857-61, ISSN 1091-6490

Pushpakom, R., Hogg, J., Woolcock, A., Angus, A., Macklem, P. & Thurlbeek, W. (1970). Experimental papain-induced emphysema in dogs. *The American Review of Respiratory Disease*, Vol.102, No.5, (Novembro 1970), pp. 778-779, ISSN: 0003-0805

Ribeiro-Paes, J., Bilaqui, A., Greco, O., Ruiz, M., Alves-de-Moraes, L., Faria, C. & Stessuk, T.(2009). Terapia celular em doenças pulmonares: Existem perspectivas? *Revista Brasileira de Hematologia e Hemoterapia*, Vol.31, (August 2009), pp. 140-148, ISSN: 1516-8484

Ribeiro-Paes, J., Bilaqui, A., Greco, O., Ruiz, Marcelino, M., Stessuk, T., Faria, C. & Lago, M. (2011). Unicentric study of cell therapy in chronic obstructive pulmonary disease/pulmonary Emphysema. *International Journal of COPD*, Vol.6, (January 2011), pp. 63-71, ISSN: 1178-2005

Rojas, M., Xu, J., Woods, C., Mora, A., Spears, W., Roman, J. & Brigham, K. (2005). Bone marrow-derived mesenchymal stem cells in repair of the injured lung. *American Journal of Respiratory Cell and Mollecular Biology*, Vol.33, No.2, (August 2005), pp. 145-52, ISSN:1044-1549

Rufino, R. & Lapa e Silva, J. (2006). Bases celulares e bioquímicas da doença pulmonar obstrutiva crônica. *Jornal Brasileiro de Pneumologia*, Vol.32, No.3, (May 2006), pp. 241-248, ISSN 1806-3713

Schrepfer, S., Deuse, T., Reichenspurner, H., Fischbein, M., Robbins, R. & Pelletier, M. (2007). Stem Cell Transplantation: The Lung Barrier. *Transplantation Proceedings*, Vol.39, No.2, (March 2007), pp. 573-576, ISSN: 0041-1345

Shapiro, S. (2000). Animal Models for COPD. *Chest*, Vol.117, pp. 223–227, ISSN: 0012-3692

Schweitzer, K., Johnstone, B., Garrison, J., Rush, N., Cooper, S., Traktuev, D., Feng, D., Adamowicz, J., Van Demark, M., Fisher, A., Kamocki, K., Brown, M., Presson, R., Broxmeyer, H., March, K. & Petrache, I. (2011). Adipose stem cell treatment in mice attenuates lung and systemic injury induced by cigarette smoking. *American Journal of Respiratory and Critical Care Medicine*, Vol.183, No.2, (January 2011), pp. 215-225, ISSN: 0003-0805

Smith, A. (2006). Glossary A glossary for stem-cell biology. *Nature*, Vol. 441, (June 2006), pp.1060, ISSN: 1476-4687

Suratt, B., Cool, C., Serls, A., Chen, L., Varella-Garcia, M., Shapall, E., Crown K. & Worthen G. (2003). Human pulmonary chimerism after hematopoetic stem cell transplantation. *American Journal of Respiratory and Critical Care Medicine*, Vol.168, No.3, (August 2003) pp. 318-322, ISSN: 0003-0805

Till, J. & Mccullough, E. (1961). A direct measurement of the radiation sensitivity of normal mouse bone marrow cells. *Radiation Research*, Vol.14, (February 1961), pp. 213-222, INSS : 0033-7587

Xu, J., Qu, J., Cao, L., Sai, Y., Chen, C., He, L. & Yu, L. (2008). Mesenchymal stem cell-based angiopoietin-1 gene therapy for acute lung injury induced by lipopolysaccharide in mice. *Journal of Pathology*, Vol. 214, No.4, (March 2008), pp. 472-81, ISSN: 1096-9896

WHO - WORLD HEALTH ORGANIZATION. (2008). Global alliance against chronic respiratory diseases (GARD). General Meeting Report, ISBN 978 92 4 1597 13 5, Istanbul, Turkey, May, 2008

Yamada, M., Kubo, H., Kobayashi, S., Ishizawa, K., Numasaki, M., Ueda, S., Suzuki, T. & Sasaki, H. (2004). Bone marrow-derived progenitors cells are important for lung repair after lipopolisaccharide-induced lung injury. *The Journal of Immunology*, Vol.172, No.2, (January 2004), pp. 1266-1272, ISSN: 1550-6606

Yuhgetsu, H., Ohno, Y., Funaguchi, N., Asai, T., Sawada, M., Takemura, G., Minatoguchi, S., Fujiwara, H., & Fujiwara, T. (2006). Beneficial effects of autologous bone marrow mononuclear cell transplantation against elastase-induced emphysema in rabbits. *Experimental Lung Research*, Vol.32, No.9, (October 2006), pp.413-426, ISSN: 1521-0499

Zheng, H., Liu, Y., Huang, T., Fang, Z., Li, G. & He, S. (2009). Development and characterization of a rat model of chronic obstructive pulmonary disease (COPD) induced by sidestream cigarette smoke. Shantou: 2009. *Toxicology Letters*, Vol. 189, (June 2009), pp.225–234, ISSN: 0378-4274

Permissions

The contributors of this book come from diverse backgrounds, making this book a truly international effort. This book will bring forth new frontiers with its revolutionizing research information and detailed analysis of the nascent developments around the world.

We would like to thank Dr Kian-Chung Ong, for lending his expertise to make the book truly unique. He has played a crucial role in the development of this book. Without his invaluable contribution this book wouldn't have been possible. He has made vital efforts to compile up to date information on the varied aspects of this subject to make this book a valuable addition to the collection of many professionals and students.

This book was conceptualized with the vision of imparting up-to-date information and advanced data in this field. To ensure the same, a matchless editorial board was set up. Every individual on the board went through rigorous rounds of assessment to prove their worth. After which they invested a large part of their time researching and compiling the most relevant data for our readers. Conferences and sessions were held from time to time between the editorial board and the contributing authors to present the data in the most comprehensible form. The editorial team has worked tirelessly to provide valuable and valid information to help people across the globe.

Every chapter published in this book has been scrutinized by our experts. Their significance has been extensively debated. The topics covered herein carry significant findings which will fuel the growth of the discipline. They may even be implemented as practical applications or may be referred to as a beginning point for another development. Chapters in this book were first published by InTech; hereby published with permission under the Creative Commons Attribution License or equivalent.

The editorial board has been involved in producing this book since its inception. They have spent rigorous hours researching and exploring the diverse topics which have resulted in the successful publishing of this book. They have passed on their knowledge of decades through this book. To expedite this challenging task, the publisher supported the team at every step. A small team of assistant editors was also appointed to further simplify the editing procedure and attain best results for the readers.

Our editorial team has been hand-picked from every corner of the world. Their multi-ethnicity adds dynamic inputs to the discussions which result in innovative outcomes. These outcomes are then further discussed with the researchers and contributors who give their valuable feedback and opinion regarding the same. The feedback is then collaborated with the researches and they are edited in a comprehensive manner to aid the understanding of the subject.

Apart from the editorial board, the designing team has also invested a significant amount of their time in understanding the subject and creating the most relevant covers. They scrutinized every image to scout for the most suitable representation of the subject and create an appropriate cover for the book.

The publishing team has been involved in this book since its early stages. They were actively engaged in every process, be it collecting the data, connecting with the contributors or procuring relevant information. The team has been an ardent support to the editorial, designing and production team. Their endless efforts to recruit the best for this project, has resulted in the accomplishment of this book. They are a veteran in the field of academics and their pool of knowledge is as vast as their experience in printing. Their expertise and guidance has proved useful at every step. Their uncompromising quality standards have made this book an exceptional effort. Their encouragement from time to time has been an inspiration for everyone.

The publisher and the editorial board hope that this book will prove to be a valuable piece of knowledge for researchers, students, practitioners and scholars across the globe.

List of Contributors

Cenk Kirakli
Izmir Dr. Suat Seren Chest Diseases and Surgery Training Hospital, Turkey

Tamas Agh and Agnes Meszaros
Semmelweis University, Hungary

Zeynep Zeren Ucar
The Department of Pulmonary Disease and Sleep Disorders, Dr Suat Seren Chest Diseases and Surgery Training and Research Hospital, Izmir, Turkey

Maria Carafa, Carlotta Marianecci and Franco Alhaique
Department of Drug Chemistry and Technologies, "Sapienza", University of Rome, Rome, Italy

Paolino Donatella
Department of Experimental and Clinical Medicine, Faculty of Medicine, University "Magna Graecia" Catanzaro, Italy

Luisa Di Marzio
Department of Drug Science, University of Chieti "G. D'Annunzio", Chieti, Italy

Christian Celia and Massimo Fresta
Department of Pharmacobiological Sciences, Faculty of Pharmacy, University "Magna Graecia" Catanzaro, Italy

R. Martín-Valero, A. I. Cuesta-Vargas and M. T. Labajos-Manzanares
School of Nursing, Physiotherapy, Podiatry and Occupational Therapy, Psyquiatry and Physiotherapy Department, Málaga University, Spain

Aimonino Ricauda Nicoletta, Tibaldi Vittoria and Bertone Paola
Hospital at Home Service, San Giovanni Battista Hospital of Torino, Italy

Isaia Giovanni Carlo
University of Torino, Department of Medical and Surgical Disciplines – Geriatric Section, S. Giovanni Battista Hospital, Italy

Angel Vila-Corcoles and Olga Ochoa-Gondar
Research Unit of the Primary Care Service of Tarragona-Valls, Institut Català de la Salut, Tarragona, Catalonia, Spain

Donrawee Leelarungrayub
Department of Physical Therapy, Faculty of Associated Medical Sciences, Chiang Mai University, Thailand

Rosanne Seguin and Nicolay Ferrari
Topigen Pharmaceuticals Inc., Part of the Pharmaxis Ltd. Group, Montréal, QC, Canada

João Tadeu Ribeiro-Paes, Talita Stessuk and Rodrigo de las Heras Kozma
Laboratory of Genetics and Cell Therapy, GenTe Cel, Department of Biological Sciences, University of the State of São Paulo – UNESP, Campus Assis, Brazil